ALTERNATIVE HEALING

ALTERNATIVE HEALING

THE COMPLETE A–Z GUIDE
TO MORE THAN 150 DIFFERENT
ALTERNATIVE THERAPIES

Mark Kastner, L.Ac., Dipl.Ac.,
and Hugh Burroughs

An Owl Book

Henry Holt and Company
New York

Henry Holt and Company, Inc.
Publishers since 1866
115 West 18th Street
New York, New York 10011

Henry Holt® is a registered
trademark of Henry Holt and Company, Inc.

Library of Congress Cataloging-in-Publication Data
Kastner, Mark.
Alternative healing: the complete A–Z guide to more than 150 different
alternative therapies / Mark Kastner and Hugh Burroughs.—1st Owl book ed.
p.   cm.
"An Owl book."
Originally published: La Mesa, Calif.: Halcyon Pub., 1993.
Includes bibliographical references and index.
1. Alternative medicine.   I. Burroughs, Hugh.
II. Burroughs, Hugh. Alternative healing.   III. Title.
R733.K376   1996   96-3082
615.5—dc20   CIP

ISBN 0-8050-4670-4

Henry Holt books are available for special promotions
and premiums. For details contact: Director, Special Markets.

Originally published in a different form in 1993 by
Halcyon Publishing.

First Owl Book Edition—1996

Designed by Betty Lew

Printed in the United States of America
All first editions are printed on acid-free paper. ∞

1   3   5   7   9   10   8   6   4   2

This book is dedicated to the health and well-being of our readers and people everywhere.

❈ ❈ ❈

Contents

Acknowledgments .... *xv*
Foreword .... *xvii*
Introduction .... *xix*

ALTERNATIVE HEALING: A–Z

Active Muscular Relaxation Techniques *1*
Acupressure Massage *2*
Acupuncture *3*
Aerobic Dance *8*
Alexander Technique *10*
Amino Acid Therapy *12*
Anticancer Diet *15*
Applied Kinesiology *17*
Applied Physiology *19*
Aromatherapy *20*
Arthritis Diet *23*
Art Therapy *23*
Aston-Patterning *25*
Autogenic Training *27*

Awareness Oriented Structural Therapy 29

Ayurveda 30

Bach Flower Remedies 32

Bates Method of Vision Training 33

Bee Venom Therapy 34

Benjamin System of Muscular Therapy 36

Bioenergetics 37

Biofeedback Training 39

Bodywork for the Childbearing Year 42

Bonnie Prudden Myotherapy 45

Burton Treatment 48

Callanetics 49

Cayce (Edgar) Therapies 51

Cayce/Reilly Massage 53

Chakra Balancing 54

Chelation Therapy 56

Chi Kung 58

Chi Nei Tsang 59

Children Massage 60

Chiropractic 61

Colon Therapy 64

Color Therapy 67

Connective Tissue Massage 70

CranioSacral Therapy 71

Creative Arts Therapy 73

Cross-Fiber Friction Massage 74

Cryotherapy 75

Crystal Therapy 76

Dance Therapy 78

Deep Compression Massage 79

Deep Tissue Massage 80

Deep Tissue Sculpting 80

DMSO Therapy 83

Dong Diet 85

Drama Therapy 87

Dream Therapy 88

Egoscue Method 90

Electrotherapy 91

Environmental Medicine 93
Exercise Therapy 94
Eye-Robics 96
Fasting 97
Feldenkrais Method 98
Fit for Life Program 100
Geriatric Massage 102
Gerson Therapy 103
Hakomi Method of Body Mind Therapy 106
Hanna Somatic Education 107
Hellerwork 109
Herbal Medicine 111
Holistic Medicine 118
Holotropic Breathwork 119
Homeopathy 120
Hoshino Therapy 123
Hoxsey Treatment 125
Hydrotherapy 126
Hyperbaric Oxygenation Therapy 128
Hypnotherapy 128
Imagery and Visualization 132
Infant Massage 133
Iridology 135
Jazzercise 137
Jin Shin Do Bodymind Acupressure 138
Jin Shin Jyutsu 139
Laban Movement Analysis 142
Life Extension 143
Live Cell Therapy 144
Livingston Treatment 145
Lomilomi Massage 146
LooyenWork 148
Macrobiotic Shiatsu 149
Macrobiotics 151
Magnetic Therapy 154
Maharishi Ayur-Veda 157
Manual Lymphatic Drainage 158
Massage Therapy 160

McDougall Diet 162

Meditation 164

Movement Therapy 165

Mucusless Diet 167

Music Therapy 168

Myofascial Release Therapy 170

Naprapathy 171

Natural Hygiene 172

Naturopathic Medicine 174

Network Chiropractic 176

Neuro/Cellular Repatterning 178

No-Nightshade Diet 179

Ortho-Bionomy 180

Orthomolecular Therapy 182

Osteopathy 184

Oxidative Therapy 186

Ozone Therapy 187

Parasympathetic Massage 188

Past Lives Therapy 189

Pfrimmer Technique 191

Physical Therapy 192

Poetry Therapy 194

Polarity Therapy 197

Postural Integration 199

Pranic Healing 201

Primal Therapy 202

Pritikin Diet 204

Pritikin Exercise 205

Proprioceptive Neuromuscular Facilitation (PNF Stretching) .. 206

Radiance Technique 207

Radionics 208

Rebirthing 211

Reflexology 213

Reichian Therapy 215

Reiki 218

Rice Diet 220

Rolfing 222

Rolfing Movement Integration 226

Rosen Method 226
Rubenfeld Synergy Method 228
Schuessler Cell Salts 231
Shamanism 232
SHEN Therapy 234
Shiatsu 236
SomatoEmotional Release 238
Sports Massage 239
St. John's Neuromuscular Therapy 241
Strain-Counterstrain Therapy 243
Structural Integration 244
Subliminal Therapy 246
Swedish Massage 247
Tai Chi Chuan 249
Thai Massage 251
Therapeutic Touch 253
Touch for Health 255
Trager Approach 256
Transcendental Meditation 259
Trigger Point Therapy 261
Tui Na Massage Therapy 263
Urine Therapy 265
Visceral Manipulation 267
Vitamin Therapy 268
Wheatgrass Diet 271
Whole Foods Diet 273
Yoga 275
Zero Balancing 277

Appendix: Illnesses and Therapies 281
   Glossary 294
   Appellations 303
   Resources 305
   Bibliography 323
   Further Reading 339
Index 341
About the Authors 357

❊ ❊ ❊

Acknowledgments

We would like to acknowledge the many therapists and practitioners, representing numerous modalities, who took the time to explain their work to us. Also, the librarians at the San Diego City and County libraries who helped us locate resource material, and all of the professional organizations that generously provided information about their modalities.

We want to thank our editor, Bryan K. Oettel, for all of his excellent suggestions and for being so accommodating and easy to work with. And, to production editor Rita Quintas, copy editor Adam Goldberger, and all of the other people at Henry Holt who contributed to the production of this book.

A special thanks goes to our agent, Wendy L. Zhorne, for all of her invaluable assistance along the way.

❊ ❊ ❊

Foreword

We have been living through a golden age of medical technology that
is dedicated to seeking cures and battling death. There has never
been a more effective medical management of the acutely ill than the quality
of care currently practiced within our emergency rooms. However, our
treatment for the chronically and terminally ill misses the mark.

Our present medical model only minimally acknowledges the innate
healing power of the human being. There is a need to reassess the concepts
of health and illness in order to extend the scope of the healing arts beyond
the present medical limits of drugs, radiation, and surgery. Even psychiatry
has not yet fully embraced the psychosocial aspects that are found within
most organic illness.

If there is psychosomatic illness, then there must be psychosomatic
health.

As the title states, *Alternative Healing* presents alternative methods to
enhance psychosomatic health and wellness. *Alternative Healing* is not a
guide to dissuade individuals from traditional Western allopathic medicine.
Rather, *Alternative Healing* is offered as a unique adjunct for those in search
of something more—a therapy that resonates with that specific individual's
psychosocial/spiritual beliefs. *Alternative Healing* serves as a therapeutic
directory consisting of a potpourri of therapeutic modalities in a simple,

concise, informative manner. The choice for personal repair is rightfully left to the reader.

Traditionally, health has implied the absence of illness and has focused on the quantity of one's life over the quality of one's existence. Many health care professionals have judged the relative states of one's bodily parts as a sine qua non of well-being or disease. Although this paradigm has its merits, it rarely honors the precept that health is also the appreciation and the acceptance of life itself, and it too often denies the importance of the family and work environment in both causing and maintaining illness.

Illness is not necessarily the enemy and more often than not serves as the prime mover guiding individuals to deeper understanding of self and a greater love for life. If the health professional can accept illness as a transformational process rather than as the enemy, then the client is more likely to draw upon his/her inner resources for repair. In this context, disease can be viewed as a grain of sand that has the potential to birth a greater understanding of what it is to be alive.

Implicit in Mark Kastner and Hugh Burroughs's book is the shared responsibility of the healer and the client in creating wellness and repair. Beyond the 150-plus alternative therapies offered in *Alternative Healing*, I would also like to add that healing can spring from a simple telephone conversation or a smile at a checkout counter. The ill can also find succor in the ancient healing arts of music, theater, dance, or play, as well as in family therapy and forgiveness. And yet the most exquisite truth: No one is completely healthy until the last person on earth is healed. To this end, each of us must rebuild the home within. *Alternative Healing* offers a variety of road maps to direct us home in our chosen way.

Paul H. Brenner, M.D., F.A.C.O.G.
Del Mar, California

❈ ❈ ❈

Introduction

Alternative Medicine is not a new idea. The major alternative therapies described in this book have had a positive impact on the health of billions of people for thousands of years. This knowledge of how to heal the human body and mind, acquired over the millennia, cannot be discounted merely because we are now living in a technologically oriented society.

Whether it is called Alternative Medicine, Natural Healing, Holistic Medicine, Alternative Healing (terms often used interchangeably), or the host of other names used to describe this movement, the basic philosophy is the same. Alternative Medicine treats people, not just their diseases. It treats causes rather than symptoms. It is interested in maintaining good health through the prevention of disease. And it understands that there is a crucial interrelationship between body, mind, and spirit.

One important concept of Alternative Healing is that the human body has an incredible capacity to heal and rejuvenate itself if given the opportunity and proper circumstances to do so. Another given is that the individual take responsibility for his own health. This requires a commitment from an individual to become at least partly involved in his own recovery, which makes healing more of a cooperative effort between the practitioner and the patient. You will find as you read on that this self-involvement in health care is paramount for Alternative Medicine.

This book was conceived out of a need for a reference work that thoroughly describes the broad spectrum of modalities that comprise Alternative Medicine. No single work available to date has been this complete.

The purpose of this book is to introduce our readers, both laypeople and professionals alike, to the wide variety of Alternative Medicine methods currently in use. *Alternative Healing* is also meant to remove the mystery sometimes associated with Alternative Medicine by providing clear, concise information on more than 150 different healing modalities.

Alternative Healing is an educational and reference tool that you may use to answer questions about various therapies you may have heard about. It is meant to be a springboard for further research.

Although we have covered a significant number of modalities, we do not maintain that we have listed every one known. We decided to choose major time-tested therapies, many of which have had historical importance, in addition to those we felt had the greatest potential benefit to our readers. From Acupuncture to Zero Balancing, we have endeavored to present each subject in as unbiased and objective a manner as possible.

Consistent with Alternative Medicine's philosophy of taking responsibility for your own health, we feel that informed individuals are more likely to take responsibility for their own health and that they will be better able to choose a practitioner or therapy that is appropriate for them and their family.

Alternative Medicine is medicine for the people. Because many alternative therapies have been developed by individuals seeking to help themselves, we have included their personal stories and the history of the therapy's development, where available.

You will read the fascinating accounts of numerous people who were given up as untreatable by conventional Western allopathic medicine. Unwilling to accept the "fate" that they would suffer the remainder of their life, these courageous people decided to take charge of their own recovery. Determined to be healthy once again, they went on to discover or develop alternative therapies that not only cured them, but cured others as well. We hope you find these stories both interesting and inspirational.

We believe that the future of health care is in the integration of Eastern and Western methods. Today, many allopathic doctors are accepting the benefits derived from Alternative Medicine, and some are incorporating facets of it into their practice. For example, some medical doctors are using guided imagery and acupuncture to control pain, while others are utilizing alternative practices such as Vitamin Therapy and Chelation Therapy to treat a wide variety of conditions.

There are many professional organizations such as the American College of Advancement in Medicine, the American Association of Medical Acupuncture, and the American Academy of Orthomolecular Medicine that represent Western allopathic physicians and other practitioners who incorporate a specific alternative therapy into their practice.

Our hope is that every Western allopathic physician will read this book and become more familiar with Alternative Medicine. We feel that it is important for doctors to have an understanding of these therapies because many of their patients are currently availing themselves of alternative medical treatments.

We do not advocate, nor would any sensible person involved in the healing arts suggest, that Western allopathic medicine should be abandoned in favor of Alternative Medicine. We have only high regard for Western allopathic medicine and believe that it, along with Alternative Medicine, should play a prominent role in the restructuring of today's health care system.

What we do believe, however, is that there should be freedom of choice in health care today, and that an individual should know about these choices.

We recommend that you read this book cover to cover. After reading about all the different modalities, we hope you will begin to see how many of them are interconnected and how the basic concepts, applications, etc., of Alternative Healing fit together.

New to this edition of *Alternative Healing* is the appendix, "Illnesses and Therapies." This section of the book cross-references common ailments/maladies/illnesses/diseases with significant alternative treatments.

Since a major objective of this book is to educate you and get you involved with making choices for your own health care, we have provided an extensive resource section with the names of more than two hundred organizations, involved with all types of Alternative Healing, that you may call or write for additional information.

Also, listed in most of the therapies are suggestions for additional reading. The complete information for most of these books including publisher, copyright date, etc., is listed in the bibliography.

One final note: For reasons of familiarity and uniformity, we have chosen to use the older Wade-Giles System, and not the Pinyin System for the spelling of Chinese words. Hence, we use *chi* throughout this book although the word can also be spelled *qi*.

We hope that you enjoy the book. And, more importantly, we hope that you learn how Alternative Medicine can benefit you.

※ ※ ※

Important Note

This book is a reference work and is presented only as general information that the authors feel should be available to the public. The material contained herein is for the purpose of acquainting or familiarizing the reader with the many alternative therapies and choices in health care available to him or her. If there are health concerns involving illness or injury, it is recommended that you consult a duly licensed health care professional for guidance in the selection of an appropriate therapeutic modality. It is a sign of wisdom to seek professional advice. The authors disclaim responsibility for any unfavorable effects resulting from the use of information contained in this book.

ALTERNATIVE HEALING A–Z

🌿 | ACTIVE MUSCULAR RELAXATION TECHNIQUES | 🌀

Active Muscular Relaxation Techniques are a powerful new approach to bodywork used for relaxing overactive muscles and managing soft tissue pain.

Overactivity in local musculature is a typical response to pain from trauma or poor posture. Active Muscular Relaxation Techniques utilize resisted isometric contractions of the overactive muscle or its antagonist (the one opposing its action). The objective of this procedure is to relax and/or lengthen (stretch) the overactive muscle.

In the past, the client's role was to remain passive while a massage therapist or other type of practitioner administered to him. With Active Muscular Relaxation Techniques the active participation of the client is a required part of the therapy.

With the client involved, a partnership is then formed with the therapist, and both individuals take responsibility for the healing process. Additionally, as the client learns the simple techniques, he is able to perform more self-treatments. Thus, the client becomes less dependent on the therapist and can deal with minor problems on his own.

Active Muscular Relaxation Techniques are based on the gentle methods of muscular relaxation that have their origin in the osteopathic work, physical therapy, and manual medicine of the late 1940s. The techniques are complementary to passive massage therapy techniques and chiropractic adjustments, but are not intended as a substitute for them.

❧ | ACUPRESSURE MASSAGE | ❧

Acupressure Massage is a type of bodywork based on the same concept as Acupuncture. Rather than inserting needles into the body for treatment, however, Acupressure uses pressure applied from the therapist's fingertip or knuckle, or with a blunt-tipped instrument called a *tei shin* to stimulate specific points on the Acupuncture meridians (energy channels) on the patient's body.

Since many of the Acupressure points are within a person's own reach, Acupressure Massage can also be self-administered. This self-treatment can be very beneficial to persons with chronic pain.

The Chinese people have used Acupressure since ancient times. The history of Acupressure has its roots in traditional Chinese medicine, which was documented over four thousand years ago in *Huang-ti Nei-Ching (The Yellow Emperor's Classic of Internal Medicine)*, but it probably goes back even further than that, to man's origin. We know that when we receive an injury to ourselves, such as a sprain, being struck by an object, a cramp, or getting burned, our instinctive reaction is to rub, massage, or hold the site of pain to get some type of relief.

For thousands of years, effective hands-on folk remedies were passed on from one generation to the next. During many years of development, the art of massage was combined and integrated with the principles and body points of Acupuncture to produce what is now called Acupressure.

The unrestricted flow of vital life energy within the body is an essential principle to Acupressure Massage, just as it is to Acupuncture. Stress within the body can be produced by many factors including illness, injury, or emotional upset, and results in muscular tension.

Muscular tension tends to accumulate around Acupressure points, causing the large muscle groups to contract, blocking the flow of vital life energy. The body wants to be in homeostasis, a state of balance or equilibrium in which the organs, glands, and all other interdependent body systems are working together in harmony. When the flow of vital energy is interrupted, the body is out of balance and its ability to effectively deal with the disrupting condition is inhibited.

Like Acupuncture, Acupressure Massage treats the whole body. Clinical evidence has shown that by applying prolonged finger pressure to various Acupressure points, specific organs, glands, and body systems can be activated and balanced in addition to relieving muscular tension. Thus, Acupressure Massage works on the various body systems (organ, glandular, etc.) as well as the musculature to help restore the flow of vital life energy through the body meridians freely from point to point, thus returning the body to homeostasis.

There are different theories as to how Acupressure relieves pain. Since the massage increases blood circulation, toxins such as carbon dioxide, histamines, and lactic acid are removed while oxygen and other nutrients are brought to the muscle and tension is thus relieved. Prolonged pressure on Acupressure points may release endorphins by stimulating the pituitary gland. Endorphins are opiate-like substances, one function of which is to control pain.

Additionally, some of the latest research has shown that with the release of endorphins, a cortisol molecule is simultaneously released. Cortisol is the body's own natural chemical that relieves inflammation to promote healing.

Acupressure Massage is used to treat a wide variety of maladies including muscular pain, migraine headaches, insomnia, backaches, gastrointestinal problems, and gynecological problems.

Treatments can also be used as preventive health care by promoting a condition of homeostasis within the body. By balancing and regulating all the body organs and systems (glandular, nervous, muscular, skeletal, etc.) through Acupressure Massage, an overall feeling of well-being can be achieved.

Specialized training for Acupressure Massage therapists begins with a basic 150-hour certification program and ranges up to 850 hours for an advanced training program. For additional information contact the Acupressure Institute or the American Oriental Bodywork Therapy Association (AOBTA).

❧ | ACUPUNCTURE | ❦

Acupuncture is a complete medical system that is used to diagnose and treat illness, manage chronic disorders, alleviate pain, and promote health through prevention and maintenance. It can be used for physical, emotional, and psychological problems.

Acupuncture is part of Traditional Oriental Medicine, the most widely used healing system in the world. Traditional Oriental Medicine is a complete medical system that combines herbs, moxabustion (a form of heating), cupping, gua sha (scraping skin to increase circulation), massage, diet, and gentle exercise along with Acupuncture to correct energy imbalances in the body.

The practice of Acupuncture is rooted in ancient China. It is mentioned in the *Huang-ti Nei-Ching (The Yellow Emperor's Classic of Internal Medicine)*, a comprehensive documentation of Traditional Chinese Medicine during the time of the Yellow Emperor, Huang-ti, who is said to have ruled from 2697 to 2595 B.C.

The *Huang-ti Nei-Ching*, one of the oldest Chinese medical books still in existence, is used today as one of the main reference books on Acupuncture theory. Since the time of the Yellow Emperor, the practice of Acupuncture has remained virtually unchanged.

Acupuncture needles dating from four thousand years ago have been found by archaeologists in China. The first needles were made from stone; later, gold, silver, or bronze was used.

From the third century B.C. to the seventh century A.D., Chinese medicine was highly influenced by the philosophy and example of Taoist sages, who believed in preventing disease through moderation.

Acupuncture spread into other Asian countries in about A.D. 1000 and was introduced into Europe about A.D. 1700.

At the turn of the century Sir William Osler (1849–1919), a Canadian physician, was using Acupuncture to treat low back pain. Dr. Osler felt that Acupuncture was the best treatment available to deal with this condition.

More recently, Acupuncture was introduced into the United States as a direct result of President Richard Nixon's trip to China in 1970. During the trip, a member of the mission became ill and required an appendectomy. What made his surgery unique was the fact that it was performed while the patient was anesthetized with Acupuncture as the only method of anesthesia.

Impressed with what he had learned of Acupuncture, President Nixon helped to organize a cultural exchange of medical practitioners between the United States and China.

Later that same year, thirty Chinese acupuncturists were invited to participate in a program at the University of California, Los Angeles Medical

School—thus Acupuncture was introduced to conventional medicine in the United States. Today, after more than twenty years of clinical usage, the UCLA Pain Center continues to use Acupuncture as one of its main modalities for the relief of pain.

Basic Acupuncture theory lies within the ancient philosophy of Taoism. The Taoists believed that the universe can be described by the dualistic concept of *yin* and *yang*. All matter is made of yin and yang, including every part of the human body. The concept of yin is described as that which is dark, cold, moist, yielding, negative in polarity, and feminine. The concept of yang is described as that which is light, warm, dry, dominant, positive in polarity, and masculine.

Although yin and yang are opposites in nature, it is their ability to interact and balance each other that creates a dynamic interplay that we call health. All diseases or conditions can be classified as either yin or yang in nature due to an imbalance of one or the other. An example of a yin disease would be a chronic, long-standing degenerative condition such as cancer. An example of a yang disease would be an acute condition of short duration such as flu or sore throat.

An equally important concept in Traditional Oriental Medicine is that of *chi* (pronounced "chee"). The Chinese have more than a thousand different representations (concepts) of what *chi* is, which makes defining it extremely difficult. For simplicity's sake, we can think of *chi* as the energetic force behind all of life. It is this concept of *chi* or vital energy that many of the alternative therapies described in this book have borrowed, and it is a mainstay of Alternative Medicine.

Related to the practice of Acupuncture, *chi* can be described more specifically as the vital energy that circulates through Acupuncture meridians.

Chinese Acupuncture theory maintains that there are twelve main meridians or energy channels that relate to the internal organs: lungs, large intestine, stomach, spleen, heart, the pericardium (the sac around the heart), known as the gate of life, small intestine, bladder, kidney, gall bladder, liver, and what is called the triple warmer, whose function is the assimilation and transportation of energy and the maintenance of body temperature.

Located along these twelve meridians, which literally run all over the body from head to toe, there are more than 461 specific Acupuncture points. Acupuncturists believe that either an excess or a deficiency of *chi* can result in the manifestation of a particular type of illness.

Thus, when an Acupuncture point is needled (a needle inserted into the point), the Acupuncturist can manipulate the needle to either build *chi* if there is a deficiency of energy, or drain *chi* if there is an excess of energy. It is through this balancing of energy that the patient's health is restored.

In addition to manual needle manipulation, the point can also be stimulated by the use of heat, cold, pressure, or electrical current. The Chinese are currently experimenting with laser light as a means of stimulating points.

Heating, which is termed *moxabustion*, is the most popular method of stimulating a point. Moxabustion can be used in conjunction with Acupuncture treatments or as a stand-alone treatment. The traditional moxabustion technique involves a practitioner placing a small pile or ball of *moxa*, the leaf of the Chinese mugwort (wormwood) tree, on the end of an inserted needle or on the skin, and igniting it. When ignited, moxa smolders without producing a flame. Today, the more commonly used form of moxa is a commercially prepared stick which is easier to work with. The ignited moxa stick is moved around the needle to produce gentle, even heating which stimulates the point.

Electrical stimulation of a point is accomplished by sending minute amounts of pulsed current into the needle. The current pulses, which can be adjusted for both frequency and intensity, are generated by a small battery-powered device.

Although some people in the United States have only recognized Acupuncture for its ability to control pain, the World Health Organization accepts Acupuncture therapy for over one hundred different diseases. Additionally, the National Institute on Drug Abuse and the National Institute on Alcohol Abuse and Alcoholism have initiated demonstration projects using Acupuncture treatment for crack cocaine detoxification and alcoholism.

Currently in the United States, Acupuncture is used to treat a wide variety of physical problems including pain, gastrointestinal problems, sinusitis, gynecological syndromes, stress management, asthma, AIDS, urogenital problems, impotence, infertility, tennis elbow, "frozen" shoulder, various forms of tendonitis, arthritis/joint problems, and many others.

Although the exact mechanism that would explain how Acupuncture works is still unknown, recent studies into the physiological reactions of the body to Acupuncture by researcher Dr. Bruce Pomeranz at the University of Toronto has provided some scientific insight into how Acupuncture affects pain.

Dr. Pomeranz's findings focused on the ability of Acupuncture to stimulate the production of endorphins, opiate-like substances produced in the brain whose function is to control pain in the body. Endorphins have been found to be nearly one thousand times stronger than morphine. Thus, there is now some scientific validation as to how Acupuncture controls pain.

Along with the release of endorphins, another substance called cortisol is simultaneously released. Cortisol is the body's own natural anti-inflammatory drug. Controlling pain and reducing inflammation helps to promote healing; this seems to explain why Acupuncture works so well for joint and structural disorders.

An Acupuncture needle is very fine, about the diameter of a thick hair, and made from stainless steel. Unlike a hypodermic needle, it is not hollow, and nothing is injected into the body. Reusable Acupuncture needles are sterilized using procedures regulated by state and federal agencies. With the arrival of the AIDS virus, however, most practitioners have adopted the use of presterilized disposable needles, which eliminate the risk of infection or disease transmission from the treatments.

For greater patient comfort, needle insertion techniques have been refined over the centuries enabling a skilled practitioner to place the needle with little or no sensation.

In China, traditional Oriental and Western medicines are used in conjunction with one another. A typical Chinese hospital will have one wing devoted to Acupuncture and another for Western allopathic medicine. Patients are moved between wings for treatment so they are able to receive the benefits provided by both modalities.

Today, Acupuncture is widely practiced throughout Asia, in the former Soviet republics, and in Europe. In the United States over the past twenty years, it has grown increasingly popular. Currently, there are approximately five thousand Acupuncture practitioners throughout the United States, with hundreds of new acupuncturists starting practice each year.

In the United States, there are currently more than thirty schools of Acupuncture in existence. Prerequisites for admission to a school of Acupuncture include courses in Western sciences such as anatomy, physiology, and chemistry. The Acupuncture curriculum consists of 2,400 hours of instruction, usually taken over a period of three to four years.

The regulation and licensing of health care professionals throughout the United States varies from state to state and some states do not regulate the practice of Acupuncture. In many states, however, acupuncturists are licensed while in other states only licensed medical doctors have the ability to practice Acupuncture.

For additional information contact the American Association of Acupuncture and Oriental Medicine, the American Academy of Medical Acupuncture, the California Acupuncture Association, the American Foundation of Traditional Chinese Medicine, or the National Commission for the Certification of Acupuncturists.

✌ | AEROBIC DANCE | ☙

Aerobic Dance is a complete physical fitness program designed for fun and enjoyment. Unlike many stop-and-start calisthenics which exercise only a particular part of the body, Aerobic Dance uses the concept of continuous activity to achieve its goals of physical conditioning and figure improvement.

Aerobic Dance puts the body through a carefully tested and well-monitored fitness workout that strengthens and develops the aerobic (cardiovascular) system while it shapes the figure and tones the muscles. Virtually every part of the body is affected during the workout.

Aerobic means "in the presence of oxygen." The sustained activity of dance movements stimulates and strengthens the heart and lungs, thereby improving the body's ability to deliver and utilize oxygen quickly and efficiently. This results in greater energy and vitality.

Aerobic Dance is not merely exercising to music or performing a series of dance exercises; rather, it is a series of carefully designed patterns (steps/movements) that are learned by the student and then danced to with music. Each pattern can have several different suggested musical selections that are appropriate for it.

Additionally, complete dances are choreographed to emotionally match the mood and beat of a specific song. It is the choreography that makes the participants become part of the music as they dance, and makes Aerobic Dancing a stimulating and enjoyable experience.

The creator of Aerobic Dance, Jacki Sorensen, loved to dance from the time she was six years old. While still a young girl, her dance teacher pointed out that she was huffing and puffing too much during a routine. Sorensen began to increase her physical endurance by jumping rope and tap-dancing for hours at a time. Before long she was able to perform her dance routine and make it look easy. This started her lifelong program of physical conditioning.

In 1969, at the age of twenty-six, Jacki Sorensen was asked to host a local television exercise program for the United States Air Force base in Puerto Rico. While preparing for the show she studied the U.S. Air Force Aerobics program and decided to take their cardiovascular fitness evaluation. After scoring "excellent" on the twelve-minute running test, though having never run before, Jacki Sorensen had a revelation: She concluded that the years of dance training not only kept her figure trim, but kept her heart and lungs in good shape as well.

Sorensen realized that her fitness was the result of years of dancing and that dance itself could be organized into an aerobic fitness program. After the dances choreographed for the television show met with a favorable response, she decided to set up a research program to test them.

The research would compare the increase in physical endurance between participants in her twelve-week Aerobic Dance program and participants in a similar jogging program. Results showed that Aerobic Dance increased endurance as well as or better than jogging. The Aerobic Dance participants, however, received a bonus in the way of improved figures.

After moving to New Jersey in 1970, Sorensen kept testing and refining the dance routines, and in 1971 she decided to see what kind of public interest her Aerobic Dance program would receive.

The first Aerobic Dance class was held in a church recreation room in East Orange, New Jersey, with only six women participating. A short time later there were two classes with twenty-five participants at the church and three other classes at a nearby YMCA. Thus Aerobic Dancing, Inc. was born.

The Aerobic Dance workout consists of several parts. It begins with the Flexibility routine, which is designed to increase the elasticity of the muscles and gently prepare the body for vigorous physical activity. It is not choreographed into patterns, nor is it intended to be a dance.

Next is the Warm-up portion, which incorporates stretching and limbering movements into a dance. This routine is designed to raise muscle temperature, making it easier for chemical reactions that take place between the muscles and nerves, and to gradually increase the heart rate.

Next come the Aerobic Dance Routines. Consisting of a series of steps, patterns, and complete choreographed dances, these routines are adapted to a wide range of music styles. This is the aerobic phase of the workout and the emphasis is on continuous motion. This phase lasts from fifteen to thirty minutes.

Last is the Cool-down. This consists of a slow dance with graceful stretching movements designed to gradually reduce the intensity of the workout, help the body wind down, and allow the heart rate to gradually return to an acceptable recovery level.

Today Aerobic Dance Routines are taught worldwide. Classes are offered in a wide variety of venues and for almost any age group. For additional information, consult Jacki Sorensen's excellent book, *Aerobic Dancing*, which explains the program in detail.

❧ | ALEXANDER TECHNIQUE | ❦

The Alexander Technique is an educational process which teaches the student improved use of his body. It also helps him to identify and change poor and inefficient physical habits which may be causing stress and fatigue.

People unconsciously misuse their body in the performance of their occupation, and while accomplishing ordinary, everyday tasks and activities.

The muscular habits involved with activities such as walking, playing tennis, dancing, standing in line, washing dishes, playing a violin, or sitting at a computer can create tension within the body. Tension interferes with the body's healthy physical and mental functioning, and restricts an individual's feeling of freedom of movement.

Because he gradually becomes accustomed to it, an individual is rarely aware of the tension he carries unless it causes pain, or some other physical symptom is manifested. Tension has a powerful impact on the ability to accomplish a wide variety of daily goals. Becoming aware of and changing the habits that interfere with these simple everyday activities builds a foundation for change.

The goal of the Alexander Technique, after a series of lessons has been completed, is to improve the student's postural habits. This improvement generally results in greater ease and freedom of movement, and increased energy. By helping the individual learn to expend the appropriate amount of effort for any particular activity, more energy is left for all other activities.

The Alexander Technique lessons provide a means of overcoming the harmful habits that cause physical and emotional stress in the body. Additionally, they allow people to learn to perform their daily activities more freely. This is achieved by releasing tension and replacing it with calm, poise, and improved coordination, which results in improved overall health, alertness, and performance.

Physical retraining teaches an individual, through simple movements, how to develop more awareness and control in their daily activities by putting the body in a state of balance and relaxation. Since the Alexander Technique is a learning process, the student must be willing to take responsibility for fully participating in the lessons and applying in his everyday life the knowledge of the technique.

Frederick Mathias Alexander (1869–1955) was born in Wynward, Tasmania, in Australia. His parents were of ample means and he spent his youth managing and training horses. At the age of seventeen he started working for a tin-mining company. At that time his main interests were the violin and amateur dramatics. In his early twenties, he went to Melbourne to live with his uncle and trained there as a reciter. In his spare time he acted in plays and also produced them.

He became a successful Shakespearean recitalist but developed vocal problems that were ruining his career. One night he lost his voice while on stage. He consulted with numerous physicians and after none of the medications or other treatments they suggested worked, he retired from the stage.

Attempting to cure his disability, Alexander spent the next ten years carefully observing and examining the way he used his body while speaking and acting. He discovered he was creating a pattern of tension that was interfering with the correct relationship between his head, neck, and back. This work became the foundation for the Alexander Technique.

After curing himself, he continued to give recitals and taught the technique to others. A friend, Dr. McKay, urged him to go to London and teach his technique. Alexander continued to teach his technique until he died at the age of eighty-six in 1955.

Many notable personalities have studied the Alexander Technique, including Lily Langtry, George Bernard Shaw, Aldous Huxley, Paul Newman, Monty Python star John Cleese, and Nobel Prize–winning scientist Nikolaas Tinbergen. The technique has also been taught in many academic and institutional settings. It is currently part of the curriculum at the Juilliard School in New York City, the American Conservatory Theater in San Francisco, Boston University, the Royal Academy of Music in London, and many other learning institutions.

Although almost anyone can benefit from lessons of the Alexander Technique, there are two general classes of people who most often utilize it. The first consists of individuals, both professional and amateur, who are required to use complex physical coordination in their profession or daily activities, and want to consistently perform as well as possible. These include athletes involved in all types of sports, dancers, musicians, actors, and others. The second comprises people who have existing pain and/or dysfunction and are seeking relief from it.

Although the Alexander Technique does not treat specific symptoms, it can aid in bringing relief from a variety of problems such as muscle and joint pain, loss of voice, or general postural imbalances.

The Alexander Technique is normally taught in private lessons lasting thirty minutes to one hour, although some teachers hold group classes and workshops. While in comfortable clothing, students are guided with gentle touch and verbal instructions through a sequence of simple movements by the teacher. The student learns to observe simple activities like sitting, bending, talking, and walking, and then to change the habits that interfere with their optimum functioning.

Even with the teacher's hands-on guidance the student's muscular habits can be resistant to change, so part of the lesson takes place on a table where the teacher can help the student change some of these habits without the interference that often comes during even the simplest acts. After a series of lessons the internal feedback system becomes more accurate so that problems can be avoided before the onset of pain or impaired performance.

Teachers of the Alexander Technique are required, but not limited to, 1,600 hours of training over a minimum three-year period at an approved school. Persons who successfully complete the training course are eligible for membership in the North American Society of the Teachers of Alexander Technique.

A list of certified Alexander teachers can be obtained from both the North American Society of the Teachers of Alexander Technique and the American Center for the Alexander Technique.

AMINO ACID THERAPY

Amino Acid Therapy is the use of "free-form" amino acids for various therapeutic purposes. Supplements of pure amino acids in the form of powder, capsules, or pills are referred to as free-form amino acids. In conjunction with vitamins and minerals, amino acid supplements can be used to treat a variety of illnesses, including many physical and mental disorders.

By definition, an amino acid is an organic acid that contains an amine (ammonia-like) chemical group. Because they are called acids, one may think amino acids are highly corrosive, like stomach acid (hydro-chloric acid). Actually, they are very weak acids and are virtually neutral in the body.

The human body has been likened to a huge chemical factory. It takes raw materials and turns them into the thousands of chemicals the body needs to function. Amino acids are essential for maintaining a healthy body and mind. Without them we could not exist as living beings.

In the body, amino acids link together like building blocks to form pro-teins and polypeptides (small proteins like hormones). The word *protein* comes from the Greek meaning "first things." Amino acids are the essential materials for growth and reproduction, and can be found in every cell in the body. Bones, muscles, organs, other tissues, and nearly all the hormones used in the body are aggregations of various amino acids. Amino acids are often combined with vitamins and minerals to make a complete entity. The body contains over fifty thousand different protein structures.

There are two types of amino acids, nonessential and essential. A nonessential amino acid refers only to the fact that the body is capable of manufacturing it internally and so it is not required in the diet. An essential amino acid cannot be made by the body and must be consumed in the diet. Reference works on the subject list the following as essential amino acids: arginine, histidine, isoleucine, leucine, lysine, methionine, phenylala-nine, threonine, tryptophan, and valine.

In nature, these essential amino acids can be found in foods such as beef, chicken, fish, eggs, cottage cheese, milk, soybeans, some vegetables, seeds, and nuts. Different foods have varying amounts of a particular amino acid.

Amino Acid Therapy is a holistic approach to health. It sees all of the chemical reactions that take place in the body as a complete, functioning, and interrelated unit. The idea is to provide the body with the proper raw materials it requires, through supplementation when necessary, to produce all the substances needed for optimal health.

An individual may be deficient in certain essential body chemicals because either he does not have the necessary amino acids to manufacture them or he is unable to properly utilize the amino acids he does have. Either of these situations can be due to a variety of causes, including poor or incomplete nutrition; pollution, chemical fertilizers, food processing, or the use of alcoholic beverages and tobacco products; the person's own bio-chemistry; or other factors.

Amino acids are not a new discovery. In 1913 researchers established the connection between pellagra, a disease characterized by scaly skin, diarrhea, and dementia (symptoms similar to schizophrenia) and a deficiency in the amino acid tryptophan. Pellagra is caused by a lack of vitamin B_3 (niacin). Although niacin can be obtained from a source such as yeast, it can also be manufactured in the body. This process begins with the amino acid tryptophan.

Amino Acid Therapy became possible in the early 1960s, when free-form amino acids became widely available. The medical establishment tended to view the taking of free-form amino acids as unnecessary. However, due to the work of researchers and the results obtained in practice by medical colleagues, doctors today are more aware of the benefits of treating people with free-form amino acids.

For example, research has shown that the release of histamine is required for physical orgasm to take place. The amino acid histidine, in the presence of vitamin B_6, is converted by the body into histamine. Men and women who are unable to achieve orgasm are usually low in histamine and are benefited by histidine supplements.

Many so-called diseases, physical problems, and emotional states are biochemical in nature. It has been shown that Amino Acid Therapy is beneficial to people who suffer from a variety of disorders such as depression, anxiety, obesity, poor memory, insomnia, heart problems, peptic ulcers, viral infections such as herpes, sexual problems, or the inability to stop using tobacco or alcohol.

In the early 1980s Durk Pearson and Sandy Shaw, in their book *Life Extension*, detailed the use of amino acids for a variety of therapeutic uses. The goal of Life Extension, a relatively new field, was to mitigate the aging process through the use of nutritional supplements including amino acids, vitamins, and minerals.

Gary Zisk, M.D., in his book *The Amino Acid Super Diet*, details how amino acids can be used for a weight-loss program. This successful program, tested over a ten-year period on more than ten thousand patients, not only helped people reduce their weight but improved their mental condition as well.

For twenty years Priscilla Slagle, M.D., suffered from intense depression. As a psychiatrist, she had undergone personal psychoanalysis. After spending several thousand dollars on five years of therapy she still suffered. Realizing she felt worse after eating some foods, Dr. Slagle became interested in a biochemical approach to the alleviation of depressive moods.

After learning how specific nutrient substances can affect specific mood-elevating brain chemicals, she began nutritional treatment on herself. By using certain amino acids, vitamins, and minerals, Dr. Slagle became depression free. This program is detailed in her book *The Way Up from Down*.

Many naturopaths are prescribing L-lysine to control skin eruptions due to the herpes virus. DL-phenylalanine is used to mitigate or control chronic pain by allowing endorphins to remain in solution. It is also used as an effective appetite suppressant. L-tyrosine used in combination with phenylalanine is used to treat depression. L-glutamine is used in alcohol rehabilitation to help stop alcohol cravings and is also effective in curbing sugar cravings.

L-tryptophan was the most popular amino acid in use. Studies have shown that when used at night, L-tryptophan is an excellent sleep inducer. *Lancet*, the British medical journal, reported that when used during the day, L-tryptophan is an excellent antidepressant with little or no side effects.

Today, Amino Acid Therapy has been severely restricted because the FDA has permanently taken all of the amino acid tryptophan off the market. This was in response to a single tainted batch produced by a small, obscure manufacturer in Japan, even though the supplies from other large manufacturers were not contaminated. Although tryptophan has been proven to be totally safe and is sold around the world, the FDA still refuses to allow tryptophan to be sold in the United States.

Tryptophan is an important amino acid used for many beneficial purposes, and it is a key element in Dr. Slagle's program for treating depression without drugs. Now, without tryptophan, her program is unavailable to people wanting to use it.

Although amino acids are not medicines or drugs, they should be used with caution. It is advisable to consult a physician knowledgeable in the use of amino acids before starting a free-form amino acid supplementation program.

There are many excellent books available in bookstores, health food stores, and libraries on the therapeutic uses of amino acids. A good one is *The Amino Revolution* by Robert Erdmann, Ph.D., with Meirion Jones.

❧ | ANTICANCER DIET | ☙

The Anticancer Diet, as it is sometimes referred to, is no more than a set of dietary guidelines recommended by the American Cancer Society, the

National Cancer Institute, and the American Institute for Cancer Research. The information published by all three organizations is very similar.

These dietary guidelines are based on the conclusions of the nation's leading experts who have carefully reviewed worldwide studies of eating habits, and the latest scientific evidence on the influence of diet and nutrition on the development of cancer.

The dietary guidelines are only *recommendations* and not a *guarantee* that following them will prevent a person from getting cancer. Cancer, with its many different forms, is still a mysterious disease not completely understood. Human biochemistry is extremely complex and varies with each individual. Add to that variable factors such as age, sex, weight, genetics, environment, and previous health history, and it is clear that both the disease and people are far too complex for that kind of assurance.

The National Cancer Institute estimates that about one-third of all cancer deaths may be related to what a person eats over a long period of time. A cancer does not just suddenly appear. It develops very slowly through different stages, some of which are reversible. The type of food a person eats can affect many or perhaps all of these stages of development, from an initial exposure to a carcinogen to the long gradual development of a tumor.

Diet and nutrition can work two ways to help prevent cancer. The first is to avoid, or consume only in moderation, foods that are known to contain significant levels of carcinogens, and foods that seem to provide the type of environment a cancer cell needs to grow in and multiply when the foods are eaten over a long period of time. The second is to consume quantities of foods which contain nutrients and other compounds which seem to augment the body's natural defense system and its ability to destroy carcinogens.

General Dietary Guidelines:

- Reduce the amount of fats consumed, especially saturated fats.
- Reduce consumption of salt-cured, smoked, and nitrate-cured foods (bacon, smoked ham, cheese, seafood, corned beef and pastrami, and luncheon meats).
- Eat high-fiber foods (whole grains, cereals, legumes, fruits, and vegetables).
- Eat foods rich in vitamin A, vitamin C, and beta-carotene (dark green

leafy vegetables, red, yellow, and orange vegetables and fruits, and citrus fruits and their juices).
• Eat cruciferous vegetables (cabbage family).
• Avoid or consume only in moderation alcoholic beverages.

Other Recommendations:

• Avoid tobacco.
• Avoid too much refined sugar and sodium.
• Avoid obesity (being 40 percent or more overweight).
• Get the proper amount of exercise.

By following the recommended dietary guidelines, the organizations that publish this information believe, an individual's chances of avoiding the disease will be improved. Also, it may reduce the chances of other illnesses such as heart disease and diabetes.

Additional information is available from the American Cancer Society, the National Cancer Institute, and the American Institute for Cancer Research.

❧ | APPLIED KINESIOLOGY | ❧

Applied Kinesiology is a healing system which evaluates and treats an individual's structural, chemical, and mental aspects. It employs muscle testing and other standard methods of diagnosis.

Applied Kinesiology therapeutically utilizes nutrition, manipulation, diet, Acupressure, exercise, and education to help restore balance and harmony in the body and maintain well-being throughout life. It is sometimes confused with standard kinesiology, which is the study of the principles of mechanics and anatomy related to human movement.

Applied Kinesiology had its beginning in 1964 when Dr. George Goodheart, a chiropractor in Detroit, Michigan, made a discovery while treating a young man with a severe muscular dysfunction which caused the scapula (shoulder blade) to protrude like a "wing."

Goodheart found that a few seconds of deep pressure on the serratus anterior muscle (located under the arm) improved its function, and the young man's problem was eliminated. He also found that other muscles could be treated in the same way to improve posture. Thus the first Applied Kinesiology procedure was developed.

Although trained as a chiropractor, Goodheart was well versed in Oriental meridian therapy, osteopathic cranial technique, anatomy, physiology, biochemistry, and clinical nutrition. He investigated the findings of an osteopath named Chapman, which demonstrated the clinical relationship between muscles, organs, and glands.

Later, nutrition and Oriental meridian therapy, or Acupressure (Acupuncture points treated by finger pressure) were correlated with muscle inhibition. Goodheart developed the hypothesis that muscles were related to other parts of the body, and muscle testing became a diagnostic tool. Eventually he developed a systematic charting-out of muscle reflexes and their effect on corresponding body organs.

A simplified version of Applied Kinesiology called "Touch for Health" was developed in the 1970s by Dr. John F. Thie, a chiropractor in Pasadena, California. Touch for Health is a practical system of self-help health care that the average person can learn and apply to her daily life.

Muscle testing is the most well known procedure in Applied Kinesiology. The idea is that a weak muscle causes tension in the opposing muscle, thus creating dysfunction in the organ corresponding to that muscle (according to Goodheart's charting).

By testing the muscles which relate to the body's twelve major organs, the procedure can help locate and correct imbalances in the body's energy system. Muscle testing can also determine whether the imbalance is nutritional, psychological, or structural.

The test is simple and consists of the practitioner applying a force to a specific location on the person's arm or leg. The person then tries to resist having her arm or leg moved by the practitioner. If the subject cannot resist, the organ related to the muscle being tested is determined to be weak.

To treat a weakened muscle and related organ, the practitioner applies firm pressure to the appropriate Acupuncture reflex point, stimulating and strengthening the weakened tissue. After several moments, the Acupuncture point is released and the muscle is rested.

In chiropractic treatment muscle testing is used to evaluate the effectiveness of adjustments. If the initial muscle test shows weakness, a chiropractic adjustment is then given. A follow-up test can determine if the adjustment has restored the nerve transmission and helped the organ regain a normal level of function.

Although Applied Kinesiology is used primarily by chiropractors, medical doctors, dentists, podiatrists, psychiatrists, and other health care professionals apply its principles when treating their patients.

Additional information and a list of Applied Kinesiology practitioners is available from the International College of Applied Kinesiology.

✿ | APPLIED PHYSIOLOGY | ✿

Applied Physiology is a powerful system of stress-management procedures, utilizing muscle monitoring and biofeedback, that allows the body to communicate what is out of balance and what it requires to correct each stress condition.

Applied Physiology was developed in the early 1980s by Richard Utt. With his own physical condition far from healthy, a friend suggested he seek help from Dr. Sheldon Deal, an expert in Applied Kinesiology. Working with Dr. Deal, Utt participated in intensive sessions of biofeedback training and began to study physiology and nutrition as he regained better health.

Utt next began to read extensively on kinesiology, learned the Touch for Health technique, and became Dr. Deal's assistant. After two and one-half years, he started his own professional practice.

One day he woke up and "saw" a blueprint in front of his eyes. His previous expertise in electrical technology and computer sciences, combined with what he had learned from Dr. Deal and his reading, helped him understand the body's electromagnetic circuitry.

Over the years Utt has created and thoroughly researched many innovative techniques. As a new system developed, he called his work Applied Physiology.

Applied Physiology uses the science and art of muscle/fascial monitoring to learn about states of stress in the body. Certain specific muscles are related to various organs and body systems through the Acupuncture meridian network. By monitoring a specific muscle, it is possible to get a "readout" of energy related to a particular organ or body system.

The use of Applied Physiology adds tremendous depth and accuracy to conventional muscle-testing techniques. Its advanced procedures allow systematic investigation and correction of stress anywhere in the body, including comprehensive monitoring of the peripheral, central, and autonomic nervous system.

Applied Physiology uses what is termed an "indicator muscle" for muscle monitoring. An indicator muscle is simply one that is in balance, or homeostasis, being neither overstressed nor understressed; there is clear communication between the muscle and the brain.

This indicator muscle provides a "clear circuit" of communication into the body's own biocomputer (the innate intelligence which coordinates the parasympathetic nervous system that controls such unconscious activities as respiration, digestion, blood pressure, and numerous other functions).

In Applied Physiology, the procedure is to test various points on the body while the clear indicator muscle is being monitored. When changes in the indicator muscle take place, important information is learned about the state of stress in tissues, organs, meridians, and emotions related to these points.

Once stress imbalances are located the Applied Physiologist works with the individual to relieve stress and return the body to a state of balance and harmony. This is accomplished by use of Applied Physiology's comprehensive Acupressure techniques based on the Five Element Theory of Chinese Acupressure.

Applied Physiology has been used to increase muscle use and coordination in muscular dystrophy and polio victims, to relieve skin conditions and stresses caused by food and the environment, to diffuse the aftereffects of accidents and trauma, and to aid those with dyslexic disabilities.

Applied physiologists receive a five-hundred-hour intensive training course. In addition, many other specialized courses are taught at the International Institute of Applied Physiology. The name of an Applied Physiology practitioner in your area is available from the institute.

❧ | AROMATHERAPY | ❦

Aromatherapy is the therapeutic use of essential oils extracted from the flowers, stems, leaves, roots, or fruits of a plant or tree. Essential oils are the most potent form of the plants available and are known for their beneficial healing properties. The physiological and psychological benefits of the essential oils are achieved by absorption through the skin and inhalation. The latter can be accomplished through either natural evaporation or some type of diffusing device.

The use of flowers and plants for their aromatic effects can be traced back five thousand years to the Egyptians. Evidence shows they used natural aromatics for embalming, cosmetics, and medicines, and in religious ceremonies. From Egypt, Aromatherapy spread to Greece, Rome, and the rest of the Mediterranean world.

In the tenth century, plants and flowers were used by the Greeks, Romans, and Persians; a Persian physician named Avicenna laid the groundwork for modern Aromatherapy by developing the process of distillation that made it possible to extract pure essential oils from aromatic plants.

In the Indian *Vedas*, cosmetic and therapeutic properties of cinnamon, ginger, myrrh, and sandalwood, to name only a few, are systematically classified.

In England in 1651 Nicholas Culpeper's book, *The Complete Herbal* (also called *The English Physician*), contained detailed information on the medicinal properties of hundreds of herbs. During the nineteenth century the popularity of Aromatherapy for therapeutic purposes waned as scientists began isolating the active ingredients in plants and synthesizing them in the laboratory.

Aromatherapy was revived in the early part of this century. A French chemist named Rene M. Gattefossé is considered the father of modern Aromatherapy. He coined the term "Aromatherapy" in the 1930s when he used it as the title of his book on the subject.

Impressed with the findings of Gattefossé, a French physician named Dr. Jean Valnet treated war injuries extensively on the field of battle during World War II with essential oils. Valnet continued his work and wrote *Aromatherapie*, published in English as *The Practice of Aromatherapy* (C. W. Daniel, 1977).

Another significant contribution to Aromatherapy was made by Margurite Muary, who revived the concept of using essential oils in conjunction with massage therapy.

There are several methods of extracting essential oils from plants, but the most common is steam distillation. Essential oils are very concentrated and it takes a considerable amount of plant material to produce a small amount of liquid oil. For example, to produce one pound of essential oil would require fifty pounds of eucalyptus, five hundred pounds of rosemary, or two thousand to three thousand pounds of rose.

Essential oils are extremely complex substances and diverse in their effects. When properly used, they can produce a wide variety of therapeutic benefits. For example, chamomile acts as an anti-inflammatory, peppermint as a stimulant, lavender as a sedative, and thyme as an antiseptic.

When aromatics are inhaled a complex chain of events within the body is put into motion. The gaseous molecules stimulate receptors in the olfactory lobe of the brain, which then triggers an electrical signal in the limbic system (the portion of the brain concerned with emotion and motivation), which in turn further influences the release of hormones and neurochemicals to produce a sense of well-being.

Essential oils readily penetrate the skin because of their molecular structure. Research in Germany has shown that once they have entered the bloodstream they can be measured in the exhaled breath after having done their therapeutic job.

Essential oils have been used worldwide for many different ailments. They aid in the healing of muscular aches, arthritis, digestive upsets, circulatory problems, menstrual difficulties, and many other physical and emotional problems. Some essential oils are antiseptic or antifungal, and over sixty are bactericidal.

For massage use, essential oils are always diluted in a vegetable oil carrier. A common ratio is twenty drops of essential oil per ounce of carrier oil. When Aromatherapy is used in conjunction with massage, a subtle interaction takes place between the elements of therapeutic touch, which communicates caring and promotes relaxation, and the essential oils themselves, which contain a variety of therapeutic properties.

As a healing art, Aromatherapy is far more complex than just adding essences to massage oil or bathwater, sniffing a bottle of essential oil, or applying an essential oil directly to the skin.

Although Aromatherapy is largely a self-help system, there are professional Aromatherapists. The complexities involved with using multiple essential oils to achieve certain effects such as an invigorating bath or treating a specific condition such as sinus congestion usually require the help of an experienced professional.

Essential oils can also be taken internally in very small quantities, but because of their potency it is recommended that laypeople not experiment with ingestion.

Numerous books on the subject are available for those who are interested in self-care. Essential oils and Aromatherapy can easily be integrated into daily life for their therapeutic and aesthetic benefits.

For additional information contact any of the Aromatherapy organizations listed in the resource section of this book.

❧ | ARTHRITIS DIET | ❧

The Arthritis Diet, as it is sometimes called, refers to nutritional therapy used to treat arthritis. A 1987 brochure published by the Arthritis Foundation states, "There are some scientific reasons to think that diet affects arthritis."

At the present time, though, due to a lack of scientific studies, the Arthritis Foundation offers no specific dietary recommendations other than that of "good balanced diet." Called the "Seven Guidelines for a Healthy Diet," the brochure includes the following recommendations: Eat a variety of foods, maintain ideal weight, avoid too much fat and cholesterol, avoid too much sugar, eat foods with enough starch and fiber, avoid too much sodium, and drink alcohol in moderation.

However, there is some anecdotal clinical evidence that has shown arthritis is more prone to attacking a person whose body is acidic in nature (referring to the acid-alkali balance that is maintained) than one that is alkaline.

All food, after it is eaten, digested, and metabolized, leaves a residue in the body that is either acid or alkali in nature and which is called acid or alkali ash. Foods that leave acid ash tend to make the body acidic.

The foods that leave high amounts of acid ash in the body include red meat, sugar, and those high in saturated fats such as dairy products. In addition, most cooked foods create acid ash. Foods such as grains, raw fruits, and vegetables produce alkali ash and tend to make the body alkaline in nature.

Two nutritional therapies used in the alternative treatment of arthritis are the Dong Diet and the No-Nightshade Diet. They are described elsewhere in this book. Additional information can also be obtained from the Arthritis Foundation.

❧ | ART THERAPY | ❧

Art Therapy is the use of art for therapeutic purposes. Therapeutic art experiences, using simple art materials, provide a means to restore, maintain, or improve an individual's physical and mental health. It is recognized as a valuable method of assessment and treatment.

Before the 1800s the mentally ill were institutionalized to segregate them from the general population. Emphasis was on isolation and custodial care rather than treatment. During their confinement the mentally ill were not allowed to participate in any normal cultural activities.

The origin of Art Therapy began in the early 1800s, when some individuals began to take a scholarly interest in the psychological significance of the arts. At this same time a movement in the United States began for "moral treatment" of the mentally ill which stressed worthwhile activities.

Although this philosophy was never really put into practice, the approach later found its way into occupational therapy, which occasionally made use of various elements of artistic activity.

Margaret Naumburg was the first person to define Art Therapy as a profession in the United States. In 1915 she founded the Walden School. As a teacher with a deep understanding of psychology, she utilized art to meet her students' psychological needs. This was the beginning of Art Therapy.

The benefits of Art Therapy began to be recognized by the 1950s. In 1961 the *Bulletin of Art Therapy* was founded by Elinor Ulman. This publication became a forum for practitioners that were independently involved in similar work.

In 1969, a year after a series of lectures on Art Therapy was presented at Hahnemann Medical College in Philadelphia, the American Art Therapy Association came into existence in Louisville, Kentucky.

Therapy through art recognizes art processes, forms, contents, and associations as reflections of an individual's development, abilities, personality, interests, and concerns. The use of Art Therapy implies that the creative process can be a means of both reconciling emotional conflicts and fostering self-awareness and personal growth.

Art Therapy involves creating "art makings" from simple art materials such as paints and brushes. This provides the client with a means of non-verbal communication and expression. However, during a session the art therapist will typically make use of verbal exploration and intervention as well.

Through observation and analysis of art behaviors, art products, and the client's communications, the art therapist formulates diagnostic assessments and treatment plans as part of a total therapy program.

The art therapist integrates personal training and experience in art and therapy with theories of human behavior, with a knowledge of visual symbol production, with an understanding of normal and abnormal behavior, and with skills in intervention methods.

Art Therapy may be used as a primary therapy or as an adjunct to other forms of psychological and physiological therapy, depending on the needs of the individual client and setting.

Therapeutic artwork can be used to treat individuals, couples, families, and groups. They include the emotionally disturbed, physically disabled, elderly, developmentally delayed, drug dependent, or those who suffer from other problems or disabilities.

Art Therapy is used in alleviating distress, reducing physical, emotional, and behavioral impairments, and promoting positive development. An art therapist may treat clients in mental health facilities, family service agencies, community mental health centers, rehabilitation centers, schools, correctional institutions, private practice, and other facilities.

The American Art Therapy Association sets educational standards for membership and registry in the profession. Art therapists will have graduated from a minimum of a two-year master's degree program or the equivalent, which includes a minimum of six hundred hours of supervised practical application experience. Art therapists registered by the American Art Therapy Association are designated A.T.R. (Art Therapist, Registered).

Today the American Art Therapy Association, which represents several thousand Art Therapy professionals and students, is involved in the progressive development of the therapeutic use of art.

For additional information regarding Art Therapy and how to locate an art therapist in your area contact the American Art Therapy Association. They also have available many books dealing with different aspects of Art Therapy.

ᴥ | ASTON-PATTERNING | ᴥ

Aston-Patterning is an integrated system that utilizes movement education, different forms of soft tissue bodywork, and environmental consultation and modifications to relieve pain and restore ease of movement and natural grace to the body.

Judith Aston became involved in the field of body therapy because of her own physical problems, as did Ida Rolf, Moshe Feldenkrais, F.M. Alexander, Tomezo Hoshino, and many others.

Born in Long Beach, California, Judith Aston as a young child was always fascinated with the mechanics of human movement and the unique way each person moved. She was also very adept at imitating the wide variety of these movement patterns, which eventually led her to study dance.

Aston earned a master's degree in dance and fine arts from the University of California, Los Angeles, and by 1965 she was teaching dance at Long Beach City College. After she sustained severe neck and back injuries in two separate auto accidents in 1967 and 1968, doctors recommended spinal fusion surgery.

During her investigation of alternatives to surgery she was led to see Ida Rolf at the Esalen Institute in Big Sur, California. After undergoing Rolf's treatment, her back condition improved immediately, and Dr. Rolf invited Aston to take the Rolfing training course.

At that time, Rolf utilized a set of exercises which were intended to maintain the changes that Rolfing produced. In 1971, while working with Rolf, Aston was asked to develop these existing exercises into a movement-maintenance program.

During the next five years Aston's work evolved, and by 1977 the differences between her work and Rolf's became so great that she left to form her own organization. Her philosophy views the body as an integrated whole and addresses physical problems by treating the whole person, not just the affected areas. Aston practitioners work to help the individual to release historical patterns within the body and to create a new ease in the body/mind.

Every human body is unique in shape and expression. The ways in which a person moves, and areas within his body that exhibit either discomfort or ease, reveal the body's history of injury, physical activity, and mental attitude. Stress or tension "held" in certain areas of the body is revealed as movement or postural "patterns" to the trained practitioner. These held patterns, often accumulated over many years, cause the body to lose natural grace, resilience, and ease of movement. The components of Aston-Patterning are designed to increase the body's grace and coordination.

As evaluation tools, Aston-Patterning uses visual observations of both static and dynamic functions and palpation of soft tissue to determine restrictions which limit movement options. The technique is threefold, and a session with a practitioner can include any one or all of the following:

• Movement education, often with the aid of a video camera, analyzes the problem, such as that of a runner who constantly gets shin splints, and then teaches alternatives to the stressful movement habits which cause it.

- A gentle, hands-on massagelike form of bodywork can relieve chronic physical and mental stress, restore flexibility, and expand range of motion.
- Environmental consultation and redesign. First, any problems with the objects an individual uses, such as chairs, tables, etc., are identified. Then, the objects or surroundings are modified to suit the body's particular needs, such as adjusting the height of a desk chair or repositioning a desk.

Aston-Patterning is a widely applicable body therapy and is used to treat back and/or neck pain, postural dysfunctions, and many other types of problems with the wide variety of techniques available. It is especially useful to athletes and dancers. In Aston-Patterning work, participation of the client is essential.

Currently, to become a certified Aston-Patterning practitioner requires completion of a sixteen-week program, over a period of fifteen months, at the Aston Training Center in Incline Village, Nevada. A list of certified Aston-Patterning practitioners is available from the Aston Training Center.

❧ | AUTOGENIC TRAINING | ❧

Autogenic Training, also known as Autogenics, is a system of simple mental (meditative) exercises which consciously focuses the creative power of the mind on relaxation and awareness.

It promotes deep relaxation, greater awareness, self-discovery, and self-regulation. It is designed to switch off the "fight or flight" response and invoke the rest, relaxation, and recreation system within the body.

Although Autogenic Training was developed in the 1930s in Berlin, Germany, by psychiatrist-neurologist Johannes Schultz, it was inspired by the work done in the 1880s by Oskar Vogt. As a brain physiologist at the Berlin Neurobiological Institute, Vogt observed that some patients could put themselves into a self-hypnotic state which seemed to have beneficial effects on their process of recuperation.

With his associate Korbinian Brodmann, Vogt began to experiment with various techniques of self-hypnosis. After patients used the techniques several times a day they experienced relief from symptoms of stress such as headaches and muscular tension.

Schultz became interested in the therapeutic value of hypnosis but wanted to develop it as a self-help tool so that patients would not require a hypnotherapist to utilize its benefits.

In developing Autogenic Training, Schultz combined elements from deep physiological relaxation with Eastern meditative practices such as Yoga and Zen. The idea was to invoke experiences associated with hypnotic states without having the individual go into a trance.

The Autogenic Training exercises, developed by Schultz and his student Wolfgang Luthe, utilize a series of six standard phrases based on the physiological processes of deep relaxation. Phrases such as "My right arm is heavy," "My right arm is warm," "My heartbeat is calm and regular," are repeated while the attention is focused on a particular body area. The sessions are ended with the return phrase, "I am refreshed and alert."

This procedure can be used to influence the autonomic functions which control such unconscious activities as respiration, blood pressure, and numerous others. These bodily functions were previously thought to be outside an individual's direct control.

The Autogenic Training process combines the advantages of focused meditation and autosuggestion. When properly used, Autogenic Training produces amazing results for the day-to-day relief of tension and fatigue.

It can also be effective in eliminating stress held in the body over a period of years. Frequently a sudden startling sensation such as pain or fear is experienced when the suppressed physical or emotional energy is released. This phenomenon is known as "Autogenic Discharge."

Autogenic Training can be practiced in different positions, including lying flat on a comfortable surface or sitting in a straight or reclining chair. It should be practiced twice a day, morning and evening, with each session being twenty minutes long. It can also be used for a few minutes during the day to accomplish specific needs such as raising energy level or calming down.

Results achieved through the use of Autogenic Training have been well documented in medical case studies. It has been used effectively as therapy for migraine headaches, diabetes, sinus problems, sexual dysfunctions, and many other problems. It is also used to treat psychosomatic disorders, to improve athletic and academic performance, and to regulate habits such as smoking, alcohol use, and overeating.

In the late 1960s Wolfgang Luthe edited a six-volume textbook, *Autogenic Therapy*, that summarized years of research and methodology. This venerable work raised Autogenic Training to the status of an internationally recognized method of therapy.

Schultz and Luthe wrote a book which was published in 1959 titled *Autogenic Training: A Psychophysiologic Approach to Psychotherapy*. For additional information on Autogenic Training contact the International Committee for Autogenic Training.

AWARENESS ORIENTED STRUCTURAL THERAPY

Awareness Oriented Structural Therapy is a psychophysical approach to bodywork involving the body/mind concept. It is an integrated therapy, combining a variety of structural bodywork techniques with various body-oriented psychological therapies.

The structural portion of the therapy mainly consists of manipulating the body's soft tissues, fascia (connective tissue), and muscle. Fascia is lengthened and softened and the muscles become more elastic. Additionally, the muscles' proprioceptors (sensory receptor sites) are stimulated to improve balance and ease the effects of gravity. Elements are taken from Structural Integration, Connective Tissue Therapy, Neuromuscular Therapy, Deep Tissue Therapies, and Polarity Therapy.

Structural bodywork can produce increased vitality, easier and freer movement, more dynamic interaction with gravity resulting in improved posture, a sense of greater stability, improved metabolic functions, and relief from physical pain.

The psychological aspects of the therapy are based on the Hakomi Method of Body Mind Therapy, Gestalt Therapy, Psychosynthesis, Sensory Awareness, Present-Centered Awareness and Therapy, and meditation practices. These therapies can produce emotional release, which can lead to personal growth and transformation.

The goal of Awareness Oriented Structural Therapy is to provide an individual with the opportunity for improved structural functioning of the body and to experience greater clarity and emotional well-being.

Awareness Oriented Structural Therapy is taught at the Florida Institute of Natural Health's Florida Massage School. Upon completion of the five-hundred-hour curriculum, a certification in Awareness Oriented Structural Therapy is granted. For additional information or to locate a practitioner trained in Awareness Oriented Structural Therapy, contact the Florida Institute of Natural Health & Florida Massage School.

༄ | AYURVEDA | ༄

Ayurveda, the ancient Indian art and science of healing and rejuvenation, is a preventive and holistic system of medicine that aims at a balanced state of inner harmony, health, and natural well-being. It provides the individual with a complete life-regimen and deals with body and mind through an integrated science of lifestyle counseling combined with the use of natural herbs, roots, and minerals.

Ayurveda is the medicine of nature and of life. Its philosophy is to present the individual's mind with the principles and power of nature and then teach him how to put these great principles and powers of health and natural living into practice.

It provides knowledge of how to care for the body in terms of diet and medicine. Ayurveda is an aspect of Yoga and is most allied with Hatha Yoga. Yoga provides exercise for physical health, flexibility, and dissolution of tension.

The word Ayurveda is a Sanskrit term meaning "science of life." It is derived from *ayur*, meaning "life," "daily living," or "longevity," and *veda*, meaning "knowing," "knowledge," "wisdom," or "science."

Ayurveda is the oldest medical system known to man and the oldest and most comprehensive spiritual teaching in the world. It has been practiced in daily life in India for more than four thousand years. It was recorded in the Vedas, one of the world's oldest existing literature. All Avurvedic literature is based on the *Samkhya* philosophy of creation. Samkhya is derived from two Sanskrit roots: *sat* meaning "truth" and *khya* meaning "to know."

Ayurveda is the science of daily living. As a system of knowledge it is derived from the practical, philosophical, and religious illumination received by *rishis*, the ancient "seers of truth" in India.

Rishis, through meditation and mystic visions, gained knowledge of the human system and how to maintain the body's health, and to be in total harmony with nature. For several thousand years their teachings were passed on orally from the teacher to the student and eventually were written in Sanskrit, the ancient language of India. Although many texts were lost through the long passage of time, a great deal of Ayurvedic knowledge has survived.

Ayurveda recognizes five basic elements: air, fire, water, earth, and ether. They manifest in the human body, condensed, as three basic elements: Vata (air and ether), Pitta (fire and water), and Kapha (water and earth). The human body is ruled by these three vital life-forces or humors. The humors are called *doshas*, which in Sanskrit means "what spoils or causes decay."

According to Ayurvedic teachings, Vata, Pitta, and Kapha, also known as *tridoshas*, are the forces that govern all the functions of the body, mind, and consciousness. When the doshas are in balance they sustain the body and when out of balance they serve to destroy it. Thus, health in the body consists of the correct balance of the creative and destructive forces of the doshas.

The healing science of Ayurveda is based totally on the knowledge of *prakruti* or the human constitution of the individual person. The basic constitution of each individual can be determined from charts using the individual's various physical and emotional characteristics. Features such as body frame, weight, skin color and complexion, hair, nails, eyes, mouth, sweat, climate preference, dreams, and personality traits are used as criteria for constitutional type evaluation. No individual constitution is made up of only one element (dosha). Each person is a combination of all three elements, with a predominant tendency toward one or more.

There are two methods of Ayurvedic treatment: constitutional and clinical. Balancing of the doshas is essential for any cure to be permanently effective.

Constitutional remedies include diet, mild herbs, specifically prepared mineral substances, and lifestyle adjustments to balance the life forces and return the body to a state of harmony.

Clinical remedies consist of strong herbs and medications, and cleansing or purification practices. Cleansing includes purgation, medicated enemas, therapeutic vomiting, nasal medication, and therapeutic bloodletting.

Ayurveda is a spiritually based medicine and primarily a self-healing system. Some say that Ayurveda works slowly, but slowness is often part of the remedy, especially when many individuals today suffer from the disease of haste. The goal of Ayurveda is to balance and rejuvenate the individual, and increase his immunity to prevent new diseases from developing.

According to Ayurvedic philosophy, an individual cannot expect to be well through natural healing methods if his everyday life is out of harmony.

There are now medical doctors, many of whom have come from India, that practice Ayurvedic medicine. Additionally, there are many excellent books available at local health food stores that cover the subject in detail.

For additional information contact the professionals at the Ayurvedic Institute. They offer a large selection of books, publications, audio- and videotapes, herbs, and other products associated with Ayurveda. Also consult the other organizations listed in the resource guide at the back of this book.

❧ | BACH FLOWER REMEDIES | ❦

Bach Flower Remedies are a set of thirty-eight different herbal remedies (plus one combination remedy) made from the specially prepared, "poten- tized" essence of the petals and heads of flowers. Each essence is made from a particular type of flower and preserved in unflavored brandy to prevent spoilage.

Bach Flower Remedies are nontoxic and nonaddictive, and utilize the mood-altering properties of the plants to harmonize and balance emotional sensitivities. The Remedies act as catalysts to alleviate the underlying causes of stress.

Dr. Edward Bach (1886–1936) was a renowned British scientist and physician. He was inspired by Samuel Hahnemann, the founder of home- opathy. After turning to homeopathy, he was appointed pathologist and bacteriologist at the London Homeopathic Hospital.

In the late 1920s Dr. Bach observed that his patients' state of mind was directly related to their physical ailments, and noted that apprehension, worry, loneliness, boredom, depression, uncertainty, hopelessness, and fear inhibited their natural healing powers and ability to prevent disease. He then realized that disease was not due to physical causes but the underlying emotional stresses, which had their origin in the mind.

After a great deal of research identifying and categorizing every negative state of mind known to man, Dr. Bach concluded that there are thirty-eight outstanding states of mind from which the sick suffer. Leaving his lucrative Harley Street practice behind, he moved to the English countryside and began researching the healing properties of flowering plants. Dr. Bach observed plants, noted the type of soil they grew in, the color and shape of their flowers, and many other details.

Dr. Bach was strongly psychic and hypersensitive. When placing his palms over a flower's petals he could "feel" the vibrations they sent out, and he realized that the flower contained the most potent healing elements of the entire plant. He would test the properties of the flower by placing a bloom on his palm or on his tongue and feeling the effects in his body. Some vitalized him, others caused pain or even made him vomit.

After numerous trial-and-error experiments he developed thirty-eight natural Remedies to alleviate every negative state of mind he identified. He also developed a combination formula called Rescue Remedy for immediate, emergency relief of stress.

To identify which Bach Remedy is needed, a list of the thirty-eight Remedy indications which describes the emotional state and personality trait that each Remedy addresses is available from Ellon USA or from retail outlets where Bach Flower Remedies are sold. You then select the remedy which most closely corresponds to your basic personality type or the emotional stress you're experiencing. It is recommended that no more than six Remedies be used at one time.

The liquid Remedies are dropped under the tongue four times a day for a week to several months to banish such feelings as fear, extreme anguish, lack of confidence, mental fatigue, etc. A common occurrence with Bach Flower Remedies usage is known as the "peeling effect." As one or more emotional difficulties are resolved, other underlying emotions are brought to the surface and other Remedies can then be taken in the process of growth.

Bach Flower Remedies have been used for sixty years by millions of health practitioners worldwide. There are many books available on Bach Flower Remedies for self-use. Also, for additional information contact Ellon USA. The remedies can be found at most health food stores or can be ordered directly from Ellon USA in Lynbrook, New York.

❧ | BATES METHOD OF VISION TRAINING | ☙

The Bates Method of Vision Training is a routine made up of specific mental and physical exercises designed to improve many vision problems in a natural, holistic way. It will not improve organic problems such as glaucoma or cataracts. This system has alternately been called the Bates Method of Vision Training, the Bates Method of Visual Reeducation, and the Bates Method of Sight Improvement.

William Horatio Bates, M.D. (1881–1931), was one of the most distinguished ophthalmologists of his day in New York City. Gradually he became disenchanted with orthodox medicine and began to question the use of glasses to correct vision problems. This sent him to the laboratory at Columbia University, where he repeated the old experiments on which ophthalmology was based.

After analyzing the eyes of twenty thousand schoolchildren Dr. Bates discovered that vision defects (refractive errors) were caused by misuse, because of weakness, of the six intrinsic eye muscles, which prevented them from focusing the lens correctly. The defect was not in the lens itself. Dr. Bates found that the main cause of weak eye muscles was stress and that once the stress and tension were removed, the eye muscles were able to focus the lens correctly.

Dr. Bates exhaustively studied the actions and reactions of the eye. He experimented with fish, birds, animals, and humans. In 1920, from the results of this work, he invented a system of exercises to strengthen eye muscles and procedures to relieve muscular tension.

He pointed out that relaxed organs function better than tense ones, and encouraged the systematic use of memory and the imagination to improve vision. Unfortunately, during this time in history, the idea of healing the body by using the mind was not well received.

Dr. Bates's techniques for relaxing the eyes were so effective that other problem conditions in the body were often cured as well. The techniques resemble meditation and incorporate certain principles that are similar to what is now known as biofeedback and stress-reduction training.

Famous author Aldous Huxley used the Bates Method in 1939 to recover from near blindness caused by a serious illness. The method was adopted by the German army, navy, and air force. Today there are Bates Method practitioners throughout the world.

BEE VENOM THERAPY

Bee Venom Therapy is the use of venom from the honeybee to treat various diseases that cause joint problems. It can be administered two different ways, either by hypodermic injection or by a sting from a live bee.

Bee venom used in the former method of administration is a pharmaceutically prepared product. The venom is extracted from bees and dried under controlled conditions. It is then added to a saline solution, filtered, packaged, and then sealed in sterile glass containers. In the latter method, a person can have a beekeeper hold a bee with forceps and let it sting the desired skin site.

Scorned by the medical profession in the United States, Bee Venom Therapy has found broad acceptance for the treatment of arthritis and rheumatism in many parts of the world. Scientists in Switzerland, France, Germany, and Great Britain have recently done research and clinical testing of this therapy. In the United States, the Arthritis Foundation has begun to study this therapy.

In his book *Curative Properties of Honey and Bee Venom*, Russian scientist Y. Yourish claims excellent results with bee venom in the many case studies cited.

Therapeutic use of bee venom has a long history. It was used by Hippocrates nearly two thousand years ago to treat arthritis-related diseases and other specific painful conditions. For centuries people of the country- side believed that bee stings were the supreme cure for rheumatism, arthritis, lumbago, and gout. Ivan the Terrible of Russia was cured of gout by bee stings.

Bee Venom Therapy works in somewhat of a "backdoor" way, by stimulating the body's immune system. The bee venom causes inflam- mation in the area where it was introduced and the body then produces anti-inflammatory hormones and other substances to help alleviate it. By deliberately injecting bee venom into an area that is already inflamed, the anti-inflammatory hormone released to deal with the bee venom is so pow- erful that it treats the original condition causing the inflammation as well.

Bee venom is a very complex substance. Analysis has shown that it con- tains formic acid, histamines, and magnesium phosphate. The active ingre- dient in bee venom is somewhat related to the active ingredient of snake venom. It also contains an alkaloid substance related to very active poisons like strychnine or belladonna.

Dr. Christopher Kim, a physician in New Jersey, has found Bee Venom Therapy to be effective in treating any chronic joint inflammation including osteoarthritis, rheumatoid arthritis, tendonitis, neuritis, and bursitis.

Bee Venom Therapy is not a "one-shot" cure and requires a series of treatments (injections or stings) because it is helping the body to heal itself. Note that some people are allergic to bee venom and a rare few may suffer fatal shock from it, although these problems are found in less than 2 percent of the population.

For additional information contact the American Apitherapy Society.

❧ | BENJAMIN SYSTEM OF MUSCULAR THERAPY | ❧

The Benjamin System of Muscular Therapy is a unique combination of treatment, exercise, and education designed to reduce chronic muscular tension and to promote physical health in the body.

The Benjamin System of Muscular Therapy was developed in 1967 by Ben E. Benjamin, Ph.D. The system was inspired and influenced by the techniques and approaches of several different people:

From Dr. Alfred Kagan came deep massage treatment of muscular pain and injury. From the F. M. Alexander Technique came posture and movement training. From the English orthopedist Dr. James H. Cyriax came injury evaluation and "deep transverse friction" treatment to prevent scar tissue. From Dr. Wilhelm Reich came the theory of physical manifestation of emotional distress which recognized the emotional side of physical tension.

While in rigorous dance training at the age of fourteen, Ben Benjamin sustained an injury that was diagnosed as serious enough to permanently end his dance career. Unwilling to accept the diagnosis, Benjamin sought out Dr. Alfred Kagan, a well-known French practitioner whose deep-massage techniques had benefited numerous dancers. Kagan diagnosed the problem as excess muscular tension and after three weeks of treatment Benjamin was able to dance again without pain.

Due to this incident, Benjamin became interested in Kagan's work, and in learning how to reduce muscular tension. At the age of eighteen he began deep-massage therapy training with Kagan. When he was nineteen, under Kagan's guidance, he began his own massage practice in New York City.

In the ensuing years, Benjamin studied and further developed Kagan's techniques and defined over seven hundred therapeutic manipulations.

He later created a program to break down tension in children using movement. He further refined these tension-release techniques and combined them with his study of voice, speech production, body alignment, and movement techniques into his own method, which he named the Benjamin System of Muscular Therapy.

According to Benjamin, there are two categories of causes for excess muscular tension—mechanical and emotional. The emotional type, chronic tightening of the muscles or armor (taken from Wilhelm Reich's concept of "armor") caused by constant repression of emotional expression, is not treatable by the Benjamin System of Muscular Therapy.

Mechanical tension can be caused by numerous factors in an individual's life, including poor posture, bad physical habits, incorrect body alignment, trauma (accident, injury, or surgery), occupation, and the environment.

The Benjamin System of Muscular Therapy includes a series of techniques and exercises designed to break down muscular tension and prevent it from returning. It incorporates deep massage, tension-release exercises, body-care techniques, and postural realignment.

Deep massage—unlike ordinary superficial massage, which only touches the superficial muscles—use finger and hand techniques to reach muscles deep within the body to release long-standing pain and tension, and to increase circulation.

The tension-release exercises are a self-help method to release tension in specific muscles and parts of the body.

Body-care techniques such as baths, deep breathing, healthy eating, and leisurely recreation help to reduce tension in a more relaxed way.

Postural alignment is essential for maintaining a relaxed body. When necessary the Benjamin System of Muscular Therapy designs a program of exercises to help the individual remain free of tension and pain.

In 1974 Ben E. Benjamin established the Muscular Therapy Institute in Cambridge, Massachusetts. Practitioners who graduate from the institute's two-year core program receive approximately 1,200 hours of training, including 500 hours of externship. A list of practitioners is available from the institute.

For additional information, Ben E. Benjamin's book, *Are You Tense? The Benjamin System of Muscular Therapy*, describes the system in detail.

❧ | BIOENERGETICS | ☙

Bioenergetics is a method of studying and understanding the human personality in terms of the body and its energetic processes. In Bioenergetic theory, it is believed that the body and the mind are functionally identical. What happens in the mind reflects what is happening in the body and vice versa.

Bioenergetics is a therapeutic technique that utilizes many bodywork methods and exercises to help an individual become aware of tensions in the body and release them through appropriate movement. Bioenergetics also involves verbal exploration of emotional conflicts and their relationship to an individual's personal history.

Bioenergetic Therapy helps an individual integrate her mind with her body. This emphasis on the body includes sexuality, breathing, moving, feeling, and self-expression.

Bioenergetics was developed by Alexander Lowen and is based on the work of Wilhelm Reich (1879–1957), a scientist and psychoanalyst who was an early collaborator with Sigmund Freud. Reich was born, raised, and trained in Austria and came to the United States in 1939.

Lowen was born in New York City in 1910. After receiving his law degree in 1936, he began to teach law. During summer vacation he worked as athletic director at several adult camps.

He found that a personal program of regular exercise and physical activity not only improved his physical health, but had positive effects on his mental state. While researching this idea, he found that studies done by Emile Jaques-Dalcroze and Edwin Jacobson confirmed his strong feeling that mental attitude could be influenced by working with the body.

In 1940 Alexander Lowen met Wilhelm Reich at the New School for Social Research in New York City. Reich then became his teacher from 1940 to 1952. Before meeting Reich, Lowen had been pursuing his own investigation of the mind-body relationship. His interest grew out of personal experience with the physical activity involved in sports and calisthenics.

In 1942 Lowen began analysis with Reich, which lasted until 1945. After Reich's book, *The Function of the Orgasm*, was published in 1941, demand for Reichian Therapy increased. In 1945 Lowen became a Reichian therapist. In 1947 he went to medical school in Geneva, Switzerland, and graduated in 1951 with an M.D.

Lowen returned to the United States and completed his medical internship in 1952. In 1953 he became associated with Dr. John C. Pierrakos, also a follower of Reich. The following year they were joined by Dr. William B. Walling, a classmate of Pierrakos. The three psychiatrists worked together presenting seminars teaching other therapists about the underlying concepts of the body approach. In 1956 the Institute for Bioenergetic Analysis was founded to carry out the aims of the seminars. It later became the International Institute for Bioenergetic Analysis.

Although he successfully completed Reichian Therapy, Lowen was aware that his body still retained many chronic muscular tensions that prevented him from experiencing the joyfulness he longed for. He went into therapy for another three years with his associate John Pierrakos. While working on himself, Lowen developed the basic positions and exercises which are now standard in Bioenergetics.

Wilhelm Reich had always emphasized the importance of character analysis. Lowen therefore knew that regardless of how important the work on muscular tension was, equally important was the careful analysis of a person's habitual mode of being and behavior. He made an intensive study of character types and published *The Physical Dynamics of Character Structure* in 1958. This book served as the foundation for all character work done in Bioenergetics.

Emotional stress from many areas of daily life such as employment, relationships, family crises, health, etc., produces tension in the body. In other words, a person reacts to stress in her life by contracting her muscular system.

Over a period of time muscular tension builds up within the body and becomes chronic. At this point it affects emotional well-being by decreasing energy level and restricting the capacity for spontaneity and self-expression, thereby interfering with the attainment of various satisfactions in life.

In Bioenergetic Therapy much attention is focused on these patterns of muscular tension and their relationship to movement, breath, posture, and emotional expression. It is believed that these characteristics of the body are directly related to a person's emotional history and reflect early childhood relationships.

Designed to reactivate the body through specific exercises, Bioenergetic Therapy has three principal aims: (1) to enable the individual to understand her personality in terms of the body; (2) to improve all functions of the personality by mobilizing the energy bound by muscular tensions; and (3) to increase the individual's capacity to experience pleasure by resolving the "characterological attitudes" that have become structured in the body and that interfere with its rhythmic and unitary movements.

A detailed description of the Bioenergetic process can be found in Alexander Lowen's book *Bioenergetics*. Also consult the Institute for Bioenergetics and Gestalt, and the International Institute for Bioenergetic Analysis.

❧ | BIOFEEDBACK TRAINING | ❧

Biofeedback Training is a process of learning various techniques to utilize information from a device called a biofeedback machine. This information is then used to monitor and gain control over so-called autonomic body functions such as blood pressure, heart rate, circulation, digestion, or perspiration. Biofeedback is feedback with biology.

In Biofeedback Training the practitioner teaches an individual how to use the many different types of biofeedback instruments available for this purpose. In addition to the professional models, there are also portable machines designed for home use.

Through the use of specialized electrodes attached to various parts of the body, a biofeedback machine can monitor and measure physical states such as muscle tone, skin temperature, the amount of sweat on the skin, brain wave activity, or other physical conditions as required.

Responses from a biofeedback machine are both auditory and visual. Information gathered from the electrodes is relayed to the user through gauges, lights, tones, or other means.

This "feedback" provides the user with a new, perceptible awareness of different body/mind processes which extend beyond his normal five senses. In short, it gives an individual information about his physiological functioning that was previously unavailable to his conscious mind.

Feedback is a term coined by early radio pioneers in the early 1900s. The word *biofeedback* was coined in the 1960s to describe laboratory procedures then being used to train experimental research subjects. Quoted in a 1970 *Scientific American*, Norbert Wiener, a mathematician and founding father of feedback research, gave it this definition: "a method of controlling a system by reinserting into it the results of its past performance."

The principle behind biofeedback is not new. In British colonial India during the eighteenth century, army physicians and civilian administrators reported that Yogis could voluntarily control so-called involuntary body functions such as heart rate and pain (lying on a bed of nails). The Yogis claimed this ability came from extensive practice of certain mental, physical, and emotional disciplines.

In the 1950s Kamiya, Brown, and Green discovered how an individual can rapidly learn voluntary control of certain physiological processes by using information gathered from physiological measuring instruments.

While Kamiya was doing research on sleep and dreaming, his subjects learned to use information from an electroencephalograph (EEG) machine to change their state of mind. They were able to achieve the alpha state, the most relaxed state possible while awake.

After moving his research to the University of California Medical Center in San Francisco, Kamiya developed a prototype which has become the standard for current alpha training machines. When attached to the machine, subjects could hear a specific tone when they achieved the alpha state. He later observed that after practice they could maintain the alpha state on their own.

In the late 1960s, Dr. Neal Miller, a scientist at Rockefeller University in New York, was able to teach laboratory rats to regulate their blood flow while they were paralyzed with a muscular relaxation drug. At the same time Dr. Elmer Green and his co-worker, Alyce (Mrs. Green), were working on experiments at the Menninger Foundation in Topeka, Kansas, teaching people to warm their hands by means of biofeedback.

Prior to these experiments it was thought the nervous system was divided into voluntary and involuntary functions. It was believed that critical functions such as heartbeat, respiration, and blood flow were unconscious or involuntary while walking, talking, or writing were under voluntary control.

The idea behind biofeedback is simple, and most people have probably used it without even knowing it. If you take your temperature or step on a scale you have used it. The thermometer tells whether you have a fever, and the scale indicates if you have gained weight. Both devices "feed back" information about your body's condition. Armed with this information you can take steps to improve your condition.

The body's built-in feedback systems enable us to live safely and comfortably in our surroundings by providing signals that tell bodily systems when to activate and when to shut down. These natural feedback systems allow us to adapt to changing environmental conditions.

Biofeedback has numerous uses in behavioral medicine and medical applications that unite body and mind. Physical therapists use biofeedback to help stroke victims regain movement in paralyzed muscles. Psychologists use it to help tense and anxious clients learn to relax. Specialists in many different fields use biofeedback to help their patients cope with pain.

Detection of stress is one area where biofeedback is very valuable. It is generally agreed that stress and tension held within the body are not healthy and contribute to so-called stress-related disorders like high blood pressure, ulcers, heart attack, and migraine headaches. Since many people are not always aware when they are under stress, biofeedback provides a method of insight otherwise unavailable.

The biofeedback machine is not a "miracle device" that an individual hooks himself up to and from which he then receives a "miracle cure." It is only meant to facilitate the process of an individual's learning how to deal with problems in his own body. This allows the person to take responsibility for his own health rather than look for a "cure" from an outside source.

The role of the biofeedback practitioner (trainer) is to guide and help the client interpret information from the biofeedback machine. The client is then able to identify and become aware of what is happening in his body at the time he is under stress.

For example, a person with a tension headache discovers which muscles are contracting to cause the pain. And, by practicing relaxation techniques while on the biofeedback machine, he can learn what it feels like to be relaxed and how to relax the particular muscles causing the pain. Through repetition and reinforcement from the practitioner, the client learns how to achieve the desired state of relaxation. The ultimate goal is to learn relaxation well enough so future sessions on the machine are unnecessary.

After Biofeedback Training, if an individual encounters an uncomfortable situation, he is able to recognize when he is becoming stressed. Knowing this, he can immediately invoke the relaxation techniques he has learned to neutralize the stress.

Today biofeedback clinicians utilize a wide variety of equipment for training, which can take place in a variety of locations, including the office of a private practitioner such as a psychologist, a hospital, an outpatient medical center, or another location.

Clinical biofeedback techniques are now widely used to treat an ever increasing variety of conditions. These include migraine headaches, tension headaches, other types of pain, stomach and intestinal disorders, cold extremities, high and low blood pressure, abnormal heartbeat rhythms, epilepsy, paralysis, and other movement disorders.

For additional information contact professionals at the Association for Applied Psychophysiology and Biofeedback, the Biofeedback Certification Institute of America, or any of the other organizations listed in the resource section. They can provide the name of a biofeedback practitioner in your area.

❧ | BODYWORK FOR THE CHILDBEARING YEAR | ❧

Bodywork for the Childbearing Year is a therapeutic approach to massage, bodywork, and movement education used to support a woman during the entire year of her pregnancy. This work is also used during labor, delivery, the postpartum period, and the baby's first year.

It is also referred to by separate names such as pregnancy massage, labor massage, postpartum massage, and infant/baby massage.

Bodywork for the Childbearing Year is not a new concept. It was started by women probably at the dawn of civilization. A search of cultural and anthropological history shows that bodywork during the childbearing period was and continues to be a prominent part of many civilizations.

Current research on the benefits of touch during this period in a family's life is providing a contemporary basis for its reintroduction to the childbearing experience in technological societies.

It has been found that the more peaceful a culture is, the more prominent the use of touch during pregnancy and early childhood. It is used extensively in the Indian and the Polynesian cultures. Massaging infants is a respected profession in India.

Midwives, who are primarily responsible for delivering babies in many countries around the world, have highly developed skills in hands-on work/massage therapy. These skills are utilized during pregnancy, labor, and for the infant after it is born. The effectiveness of this type of work is well known globally.

In 1980 Kate Jordan and Carole Osborne-Sheets began to develop the Bodywork for the Childbearing Year training program currently taught. At that time both Jordan and Osborne-Sheets were instructors at the International Professional School of Bodywork in San Diego, California, and they were both pregnant.

Jordan was pregnant with her second child. Through previous experience with her own self-care and private massage practice, she had been exploring the use of massage and bodywork during pregnancy.

During that year Osborne-Sheets, pregnant for the first time, experienced an influx of pregnant women, including thirteen friends, into her private massage practice. Wanting to make pregnancy a more positive physical and emotional experience for herself, her friends, and her clients prompted Osborne-Sheets's interest in the application of massage during pregnancy.

Together Jordan and Osborne-Sheets began to investigate how the different types of bodywork and massage techniques they were already using with nonpregnant people would apply to pregnancy.

Each had her own areas of expertise. Osborne-Sheets was involved with structural myofascial (massage involving muscle, fascia, and skeleton) and deep tissue work, and Jordan was doing lymphatic drainage, foot zone therapy, and neuromuscular and cross-fiber work.

Added to their knowledge was input from their physicians on the medical implications of the work. After their children were born, they began to teach infant massage techniques to parents and perinatal professionals in San Diego area hospitals.

In 1982 Kate Jordan and Carole Osborne-Sheets began teaching the Bodywork for the Childbearing Year training in San Diego. They see this work as a way of making a contribution to the health and vitality of humanity from the very beginning.

Bodywork for the Childbearing Year is a compilation of many different modalities. Each one was chosen because it worked best to accomplish a specific purpose. Some of the modalities commonly used include deep tissue work (muscle sculpting, cross-fiber friction massage, and structural integration), Swedish massage, lymphatic drainage, joint mobilization therapy, zone therapy, connective tissue massage, trigger point therapy, infant massage, and others.

Bodywork for the Childbearing Year can be utilized by any woman having a low-risk, uncomplicated, normal pregnancy. If the pregnancy does not fall into this category, then it should only be done under the supervision of a physician after her individual case has been reviewed. In any case, it is always appropriate for a pregnant woman to receive her physician's release before having this type of work done.

The potential benefits of Bodywork for the Childbearing Year during pregnancy include increased circulation of fluids (blood and lymph) through the body; reduced swelling; prevention or alleviation of varicose veins; alleviation of stress on weight-bearing joints, and on muscles, ligaments, and fascial structures; reduction of neck and back pain caused by improper posture, muscle weakness, tension, or imbalance from the shift in the center of gravity; increased body awareness; and preparation of the birthing muscles for release and support during childbirth.

Learning proper movement techniques is also very important during pregnancy. Knowledge of how to correctly use the body during normal activities such as lifting a chair or carrying a child can prevent unnecessary strain from occurring.

Documented studies done at the University of Pittsburgh in 1972 showed that a woman touched lovingly and nurturingly during the last few months of pregnancy will touch her baby more frequently, more lovingly, and with more sensitivity than a woman who has not received such touch.

Further research published in 1992 showed that if a woman is touched in a loving and caring way during labor, it will make the process much easier. When a woman is touched appropriately by a person singularly devoted to that task, the need for forceps during delivery is reduced by more than 50 percent.

After giving birth (postpartum period), massage therapy can help restore the body to its prepregnancy state in terms of eliminating excess fluids, cleansing metabolic waste products from labor, restoring tone to the abdominal fascia, and restoring the function of other muscles due to the change in the center of gravity. The recovery process of the post–cesarean section mother can also be facilitated with massage therapy.

Bodywork for the Childbearing Year also teaches infant movement activities and massage routines which support the bonding process between parents and newborn.

During a session of Bodywork for the Childbearing Year a woman lies on her side or in a semireclining position, partially clothed and properly draped, on the massage table. Pillows or support cushions are used to keep her in position while she is being worked on. Being positioned on the back or abdomen is not recommended.

Current training for Bodywork for the Childbearing Year is a thirty-two-hour intensive program given over four days which includes anatomy, physiology, medical complications, specific techniques, and appropriate procedures.

It is desired that students have five hundred to one thousand hours or more of prior massage training before enrolling in the program. Upon completion of the program, hands-on and written examinations are given. A certificate is awarded to those who pass. The training program is offered at various locations throughout the United States by the Somatic Learning Associates.

The National Association of Pregnancy Massage Therapists offers a referral service to help locate a member therapist in your area.

✌ | BONNIE PRUDDEN MYOTHERAPY | ✍

Bonnie Prudden Myotherapy, also known as the Bonnie Prudden Technique, is a method of relieving muscular pain by the application of pressure to an area within the muscle known as the trigger point. Trigger points can be located throughout the body, literally from head to foot.

Though trigger points are not fully understood, they do exist. They are found in muscles that have been damaged (or "insulted," in correct medical terms). This damage to a muscle can occur at any time in life, even before birth.

A trigger point may lie dormant in a muscle for a period of time, sometimes years; then, due to a particular physical action or an emotional stress, it is activated. When this happens the muscle in which the trigger point dwells tightens and the result is pain. The trigger point may calm down and the pain may leave but it is still there and will reactivate when the stress level is raised again.

Myotherapy was discovered somewhat accidentally by Bonnie Prudden, one of the world's leading authorities on physical fitness and the author of numerous books and articles on exercise and health.

Myotherapy is derived directly from several sources, including a treatise on the insertion of needles into muscles under the skin written by Huang Fu in A.D. 300; the work of German physiologist Max Lange in the early 1930s, which located areas of muscle resistance; and the extensive clinical work done on trigger points by Dr. Janet Travel beginning in the 1940s.

Dr. Janet Travel is well known for treating John F. Kennedy's back pain while he was a senator, and later as his private physician when he became president.

Also vital to the development of Myotherapy was Prudden's association with three pioneers in the field of trigger point work: Dr. Hans Kraus, Dr. Desmond Tivy, and the aforementioned Dr. Janet Travel.

The first insight into what became Myotherapy happened during a mountain climb when Prudden awoke with a painful stiff neck, the result of a fall from a horse several years earlier. One of the climbers, Dr. Kraus, put his thumb into the back of her neck and pressed down with great force. This procedure was quite painful but when he let up her neck was free of pain.

A second insight came with the work of Dr. Travel. She pioneered a medical discipline called Trigger Point Injection Therapy, in which the physician palpates an area to locate a tender spot indicating a trigger point, and then injects a medication into it. The injection is followed by a gentle passive stretch of the muscle, and then the area is sprayed with a coolant.

This procedure, known as spray and stretch, is used extensively in physical therapy.

For many years Prudden had been doing corrective exercise work with patients, referred by physicians, after surgery or Trigger Point Injection Therapy. She then began to work mostly with back patients after they received Trigger Point Injection Therapy from Dr. Tivy.

In 1976 it all came together. At this time Prudden was locating trigger points on patients, marking them in ink, and then sending them to Dr. Tivy for injection. While palpating the neck of a woman, she found a tender spot and the woman let out a yell. To the surprise of Prudden, the woman's neck was now straight and free of stiffness.

Prudden contemplated the possibility that pressure alone, without injection, could release trigger points. Determined to find out if this was so, she used this procedure on other patients with success, and felt she had made an important discovery.

At her Myotherapy Institute she found that pain which took weeks of exercise and injections to alleviate could be eliminated in only a few sessions, and sometimes only one.

When a trigger point is activated it causes the muscle to spasm, and pain is initiated. This in turn causes the body's self-protective mechanism to engage and further spasm the muscle for protection. This cycle of pain and spasm continues over and over until it is broken when the muscle releases and remains in a relaxed state. After pressure is applied to a trigger point for about seven seconds, it loses its ability to cause pain.

There are numerous ways to break the pain-spasm-pain cycle, including prescription and nonprescription painkillers, heat, cold, liniments, rest, etc. Unfortunately, after the pain is relieved the trigger point is still there, ready to be activated once again. The real benefit of the Bonnie Prudden Technique is that it eliminates the trigger point, not just the symptomatic pain.

Some of the major causes of trigger points are the birth process, accidents of all types, sports injuries, diseases such as arthritis and multiple sclerosis, and occupations that cause abuse of the body. Myotherapy has been found to be helpful to athletes, musicians, singers, and dancers, as well as the general public.

Two excellent books written by Bonnie Prudden, *Pain Erasure the Bonnie Prudden Way* and *Myotherapy: Bonnie Prudden's Complete Guide to Pain-Free Living* are available at bookstores and many libraries.

In 1979 Bonnie Prudden founded the Bonnie Prudden School for

Physical Fitness and Myotherapy. Today it offers an educational program leading to certification as a Bonnie Prudden Myotherapist. A list of Bonnie Prudden Myotherapy Clinics and certified Bonnie Prudden Myotherapists, located throughout the United States and Canada, is available from the school.

BURTON TREATMENT

The Burton Treatment, or Immuno-Augmentative Therapy (IAT), is an alternative cancer therapy which is designed to restore the body's natural immune defenses against the disease. It is not represented as a cure for cancer.

According to IAT, Ltd., cancer is a disease of immunosuppression (suppressed immune system) or immune deficiency. Immuo-Augmentative Therapy, unlike radiation or chemotherapy, does not "attack" cancer, but restores the immune system's natural ability to seek out and destroy cancer cells.

The goal of standard immunotherapy is to stimulate the immune system as a whole. However, Immuno-Augmentative Therapy differs from this generally accepted definition. IAT involves a two-step procedure consisting of evaluation and therapy. First, deficiencies of the immune system are determined by the quantitative analysis of four specific proteins found in the blood. Second, based on the blood analysis, deficiencies are calculated and the proper amount of each protein is administered or "replenished" in the patient.

Lawrence Burton, Ph.D., developer of Immuno-Augmentative Therapy, has been studying the immune mechanism and cancer since the early 1950s when he was a postgraduate student.

Born in 1926 in the Bronx, New York, Burton received his B.S. in 1949 from Brooklyn College, Brooklyn, New York. In 1952 he received his M.S., and in 1955 his Ph.D. from New York University in New York City. He completed a postdoctoral fellowship and a term as a research associate at the California Institute of Technology in Pasadena, California, in 1957. In 1958 Burton joined St. Vincent's Hospital in New York and during the next fifteen years served in a number of different positions.

During the late 1950s Dr. Burton and a team of medical researchers began an investigation of mammalian carcinogenesis. They discovered an inhibitory protein which induced long-term remission in mice with leukemia. After further research, a therapy was developed which produced rapid antitumor effects in mice with breast tumors.

From this research Dr. Burton realized that in order for the immune system to function properly and thwart the development of cancer cells, four specific proteins must be present in the blood. These four substances are isolated and extracted from a blood sample using procedures which are patented in the United States by Burton and others.

Each of the four proteins has a specific function within the immune system's process of identification and destruction of cancer cells in the body. Immuno-Augmentative Therapy provides cancer patients with any of the four blood components which they are lacking. The four proteins are prepared for use in a laboratory from donor blood.

After daily blood tests determine the amount of each protein they require, patients are replenished by injection. Since the injections contain proteins that are naturally occurring in the body, they cause none of the side effects of other invasive cancer therapies.

Immuno-Augmentative Therapy may serve as an adjunct to conventional cancer therapies (surgery, chemotherapy, and radiation) by enhancing their effect while protecting normal body tissues from deleterious effects.

In 1977 Dr. Lawrence Burton moved to the Bahamas so that he could continue his research unhindered by U.S. regulations, and also to provide therapy for patients who chose his method of cancer control. Since then he has been director of the Immunology Research Center and IAT, Ltd. Centre, a treatment facility located in the Rand Memorial Hospital in Freeport, Grand Bahama Island.

✍ | CALLANETICS | ✍

Callanetics is an exercise program in which the largest and deepest muscles in the body are activated by executing small and delicate movements.

Each set of exercises is designed to work on a specific part of the body. Callanetics can be safely used by individuals in almost any degree of physical condition. They are enjoyed by both men and women ranging in age from childhood to eighty and beyond. The exercises are performed without any music or cadence from an instructor.

Callan Pinckney, the developer of Callanetics, grew up in and around Savannah, Georgia. Always interested in travel and foreign lands, in 1961 she boarded a freighter to Germany and began a ten-year odyssey around the world. She lived and worked in such distant parts of the globe as England, Japan, India, Africa, and Ceylon (now Sri Lanka).

Because of less than ideal living conditions, disease, the types of menial work she performed, and carrying a heavy pack for so many years, her body had been terribly abused and was in need of earnest care.

After returning to the United States in 1972 she began working at an exercise salon in New York City. Pinckney found that some of the exercises she performed hurt her back. After confronting the management about the types of exercises they were using, she developed a conflict with salon policy and departed.

Pinckney was born with congenital back problems, scoliosis (lateral curvature of the spine), and lordosis (swayback). Also, her feet were so distorted that she was required to wear leg braces for many years during her childhood. Amazingly, she later went on to study classical ballet for twelve years.

She began to experiment on her own with different techniques and various movements learned during her ballet study. Trying to avoid back pain, she found that slight adjustments in position would make the difference between experiencing pain and not.

After performing the precise and delicate movements she developed for a short period of time, Pinckney noticed that her back pain was gone and her body had become firm and tight. Amazed at how good she looked and felt after exercising for such a short period of time, she concluded that these movements were the key to successful exercising.

What sets Callanetics apart from other exercise programs is the rapid results that can be achieved. This is well summarized in the title of Callan Pinckney's book, *Callanetics: 10 Years Younger in 10 Hours.* She states that "an hour of these exercises equals approximately seven hours of conventional exercise and 20 hours of aerobic dancing, as far as firming the body and pulling it up is concerned."

In general, exercise promotes strength, endurance, and flexibility in the body. Callanetics adds many additional benefits which include coordination, balance, body awareness, discipline, speed, physical and mental relaxation, building of stamina, and decrease in appetite.

A Callanetics workout takes about one hour, with each set of exercises designed to work on a specific part of the body. Delicate movements and deep muscular contractions give the exercises their power. Not only does Callanetics remove inches, it recontours the body as well.

Today, the Callanetics program is taught throughout the United States.

❧ | CAYCE (EDGAR) THERAPIES | ☙

The Edgar Cayce Therapies are an almost bewildering number of treatments, both in quantity and variety, for hundreds of different diseases, disabilities, and other physical conditions. These therapies are derived from the 8,976 psychic readings Edgar Cayce made for several thousand people with a wide variety of physical ailments.

Edgar Cayce was born in Hopkinsville, Kentucky, on March 18, 1877. As a young man he left Hopkinsville for Louisville to become a clerk in a bookstore. Leaving the bookstore to become a salesman and insurance agent, Cayce traveled throughout western Kentucky.

Cayce then developed a hoarseness and his voice faded to a faint whisper. The condition went on for months. When doctors in Hopkinsville were unable to do anything, he realized his condition was incurable and he would never again be able to speak above a whisper. No longer able to be a salesman, Edgar Cayce became a photographer's apprentice.

A hypnotist named Hart, traveling with a show performing in Hopkinsville, heard of Cayce's hoarseness and accepted it as a challenge. Hart said that for two hundred dollars he could cure Cayce and that if he did not, no money would be owed to him. Cayce tried the hypnosis. While in the trance he spoke fine, but would not take Hart's postsuggestion and remained hoarse after coming out of the trance. Another hypnotist, Dr. Quackenboss from New York, put Cayce into a very deep sleep that lasted twenty-four hours, still with no relief of the hoarseness.

Dr. Quackenboss then suggested that Cayce be asked to describe his own condition while under trance. This technique had been used in France years before, and patients had shown powers of clairvoyance through its use. Cayce decided to try this procedure and enlisted the help of hypnotist Al Layne.

As a child Cayce would go to "sleep" with his head lying on schoolbooks; he developed a type of photographic memory which allowed him to retain the contents of the book.

On March 31, 1901, with Al Layne present to ask questions, Cayce put himself into the "sleep" he had used as a child to learn schoolbooks. As

Layne watched his breathing deepen, the body appeared to sleep. He asked Cayce to see his body and describe the trouble in his throat and to speak in a normal tone.

After a few minutes Cayce began to mumble. He cleared his throat and began to speak in a clear, natural voice. "Yes," he said, "we can see the body." He went on to describe the problem and how to cure it. Edgar Cayce went on to regain full use of his voice and thus began his career as a clairvoyant.

For the next forty-three years Cayce gave over thirty thousand diagnoses that were stenographically recorded. After his death on January 3, 1945, copies of these readings were given to the Association for Research and Enlightenment (ARE) in Virginia Beach, Virginia.

Additionally, hundreds of complete case reports containing patient affidavits and reports by physicians verified the accuracy of his diagnoses and the effectiveness of his suggestions for treatment. It is this information that forms the basis for the Edgar Cayce Therapies.

During each reading, Cayce, while in a trance state, diagnosed the physical problems for a specific individual and recommended treatment that could include one or more of the therapeutic tools available at that time.

Cayce used Osteopathy, Chiropractic, massage, exercise, sophisticated nutrition and diet, every known form of Hydrotherapy, sweat baths, fume baths, colonics, a large variety of packs, Electrotherapy, and even conventional medicine and surgery.

He also used an incredible variety of herbs, common chemicals such as sulfur and cream of tartar, every type of oil imaginable, lights, colors, and original appliances of his invention.

Cayce's philosophy on health is truly holistic as it is more concerned with keeping people well and finding causes of illness than in curing symptoms. Many of the recommendations from the readings deal with therapies people can take responsibility for themselves.

Other therapies such as massage or osteopathic manipulation, which required help from another person, were utilized to help the body help itself. The therapies of Edgar Cayce deal with methods an individual can use to regain physical, mental, and spiritual stability.

Today the ARE Medical Clinic in Phoenix, Arizona, uses the healing concepts of the Edgar Cayce readings to complement conventional medicine. For self-help, an excellent book, *The Edgar Cayce Handbook for Health through Drugless Therapy* by Dr. Harold J. Reilly (ARE Press, 1975) is available. Also, the Reilly School of Massotherapy is located at ARE head-quarters in Virginia Beach, Virginia.

Dr. Reilly (1895–1987) was one of the world's most renowned physio-therapists and proponents of drugless, natural physical therapy. He person-ally worked with referrals from Edgar Cayce for fifteen years until Cayce's death. For the following thirty years he used Cayce Therapies at his clinic in New York City until his retirement.

The valuable information contained in the thousands of Cayce medical readings has been sorted and indexed over the years and is available from the Association for Research and Enlightenment (ARE) in Virginia Beach, Virginia.

✍ | CAYCE/REILLY MASSAGE | ✍

Cayce/Reilly Massage, also called the Cayce/Reilly Massage Technique, incorporates specific massage moves recommended in the trance-readings of Edgar Cayce combined with unique methods developed by Dr. Harold J. Reilly.

During a period of forty-three years, Edgar Cayce, often called the "Sleeping Prophet," gave over thirty thousand diagnoses that were stenographically recorded. While in a trance state, Cayce would diagnose the physical problems of a specific individual and recommend treat-ment. Although massage was frequently recommended, it was rarely used alone. It was only one of the many therapies used to help the body help itself.

Dr. Harold J. Reilly, a noted physiotherapist, has impressive credentials with some eight degrees, including a doctor of physiotherapy from Van Norman University in California. During the more than thirty years he operated the Reilly Health Institute in New York City, his list of clients included heads of state, government leaders, business tycoons, famous actors, writers, and opera singers from around the world.

Cayce began referring people to Dr. Reilly in 1930, nearly two years before the two met. During their fifteen years of association, Cayce men-tioned Dr. Reilly specifically by name hundreds of times while giving trance-readings. By 1945, the year of Cayce's death, Dr. Reilly had worked with more than one thousand people sent to his New York clinic by the "Sleeping Prophet." Until his retirement in 1965, Dr. Reilly continued to use Cayce Therapies in addition to his own physiotherapy techniques at his clinic.

Edgar Cayce and Harold J. Reilly shared the same philosophy on health. It was truly holistic—more concerned with keeping people well and finding causes of illness than in curing symptoms.

In his readings, Cayce recommended almost every known type of massage available in America during that period of time. These included Swedish massage, osteopathic massage, general massage, deep massage, vibratory massage, spinal massage, neuropathic massage, and massage of specific localized body areas.

Over a period of years Dr. Reilly evolved the Swedish style of massage, in which he was trained, to include adaptations and variations on basic massage strokes such as petrissage (kneading movement) and effleurage (light stroking, either superficial or deep). He developed new ways of working with specific body areas, such as the abdomen, as well as a procedure to gently stimulate certain endocrine glands. Dr. Reilly also used specific techniques of spinal massage detailed in the Cayce readings.

Two books that provide more detailed information are *The Edgar Cayce Handbook for Health through Drugless Therapy* by Dr. Harold J. Reilly and Ruth Hagy Brod, and *Edgar Cayce's Massage, Hydrotherapy and Healing Oils* by Joseph Duggan, Ms.T. and Sandra Duggan, RN, Ms.T. Both are available from the Association for Research and Enlightenment (the Edgar Cayce Foundation).

For additional information contact the Reilly School of Massotherapy located at ARE headquarters in Virginia Beach, Virginia. Workshops in the Cayce/Reilly Massage Technique are taught here, and they can provide the names of massage therapists in your area trained in this method.

❧ | CHAKRA BALANCING | ❧

Chakra Balancing is the clearing of energy blocks from the *chakras*. By utilizing various methods, the obstructed energy in the chakras can be balanced and harmonized.

In Sanskrit, the ancient language of India, *chakra* means "what revolves" or "wheel," indicating that these force centers are wheels of energy. According to traditional yoga philosophy, the chakras are the subtle force centers that vitalize and control the physical body.

Chakras are like relay stations for the vital life force energy, and serve as channels of communication between an individual's inner nature or subtle body and the physical body. There are seven chakras and each has a variety of functions. Each chakra relates to a specific color, a particular gland, organ, or area of the body, and a mental, emotional, or spiritual feeling. The following are brief, concise descriptions of each chakra.

The first chakra, the basic or root chakra, is located at the base of the spine. It is associated with the color red and governs the survival instinct.

The second chakra, the sex center, is located in the area behind the navel. It is associated with the color orange, the spleen, and sex organs, and governs the sex instinct and the emotion of desire.

The third chakra, the solar plexus, is a point below the heart. It is associated with the color yellow and the adrenal glands, and has to do with personal power, anger, and the way one presents oneself to the world.

The fourth chakra is the heart center. It is associated with the color green and relates to the circulatory system and the emotion of love.

The fifth chakra is the throat center. It is associated with the color blue and the thyroid gland, and relates to higher intelligence and the power of communication.

The sixth chakra, the third eye, is located between the eyes and behind the brow. It is associated with the color indigo (deep blue) and the pituitary gland, and relates to the mind, individual self, and the power of perception.

The seventh chakra, the crown chakra, is located at the top of the head. It is associated with the color violet (purple) and the pineal gland, and relates to the cosmic or universal self.

Energy blocks are usually formed by a variety of different stimuli that originate either from within the body or from external sources. Physical and emotional trauma can also cause energy blocks. These obstructions slow down vital life force energy or prevent it from flowing freely within the body.

An imbalance or block in a chakra causes physical dysfunction in the organ, gland, or part of the body that it relates to. It can also cause emotional or mental problems relating to that chakra. For example, a blockage in the fifth chakra, the throat center, can cause a physical problem with the body's metabolism due to a dysfunctional thyroid gland, and a mental/emotional problem with the voice, speech, or the ability to communicate.

There are professional practitioners that practice chakra balancing. Some of the methods they use to clear the chakras include Color Therapy, Crystal and Gem Therapy, visualizations, sounds, meditation, and Acupuncture.

Many of these methods can be used as self-help techniques by an individual to balance his chakras himself.

For example, color can be used in various forms such as lighting in a room, clothing worn (both outer and undergarments), drinking glasses and dishes, or tinted eyeglasses. Gems and crystals can be applied directly to the body at the chakra site. Vibrations can be received by listening to the intonation of vowel sounds. Visualization can be used to "see" the energy in a chakra moving smoothly and freely without any obstruction.

A single purpose lies behind all of these methods of chakra balancing: to allow vital life energy to flow without restriction throughout the body, which helps the body in healing itself.

☙ | CHELATION THERAPY | ❧

Chelation Therapy is a safe, painless, nonsurgical medical procedure used to remove undesirable heavy metals such as lead, mercury, nickel, copper, cadmium, and others from the body.

More recently Chelation Therapy has also been used to reverse symptoms of atherosclerosis or arteriosclerosis (hardening of the arteries) by removing the obstructive plaque that has built up in the circulatory system. Atherosclerosis is caused by many complex factors, including the abnormal accumulation of metallic elements in the body.

In atherosclerosis the formation of plaque within the arteries restricts the flow of blood, which leads to other problems such as angina and heart attack. Plaque is a fibrous tissue composed of fatty substances and cholesterol bound together (chelated) with calcium and other binding metals.

Without surgery, Chelation Therapy directly counteracts the harmful effects of calcium by removing it from the plaque. With the calcium and other binding metals out of the plaque, its remaining ingredients are loosened and carried to the liver for eventual excretion from the body. The symptoms of atherosclerosis are improved as the inside diameter of the blood vessel is increased and new elasticity is restored to the blood vessel wall, allowing greater blood flow.

Chelation comes from the Greek word *chele* meaning "claw" (as in the pincers of a crab or lobster). The chelating agent, a synthetic amino acid called ethylenediaminetetraacetic acid (EDTA) has the capacity to attach and bind metal molecules it contacts.

Utilizing the pincer effect, metal molecules are held to the EDTA molecules in such a way that an entirely new and different chelated compound is formed. This new stable compound, the atoms of which are firmly held together, can then be excreted from the body through the kidneys.

Chelation Therapy is administered by intravenous infusion. A slow drip of EDTA solution, in the appropriate strength and quantity, is injected directly into the bloodstream. This is a slow but painless procedure which takes three to four hours to complete.

A complete program of Chelation Therapy involves a broad-based health care program of regular exercise, vitamin and mineral supplements, and dietary changes.

In 1893 Alfred Werner, a Swiss Nobel Laureate, proposed the theory of metal binding which provided the foundation for modern chelation chemistry. In 1920 Messrs. Morgan and Drew specifically defined chelation as "the incorporation of a metal ion into a heterocyclic ring structure."

EDTA was first synthesized in Germany by F. Munz around 1934–35. Munz was trying to develop a substitute for citric acid, a chelating agent used by the textile industry to remove calcium from hard water. The presence of calcium in water tended to form stains with mordant dyes which were unacceptable to the makers of clothing and textile.

A different process for synthesizing EDTA was developed in the United States by Frederick C. Bernsworth in the early 1930s and was patented by him in 1941. Chelation Therapy itself was introduced into the United States in 1948.

Between 1950 and 1990, numerous clinical studies have shown the benefits of Chelation Therapy. It is recognized by medical authorities around the world as the definitive treatment for heavy metal toxicity, radiation toxicity, snake venom poisoning, digitalis intoxication, and heart arrhythmia.

The benefit of increased blood flow due to chelation therapy was detected by Dr. Norman E. Clarke in the 1950s. While treating patients for lead poisoning he observed that their general health improved. One of them, suffering from coronary artery disease, had his symptoms of angina disappear. Because proper circulation is a prerequisite to health regardless of what an individual's physical problem is, chelation is an effective adjunctive therapy to the treatment of all chronic degenerative diseases.

Clarke was aware of the connection between calcium and plaque formation and speculated that removing the calcium might be beneficial to patients suffering from atherosclerosis and its attendant symptoms. He and his colleagues then treated other heart patients with EDTA, reporting their findings in the *American Journal of Medical Science*.

Unfortunately, the most beneficial effects of Chelation Therapy, those of preventing and reversing the problems of degenerative diseases caused by diminished blood circulation, are not currently recognized by the medical establishment. These include diabetes, gallstones, kidney disease from poor circulation, stroke, emphysema, Parkinson's disease, cataracts, senility, osteoporosis, and hypertension.

Although intravenous injection Chelation Therapy can be legally administered by any licensed physician, it is important that she be trained in this medical specialty.

Today, the American College of Advancement in Medicine trains and certifies physicians in the safe use of Chelation Therapy and maintains a list of qualified physicians throughout the United States who offer this medical specialty as part of their practice.

❧ | CHI KUNG | ☙

Chi Kung (sometimes spelled Qi Gong) is the "heal thyself" tradition of the ancient Chinese masters. In Chinese it literally means "breathing exercise." In its simplest form it is a system of self-applied health enhancements. In its more elevated form it is a remarkable personal development art. Although it combines other elements, it is best described as an exercise which balances and amplifies the *chi* or vital energy force within the body. It has been used for centuries in China to promote health, fitness, and longevity, and to cure illness.

Although the contents of Chi Kung are varied, the main elements of all forms are regulation of body (posture), regulation of mind, and regulation of breath. These three elements interact with one another. Some forms additionally use self-massage, and movement of the arms and legs with the torso.

Chi Kung is over two thousand years old. Records of breathing exercises go back to the Zhou dynasty (c. 1100–221 B.C.). At that time a form of fitness exercise called *daoyin* was popular. It combined regulated breathing with various body movements.

Chi Kung was developed in both theory and practice after the Eastern Han dynasty (A.D. 25–220). During that time Indian Yoga, brought to

China with the introduction of Buddhism, was integrated with the ancient custom of daoyin.

It developed over the centuries and was widely used as a medical treatment to cure disease. Because of links to mysticism and superstition, its use grew less popular. Currently in China, interest in Chi Kung has grown once again, and a great deal of scientific research has been dedicated to the physiological aspects of it.

The three most common Chi Kung exercises are the relaxation exercise, the strengthening exercise, and the inward training exercise. Depending on the exercise, they are performed in a standing, sitting, or lying-down position. When movement is included, it is done with gentle circular and stretching movements.

By stimulating gastrointestinal movements and the secretion of digestive juice, better digestion is achieved. In China Chi Kung has proved effective in treatment of stomach and duodenal ulcers, constipation, and high blood pressure.

During the exercise, in a relaxed, tranquil state, subjects have shown decreased heart rate, respiration frequency, and oxygen consumption.

For additional information, contact the American Foundation of Traditional Chinese Medicine or the Qi Gong Institute/East-West Academy of the Healing Arts.

❧ | CHI NEI TSANG | ❧

Chi Nei Tsang, or Internal Organ Massage, is a traditional Taoist massage technique applied in the abdomen, especially around the navel and directly to the internal organs, to balance their energies. Translated it means "internal organ energy transformation."

Chi Nei Tsang is intimately linked with Taoist-based theory and philosophy. Taoists discovered that the area of the stomach around and behind the navel is the most powerful and vitally important energy center in the body. Here, chi (vital life energy) is generated, stored, and distributed to the entire system. Tension causes the flow of energy to become blocked, causing problems in other areas of the body.

Through direct stimulation and manipulation of muscles, tendons, fascia (connective tissue), intestines, the lymphatic system, the nervous system, and organs (pancreas, spleen, gall bladder, stomach, liver, uterus, lungs), Chi Nei

Tsang works to dissolve the knots and entanglements resulting from stress and tension. Stagnation in the abdomen is broken up, fresh blood is allowed to circulate, the tissues become soft and pliable, and the free flow of energy is restored.

As the area is progressively relaxed, deeper and deeper levels of the abdomen can be reached. This allows detoxification of the system's largest lymph nodes, improvement in the immune system's function, a raise in metabolism to its full potential, and harmony of the emotions.

Chi Nei Tsang is a massage technique that can be used on oneself. It is not therapy and practitioners do not heal; they teach the patient to heal himself.

For additional information consult the book *Chi Nei Tsang* by Mantak Chia, published by Healing Tao Books, Huntington, New York.

CHILDREN MASSAGE

Children Massage, or massage for children, is the use of various massage techniques to ease some of the physical and emotional difficulties experienced in childhood. Besides being therapeutic, massage has the advantage of being emotionally supportive as well as deeply relaxing.

Professional massage therapists regularly work with children to improve a wide variety of physical problems, including those related to birth defects, handicaps, traumatic injury, and disease. In addition to its therapeutic benefits, massage is a particularly effective way to give comfort and reassurance to a child, as children respond to touch more readily than to talk.

In today's society childhood is not the carefree, easygoing, stress-free life many adults assume it is. According to John Killinger, author of *The Loneliness of Children*, "Childhood is a very difficult time of life. For many children, it is filled with fears, anxieties, and confusion. . . . Adults often forget how hard it is to be a child."

Although the kinds of stress encountered by children are different than those faced by adults, the physiological response to them is the same. The "fight-or-flight" syndrome is invoked and the body responds with the release of adrenaline and various other hormones, the heartbeat becomes stronger and faster, and muscle tension is increased.

A child under constant stress will develop a buildup of muscular tension causing external muscles to become hard and knotted and/or the inner muscles that control the eyes, stomach, and intestines to become very tense.

This excessive stress and tension causes physical and emotional fatigue, which can lead to numerous physical illnesses.

Massaging children produces the same physiological effects as it does with adults. It stimulates the nervous system, relieves muscle spasm, and aids the movement of blood and lymphatic fluid in the tense area. Massage can help children reach a deep level of relaxation by releasing the stored tension. In addition, it helps the child learn to identify where the stress is stored in the body and how he feels when the body is relaxed.

Since the beginning of time, it has been a mother's natural instinct to touch or rub a child that is crying. To help a child go to sleep, rubbing or massaging his back is an instinctive act.

An infant is held, touched, and rubbed much of the time because he is relatively immobile and requires a great deal of care and attention. After the infant becomes a child he is more mobile, more independent, and able to do more things for himself. Consequently, the touch and contact with the parent or caregiver is greatly diminished during childhood compared to that experienced during infancy.

Massage provides a way to counteract this natural reduction of touch contact during childhood and to strengthen the parent-child bond. Also, massage during these formative years can be a powerful way to teach children positive lessons about touch, body awareness, and intimacy.

Some of the minor massage treatments commonly used by parents and caregivers today include rubbing the gums of a teething baby, massaging away leg cramps at night, and rubbing an area that has received a blow or an impact from a fall, to keep a bruise from forming. Massage can also offer relief of musculoskeletal aches and pains such as strains, sprains, and tension headaches.

Parents can easily learn the sensitive and nurturing massage techniques necessary to work with their own children. There are many good books available that adequately teach the basic elements. Also, there are many massage schools, colleges, and universities that offer classes and workshops in massage techniques.

CHIROPRACTIC

Chiropractic is a health care system that deals with the relationship between the spinal column and the nervous system. Its philosophy: For a person to experience harmony, vitality, and good health there must be an unobstructed flow of nerve impulses from the brain through the spinal nerves and out to every part of the body.

It is based on the major premise that the vertebrae of the spine can, and frequently do, become misaligned for a variety of reasons, including poor posture, poor muscle tone, injury, and stress. These misalignments of the vertebrae, or subluxations as they are called, cause interference in the transmission of nerve impulses from the brain to organs and other tissues of the body.

Although most misalignments are self-corrected through normal body movement, some remain fixed. When nerve transmission to a particular organ or part of the body is interrupted for long periods of time it causes impaired bodily function and results in pain and illness.

Chiropractic does not diagnose or treat diseases and ailments. The treatments (adjustments) are not therapeutic. Chiropractic subscribes to the basic principle that the human body has tremendous recuperative powers and when it is operating at its full potential is capable of maintaining perfect health. By allowing the immune system to function at peak efficiency, disease is not allowed to gain a foothold in the body.

It is the largest drugless, nonsurgical health system in the Western world. In the United States it is the largest alternative and natural healing art practiced and second largest health care system in North America after conventional (allopathic) medical care.

The origin of Chiropractic principles dates back to ancient times. Healers in India, Greece, China, Egypt, and Rome, many years before the time of Christ, were aware of the detrimental effects of spinal misalignment. Hippocrates, in one of his many books, stated, "Look well to the spine, for many diseases have their origin in dislocations of the vertebral column."

Native American peoples—Sioux, Creek, and Winnebago—practiced spinal manipulation, as did the Incas, Maya, and Aztecs, who used it for back pain and illness. With the fall of the Roman Empire in A.D. 476 and the ensuing period known as the Dark Ages in Europe, the development of spinal manipulation was curtailed due to superstition. The practice remained alive, often in secret, mainly through the efforts of unschooled physicians in the area now known as Germany. Natives of the Polynesian Islands let children walk on the backs of afflicted adults to adjust bones and reduce the swelling they believed impaired normal functioning.

Late in the Middle Ages spinal manipulation resurfaced, and during the Renaissance it enjoyed popularity under the name *bonesetting*. Early bonesetters were regarded as gifted healers treating a wide variety of illnesses by manipulating bones into place. By the eighteenth century it had spread throughout Europe. It did not become popular in America until the nineteenth century, when it followed westward expansion.

Daniel David Palmer (1845–1913), born of English-German parents in Port Perry, near Ontario, Canada, showed an early interest in healing. As a boy he would bring home and splint small animals with broken limbs. In 1865 he left Ontario with his brother Tom and moved to the United States. Palmer met a magnetic healer named Paul Caster in Burlington, Iowa, and became his student. He rediscovered his early talents in healing and later opened his own office. During his nine years as a magnetic healer Palmer read numerous books on anatomy and physiology, concentrating on the spine. He then concluded that misaligned vertebrae could be the cause of disease.

On a September day in 1895, in the town of Davenport, Iowa, D. D. Palmer made history. A janitor, Harvey Lillard, in the building where he maintained his magnetic healing office explained to Palmer that he had been deaf for seventeen years. It happened when something gave out in his back while exerting in a cramped, stooped position.

Palmer examined the man and found one of his vertebrae out of position and proceeded to put it back into normal position. The janitor soon regained his hearing and Palmer had discovered Chiropractic.

Encouraged by his accomplishment with Lillard, Palmer practiced on more patients and observed that other disorders responded to repositioning of the spinal bones. He began to refine his technique and formulated a philosophy for the newfound healing art. At the urging of his son, Bartlett Joshua Palmer (1881–1961), D. D. Palmer opened the first Chiropractic school in Davenport in 1897.

Chiropractic adjustments have become greatly refined since 1895. When properly administered they are safe, even during pregnancy, and normally painless. A wide variety of ailments, classified as musculoskeletal disorders and organic conditions, respond favorably to Chiropractic care.

Musculoskeletal disorders include whiplash injuries, low back sprain and strain, neck problems, sciatica, arthritic conditions, and bursitis. Organic conditions include high blood pressure, migraine headaches, neuritis, headache, and nervous disorders. The age of patients ranges from preschool children to retired adults.

Under the framework of Chiropractic there are different philosophies as to the scope of the modality, and proponents are usually classified as "straight" or "mixers." Straight Chiropractic is narrow in scope and deals only with spinal adjustments to correct vertebral subluxations and restore nerve function.

A broader and more liberal scope is taken by the mixer. As the name implies it is a mix of straight Chiropractic and other therapeutic methods. It is holistic in nature and utilizes adjunctive therapies such as massage, applied kinesiology, acupressure, physical therapy, ultrasound, vitamin therapy, nutritional counseling, traction, and other methods to provide comprehensive health care.

The Chiropractic educational program consists of a four-year postgraduate program similar in hours to medical school. Most Chiropractic schools in the United States require approximately two years of college credits with emphasis on biology, chemistry, and physics for admission. In order to be licensed, chiropractors must pass written and oral examinations administered by the state in which they are going to practice and by national boards.

Additional information may be obtained by contacting any of the Chiropractic professional organizations listed in the resource section.

❧ | COLON THERAPY | ❧

Colon Therapy is the cleansing and detoxification of the large intestine or colon by removing accumulated waste matter. This is accomplished by flushing the colon with water (colon hydrotherapy) or by ingesting herbs or various other substances.

The use of colon irrigation goes back to the 1890s. Dr. Elmer Lee's irrigating apparatus for cholera stations was described in *The Principles and Practice of Hydrotherapy: A Guide to the Application of Water in Disease* by Simon Baruch, M.D., published in 1898.

During the 1920s and 1930s Colon Therapy was used by physicians to treat such diseases as arthritis, heart disease, high blood pressure, and depression.

During the 1940s, after the discovery of antibiotics and the emphasis on allopathic drug-centered treatment, colonic irrigation fell into disuse. Today colonics are used by naturopathic physicians and some chiropractors, osteopaths, medical doctors, and natural health clinics.

Colonic irrigation can be used as a stand-alone therapy or in combination with colon-cleansing herbs and other substances.

The forerunner to modern colonic irrigation was the enema. The therapeutic use of enemas, the injection of water into the rectum using only gravity pressure, is well documented throughout history.

About 1500 B.C., accounts of the ancient Egyptians using a reed to introduce aqueous substances into the body via the rectum were documented in a work called the *Ebers Papyrus*.

The use of enemas was described by two ancient Greek physicians. In the fourth century B.C., Hippocrates mentioned the use of enemas as a treatment to reduce fever. Galen, a physician and writer during the second century B.C., referred to the use of enemas.

During the time of the Roman Empire, noble citizens of Rome, with their obsession for baths, found the enema to be a kind of internal bath. In the New Testament references are made to the Essenes' use of reeds and gourds to administer enemas. They used the procedure to cleanse the body, which they believed to be a temple for the soul.

The large intestine, which starts at the end of the small intestine, consists of three sections: cecum (blind pouch where it begins), colon, and rectum. Although the large intestine serves several purposes, one of its major functions is to absorb water from the liquid residue of digested food that empties into it.

The colon, which extends from the cecum to the rectum, is made up of three connected segments totaling some five feet in length. The *ascending colon* extends up the right side of the abdomen, the *transverse colon* runs horizontally across the abdomen, and the *descending colon* extends down the left side of the abdomen and then turns toward the center of the body. As water is absorbed by the colon, the fecal matter is formed into solid stools and moves toward the rectum by muscular contractions called peristalsis. It is then discharged from the body through the anal opening.

In a true carnivore (meat eater), such as a lion, the colon is very short in comparison to that of a human. This allows the meat eaten by a carnivore to be out of its body before it has had time to putrefy, usually twenty-four hours or less. In humans this process can take up to forty-eight hours or more.

Because the typical diet of modern-day industrialized societies is low in fiber and high in mucoid-forming foods such as meats and fats, the once watery residue becomes slimy as moisture is absorbed, and its rate of movement through the large intestine is slowed down. The slimy medium then becomes gluelike as more moisture is removed from it.

Colon Therapy theory maintains that this gluey substance forms a layer along the colon wall as it passes through. Peristalsis can cause the colon wall to fold over on itself, forming pockets called diverticula that trap the gluey substance. Over a period of time, layer upon layer of gluey, putrefied feces build up in the colon, often becoming tough and rubbery. This "lining" in the colon of stagnant decaying matter causes a condition called *autointoxication.*

Autointoxication is a process whereby toxins produced by the decaying matter are released into the bloodstream and make their way to all parts of the body; the body literally poisons itself. Colon Therapists believe this condition contributes to a multitude of disease states, including colon cancer.

The reason fiber is so important in the diet is that it roughs up this gluey substance and "sweeps" it on through the large intestine. Without fiber in the diet, or without Colon Therapy, the tough rubbery lining of the colon will continue to build up. Autopsies have shown a colon that was nine inches in diameter with a passage through it no larger than a pencil. Another autopsy revealed a colon full of stagnant decaying matter that weighed nearly forty pounds.

In many naturopathic modalities, Colon Therapy is integral to the healing process because of autointoxication. Although Colon Therapy is not a specific cure for any disease, Colon Therapists believe that it helps the body overcome difficulties more readily by removing a source of toxins, thus allowing its natural healing ability to function properly.

There are two different approaches to Colon Therapy, or colon cleansing, each using the opposite end of the alimentary canal to accomplish its task. The first approach is the introduction of water into the rectum and colon by means of a colonic irrigation or enema. The second approach utilizes herbs and other organic and inorganic substances, taken orally, to cleanse the colon.

Colonic irrigation is a therapeutic process used to loosen and remove accumulated, stagnated waste from the colon, and detoxify the system. Filtered water under gentle pressure flows into the rectum until the colon is filled. The Colon Therapist massages the colon through the abdomen to help break up the accumulated gluelike material on the colon walls. The therapist can also massage foot reflexology points. The water is then allowed to flow out, the waste flushed out and removed. This process is repeated many times during the session, which generally lasts forty-five to sixty minutes.

Although plain water is customarily used, herbs and other substances can be added to adjust the acid/alkaline balance in the colon to maintain and encourage the growth of "friendly" bacteria.

Enemas containing a variety of substances such as herbs, wheatgrass, bentonite, and clay can also be used therapeutically. Proponents of the Gerson Therapy, in fact, believe that coffee enemas cause stimulation of enzyme systems of the gut wall and liver to promote excretion of toxic bile.

Although there are some units manufactured for home use, professional colonic irrigation requires specialized equipment which costs several thousands of dollars and requires a trained operator to administer. Because of the threat of the transmission of AIDS and other diseases, the design of modern colonic irrigation machines allows critical parts to be sterilized. Additionally, disposable hoses and speculums are available.

Because a colonic irrigation can only reach about half of the large intestine's five feet of length, a more complete method of colon cleansing is the ingestion of certain herbs, combinations of herbs, or certain other organic and inorganic substances.

These ingested remedies work to soften, loosen, break up, or dissolve the stagnant, hardened mucoid material buildup in the colon. The use of bentonite and pumice (special types of volcanic ash), some varieties of clay, and psyllium seed is very effective in removing stagnant material.

To be most effective, any type of Colon Therapy works better with a change in dietary habits. It is advisable to eat a diet containing more raw fruits and vegetables and less mucus-producing foods such as meat and dairy products.

Two good books on the subject are *The Colon Health Handbook: New Health through Colon Rejuvenation* by Robert Gray, and *Healing Within: The Complete Colon Health Guide* by Stanley Weinberger.

Additional information may be obtained by contacting any of the professional organizations listed in the resource section.

❧ | COLOR THERAPY | ❧

Color Therapy, or Color Healing, is the therapeutic use of various forms of color and light for physical, emotional, and spiritual benefit to the human body.

Color Healing can be traced back to ancient Egypt and other premodern societies. Egyptian priests left manuscripts showing their system of color science, and Indian and Chinese mystics had knowledge of color in their secret doctrines.

In ancient Egypt and Greece, color temples were built with seven compartments, each containing one of the seven colors of the rainbow. People were brought to the temples and put into specific compartments, depending on their need, for physical healing and spiritual uplifting. Pythagoras, the Greek mathematician and philosopher, used color for healing.

In 1666 Sir Isaac Newton developed the first valuable theory of color when he admitted sunlight through a prism. Newton established the presence of seven basic colors in the spectrum.

For centuries the healing profession has recognized that color is a force of immeasurable and infinite power, exerting a tremendous psychological and physiological influence on people.

In Europe during the late 1800s and early 1900s, psychologists working in mental hospitals researched the effect of color on patients. By utilizing different colored walls and lights it was found that depressive patients put into rooms with red or bright yellow walls, and hyperactive patients put into rooms with blue or green walls, were both calmed by the respective colors.

Black is a color associated with tragedy and death. Blackfriars Bridge, in London, was a gloomy black structure known for its high rate of suicide. After the bridge was painted green, the suicide rate declined by one-third.

The use of color has numerous applications in industry. Experiments have shown that muscular reaction time is much quicker under the influence of red light than green light, which has application on an assembly line. The colors used on factory walls and machinery affect employee morale, efficiency, absenteeism, and accident rates.

In sports, a locker room painted in colors on the red side of the spectrum is known to stimulate the team members. Uniform color can also influence a team's performance; thus, many professional football teams use red or orange as some part of the team colors.

Color is used extensively in interior design to create a certain feeling or mood, and to influence behavior. For example, red rooms cause an over-estimate of time. This is a particularly effective color for restaurants that want to make an individual feel she has spent more time there than she actually has. This allows the restaurant to seat more people in a given time period.

Restaurants and food processors use color to make food more attractive and appetizing. It has been suggested that consuming naturally colored foods and beverages is an excellent way of getting color into the body for the improvement of health.

Some Color Therapists believe colors contain energy vibrations with healing properties. Exposure to a color and its vibrations can be used to assist the body's natural healing and recuperative powers to achieve and maintain health and well-being.

There are seven natural colors in the visible light spectrum (rainbow): red, orange, yellow, green, blue, indigo, and violet. Each color vibrates at its own individual frequency. In Color Therapy each color corresponds to one of the seven chakras (energy centers in the body), which in turn can influence a specific gland, organ, or tissue of the body. For example, the color red, which corresponds to the root or base chakra, can be used for problems with the adrenal glands, kidney, and bladder.

A Color Therapist may use a variety of methods to influence healing. Some of these include immersion in colored light, wearing colored clothing and/or underwear, eating certain colored foods, drinking water that has been in a colored glass, or wearing colored eyeglasses.

Color Therapy is a part of Ayurvedic medicine, the ancient Indian art and science of healing and rejuvenation. The healing properties of certain basic natural colors are used to treat imbalances of the three *doshas* or *tridoshas*, which are the forces that govern all the functions of the body, mind, and consciousness.

We all use Color Therapy whether we are aware of it or not. Color is an integral part of our life, woven into virtually every facet of it. We choose the color of the clothing we wear, the color of the car we drive, the color of the walls, furniture, carpet, and towels in our homes. All of these colors have a psychological and physiological effect on our daily lives.

There are numerous books available on the use of color for healing. Many books dealing primarily with other subjects such as chakras and Ayurveda contain sections dealing with Color Therapy. Two good books are *The Ancient Art of Color Therapy* by Linda Clark, which covers the subject in general, and *Ayurveda: The Science of Self-Healing* by Dr. Vasant Lad, which has a section on the use of color for healing.

❦ | CONNECTIVE TISSUE MASSAGE | ❧

Connective Tissue Massage, or *Bindegewebsmassage*, is a type of German bodywork. It is a noninvasive, specialized massage technique used to relieve pain and treat a wide variety of problems.

Connective Tissue Massage was developed in Germany by Elizabeth Dicke. Suffering from a serious medical problem, Dicke was facing amputation of one leg. Unwilling to accept this consequence, she experimented with different types of massage on herself and discovered a new technique which eventually cured her.

Dicke found that dragging a crooked finger, with a fairly light pressure, through the skin and connective tissue in one area of the body had an effect on a distant site. In other words, if you stimulate a specific area on the skin it will affect the tissues and internal organs in distant areas of the body. She later devised a system for treating various illnesses and organic imbalances as well as structural problems through the use of this technique.

Connective Tissue Massage works on a principle similar to trigger points (hypersensitive areas in the muscle and connective tissue which are painful to touch). Stimulation of a trigger point "refers" a sensation of pain to some other part of the body. This neuromuscular mechanism is the result of nerve connections that developed embryologically between the skin, muscles, and internal organs.

The technique consists of the massage therapist subtly hooking her fingers into the skin and superficial connective tissue while performing a dragging or pulling stroke that stretches the skin somewhat. Connective Tissue Massage leaves a visible mark that looks something like an abrasion or burn, but which goes away without leaving a scar.

Research has shown that Connective Tissue Massage may tend to stimulate the parasympathetic nervous system, which relaxes the body and is also responsible for pain relief and healing in the body.

Connective Tissue Massage is a well-developed physical therapy technique in Germany, and in some parts of Europe it is considered a medical technique. In the United States, the technique is taught at various massage schools, and the technique is part of the armamentarium of many qualified massage therapists.

For additional information on Connective Tissue Massage, consult *A Manual . . . of the Connective Tissue (Connective Tissue Massage) "Bindegewebsmas-*

sage" by E. Dicke, H. Schliack, and A. Wolff (Scarsdale, N.Y.: Sidney S. Simon, 1978).

🕊 | CRANIOSACRAL THERAPY | 🐦

CranioSacral Therapy is a gentle, noninvasive, hands-on manipulative technique that helps to detect and correct imbalances in the Cranio-Sacral System, which may cause various sensory, motor, or intellectual dysfunctions.

The CranioSacral System is a physiological system found in the human body and in animals that have a brain and spinal cord. It is comprised of the brain, spinal cord, cerebrospinal fluid, cranial dural membrane, cranial bones, and sacrum. It is a closed hydraulic system that moves with slight but perceptible rhythmic fluctuation.

Early in the 1900s, William G. Sutherland, an osteopathic student in Kirkland, Missouri, was struck by an idea. He observed that certain bones in the skull had a distinct bevel. He reasoned that these skull bones were designed to move in relation to one another.

For more than twenty years Dr. Sutherland contemplated movable skull bones in adult humans and experimented on himself by applying pressure to various parts of his head with a helmetlike device. During these experiments his wife would describe his reactions to the different duration and intensity of pressure.

He then developed a system of examination and treatment for the bones of the skull. Sutherland's system became known as Cranial Osteopathy. Although patient success was recorded, and was sometimes even miraculous, it acquired a cultist reputation. Because it was not well understood, it became something of an embarrassment to the osteopathic medical profession.

In 1970 John E. Upledger, D.O., F.A.A.O., while observing neck surgery, noted the rythmic movement of a membranous boundary of what appeared to be a fluid system. Neither medical books nor colleagues could explain his observation. Then in 1972, while attending a seminar on Sutherland's Cranial Osteopathy techniques of evaluation and treatment, Dr. Upledger put the pieces together. He understood how a fluid system could function within a membrane sac encased in the skull and the spinal column canal. This became known as the CranioSacral System.

It is believed that within the CranioSacral System, the brain expands and contracts as a means of transporting cerebrospinal fluid throughout the brain and spine. Through this mechanism of pumping and draining, nerve cells continually receive a fresh supply of nutrients to keep them healthy, similar to the way muscles receive nutrients via the bloodstream.

At Michigan State University in 1975, Dr. Upledger and a team of researchers set about to establish a scientific basis for a CranioSacral System and to explain the function of the system in both practical and scientific terms. They showed how the system could be used to evaluate and treat innumerable health problems.

CranioSacral Therapy is used by many health care professionals, including medical doctors, dentists, chiropractors, osteopaths, physical therapists, acupuncturists, occupational therapists, and licensed bodyworkers.

Evaluation and treatment of the patient can be accomplished by hand palpation. Although all the bones of the spine and pelvis can be used for examination, CranioSacral motion is most easily felt in the bones of the skull, sacrum, and coccyx because they are attached to the membranes which encase the cerebrospinal fluid. To a trained practitioner, the rhythm of the CranioSacral System can be felt as clearly as the rhythms of the cardiovascular and respiratory systems.

The positive effects of CranioSacral Therapy are dependent to a great extent upon the practitioner's ability to sense and follow the subtle movements of the CranioSacral System. Through light touch and gentle manipulations, the practitioner makes subtle adjustments to release tension within this intricate system; this aids the body's inherent, self-corrective physiological activities to help the CranioSacral System work more efficiently.

CranioSacral Therapists use CranioSacral Therapy to treat a host of health problems. They frequently combine it with neck or spine therapy to help relieve headaches, stiffness in the neck and spine, and whiplash. It can also be used to alleviate TMJ (Tempromandibular Joint) syndrome, ear and eye problems, balance or learning difficulties, dyslexia, hyperactivity, and others. It is especially beneficial for those who have had a head or neck injury (car, sports, falls, work accidents).

More advanced practitioners of CranioSacral Therapy can utilize an effect known as "unwinding," which allows the body to release a specific trauma by recreating the same position it was in when the trauma occurred. Once the tension is released, the dysfunctional or painful part of the body is returned to its normal state. Unwinding acts like a self-correcting mechanism.

Practitioners discovered that the unwinding effect occurs spontaneously if they are able to physically support the client and follow his movement while, at the same time, maintaining contact with the client's CranioSacral rhythm.

Unwinding can occur in any position. For the sensitive practitioner, following the client's movements and staying in touch with his CranioSacral rhythm simultaneously can be like Tai Chi Chuan movements or dancing. This process requires a certain amount of agility and a great deal of sensitivity on the part of the practitioner. If the client perceives that the practitioner is following his movements accurately, he will go into the unwinding and release these traumas.

Also, during the unwinding process, there is frequently some emotional realization or memory triggered at the moment the body attains the identical position it was in when the trauma occurred. As the energy stored in the body from the trauma begins to release, its blocking effect, which causes dysfunction, begins to unravel.

For additional information which explains in detail the functioning of the CranioSacral System, consult the three textbooks written by Dr. Upledger: *CranioSacral Therapy, CranioSacral Therapy II,* and *SomatoEmotional Release and Beyond.*

The Upledger Institute offers workshops to train health care professionals such as physicians, chiropractors, massage therapists, physical therapists, and others in the benefits of CranioSacral Therapy.

To locate licensed health care professionals who are alumni and incorporate CranioSacral Therapy into their practice, contact the Upledger Institute.

In addition, the Upledger Institute maintains the HealthPlex Clinic at their Palm Beach Gardens, Florida, headquarters; the clinic offers various health care programs. For additional information contact the Upledger Institute.

❧ | CREATIVE ARTS THERAPY | ☙

Creative Arts Therapy, used in the field of mental health treatment, is a nonverbal, nonthreatening type of therapy based on natural forms of patient expression. It includes Music Therapy, Dance Therapy, Art Therapy, Poetry

Therapy, and Drama Therapy. The nature of many patients' inner conflicts makes verbal communication extremely difficult. With Creative Arts Therapy patients can choose such media as voice, instrument, dance, fine arts, poetry, or drama to create, to learn, to express themselves, and to heal.

❧ | CROSS-FIBER FRICTION MASSAGE | ❧

Cross-Fiber Friction Massage is a massage technique in which the massage therapist applies friction to the muscle by rubbing across or perpendicularly to the muscle fibers. Skeletal muscle is comprised of fibers, grouped into bundles, that all run in the same direction. This is called striated muscle. Most other massage techniques stroke the muscle in the same direction as the fibers.

Also called Deep Transverse Friction Massage, the technique was developed by English orthopedist Dr. James H. Cyriax. Cross-Fiber Friction Massage is classified as a deep-tissue massage.

Cross-Fiber Friction Massage also falls into the category of a mechanical proprioceptor reset. Proprioceptors are neurological receptive mechanisms (sensory receptors) located throughout the body. Found primarily in the soft tissue, proprioceptors function at the subconscious level to monitor every body movement. This information is conveyed through the nervous system to the brain, which is then able to tell us exactly where our body is situated in space.

Proprioceptors in soft tissues are continuously relaying information concerning the status of that soft tissue to the brain. The information includes the amount of pressure on the muscle, its state of contraction, how much tension is on the muscle tissue, etc. In essence, the proprioceptors relay essential information to the brain so that we can coordinate all the actions necessary for any movement we want to make.

Some health care professionals believe the proprioceptors that control tension in the muscles and induce them to relax are directly stimulated by Cross-Fiber Friction Massage.

Rubbing across the muscle tends to break up adhesions in the connective tissue (fascia) which permeates the muscle fibers. It also works well around the origin and insertion of the muscle. Cross-Fiber Friction Massage technique is used extensively in physical therapy and sports massage, and as a treatment to prevent or reduce the formation of scar tissue.

When a massage therapist determines that stroking in the same direction as the muscle fibers is not appropriate for some reason, Cross-Fiber Friction Massage can be a useful technique because it offers another approach. In essence, the innate wisdom of the body intuitively knows what needs to be done to make it well or whole.

Depending on the type of injury or physical problem Cross-Fiber Friction Massage can produce many benefits. In sports massage it is used on trigger points and to treat tendonitis.

Muscle trauma or muscular tension from stress and other factors will cause a buildup of lactic and carbonic acid within the muscle. When these toxic waste products are not removed by the body, a "knot" or painful spasm in the muscle results. Massage increases blood circulation to a specific area, which brings fresh oxygen and nutrients while it removes waste products. Cross-Fiber Friction Massage appears to help the muscle regain function and release the buildup of toxins more readily than some other massage techniques.

One of the keys to successful massage therapy is using the right technique at the right time on the body, and Cross-Fiber Friction Massage offers another method to accomplish this. It can be used alone or in combination with other massage strokes. Massage therapists who specialize in sports massage and physical therapists are two types of practitioners who utilize Cross-Fiber Friction Massage.

❧ | CRYOTHERAPY | ❧

Cryotherapy, also known as Ice Therapy, is the application of cold to various parts of the body for therapeutic purposes. The source of the cold can range from immersion in ice water (especially effective for the limbs) to the application of ice cubes, crushed ice (in containers), or frozen commercial gel packs directly to the problem site. Additionally, an ice cube can be rubbed over an area to gradually numb it.

The use of cold for treating physical problems has been in use since the time of Hippocrates. It has been a common practice to apply ice or cold cloths to the body or to immerse the body in cold water to reduce fever and treat heat exhaustion. Many parents have rubbed the gums of teething children with ice or put ice on a minor burn to reduce discomfort and pain.

Seemingly the opposite of heat, Cryotherapy is surprisingly similar in effect for increasing circulation and relieving pain. Although the ice initially slows circulation and metabolism in the area of application, after it is removed a rapid recovery and circulatory increase take place.

Cryotherapy is especially effective in treating a trauma injury such as a sprained ankle. Quick application of ice after the incident lessens swelling, pain, and loss of range of motion. Ice is also useful to cool and reduce inflammation. Because of its numbing effect it can be used before certain types of deep muscle massage procedures to diminish discomfort.

Ice used alternately with heat is extremely effective to increase circulation and "flush" an area. This flushing effect helps remove metabolic wastes and supplies oxygenated blood and nutrients to the area, speeding tissue growth and repair. The procedure always begins and ends with the application of ice. Usually ice is applied for fifteen to twenty minutes, followed by the application of heat for five to ten minutes, and then ice for fifteen to twenty minutes again.

Because it is so effective, simple, and inexpensive, the application of ice or ice and heat can easily be used by individuals for self-care therapy.

❧ | CRYSTAL THERAPY | ☙

Crystal Therapy, sometimes referred to as Gem Therapy or Crystal Healing, is the use of quartz crystals, gemstones, and other types of crystals and stones for therapeutic and healing purposes. Stones and crystals are also used with Chakra Balancing and Color Therapy (see elsewhere in this book).

Crystals and gemstones, like the human body, are known to have electromagnetic energy. They emit vibrations and frequencies that have the very powerful potential to affect the whole being—body, mind, and spirit.

Throughout history people have been attracted to the beauty of various types of rocks, stones, crystals, and gems. It is natural for an individual to want to pick up a beautiful rock, stone, or crystal and carry it with him. Eventually it became known that certain types of crystals and stones had the potential to create or produce certain effects on the body. Jewels and precious stones have always possessed mystical qualities and have been valued by both primitive and civilized cultures. Many Native American tribes used crystal healing.

In the United States during the early 1980s the crystal-awareness phenomenon swept across the country. People attracted to crystals and stones began to incorporate them into their daily life. Certain crystals and stones were worn on the body while others were used in the home to produce desired emotional effects.

For self-healing and other beneficial effects, the energy vibrations and inherent healing properties of crystals and gemstones can be utilized in various ways. An individual might wear them as an ornament or jewelry, place loose crystals and stones directly on her body while sitting or lying down, keep them in her pockets, or have them in different rooms of her home and in her office. Crystals and stones make people feel good, and their beneficial effects may be due to a person's belief that they will have positive effects on her.

Crystals and gemstones are commonly incorporated into items such as necklaces, bracelets, rings, earrings, headbands, crowns, headpieces, belts, waistbands, and anklets. Also, loose crystals and gemstones can be kept in a pouch and hung from the body. Crystal and gemstone jewelry is generally worn over the body's energy meridians, and on or near the chakra points. This tends to open up and increase the flow of energy in the area that is either in direct contact with or in the immediate vicinity of the stone.

Emotions are thought to be evoked by being near certain types of crystals. For example, rose quartz, a popular healing stone which corresponds to the heart area of the body, when placed in various rooms throughout the home contributes to the thought of self-love and nurturing, while the stone pink tourmaline contributes to the dynamic expression of love.

Many physical problems and diseases result from blockages of the vital life energy within the body. Crystals and gemstones can be used to regulate the flow of energy in and around the human body. By removing the energy blocks and increasing the free flow of energy, balance is restored to the body's energy system. This in turn harmonizes body, mind, and spirit. Depending on the type of stone used, an individual can be calmed, be revitalized, or have an inspiring or stimulating experience.

In the ancient art of "laying-on of stones," practitioners place crystals and gemstones on various parts of the body, corresponding to chakra points, to balance energy flow. As an example, malachite (a green stone composed of copper carbonate) placed at the solar plexus will draw out suppressed emotions so that the heart chakra can open.

Crystals and gemstones should be "cleared" before use, especially if they are to be used for healing. They can accumulate vibrations and other imprints from those individuals having previous contact with them. Sources such as sounds, light, emotions, thoughts, and the physical environment can leave their energy in the crystal. If the individual who previously had possession of the crystal was ill or had very negative thoughts, these vibrations could be passed on to the next person using the crystal if it is not cleared.

Clearing can be accomplished by several methods, including soaking the crystals and stones in sea-salt water, packing them in sea salt, passing them through a flame or smoke, holding them under running water, or burying them in earth for a period of time.

Most work with crystals is done in a self-help (healing and self-development) context, although there are many practitioners that practice crystal healing. Many good books on the subject are available at bookstores and most libraries. Crystals and gemstones are readily available from a variety of sources, both retail and mail order.

❧ | DANCE THERAPY | ❧

Dance Therapy is a nonverbal, action-oriented method of helping people become aware of their feelings by experiencing the direct sensation of movement.

The goal of Dance Therapy is to improve or restore the integration of body and mind, and to help an individual regain a sense of identity and build self-esteem. It is used to aid and support verbal psychotherapy, physical therapy, and medical therapy.

In 1966 the American Dance Therapy Association was founded to establish standards for professional education and qualifications for individuals who practice this therapy. Prior to the formation of the association, each individual practitioner would go through a trial-and-error process to develop a personalized method utilizing his own knowledge and experience.

Today professional Dance Therapy training occurs on the graduate level. Studies include courses such as dance/movement therapy theory and practice, psychopathology, human development, observation and research skills, and a supervised internship in a clinical setting.

Dance Therapy is used in a variety of settings, such as psychiatric hospitals, clinics, day care centers, community mental health centers, developmental centers, correctional facilities, special schools, and rehabilitation centers.

Dance Therapy can be used to treat a variety of conditions including some geriatric-related difficulties, physical disability, and behavioral problems such as psychosis, neurosis, autism, regression, and substance abuse.

Elderly people who are confined to a bed or sit all day often suffer from loss of self-esteem. The dance therapist, by providing an opportunity for freedom of expression through movement, can help the person improve her self-image and regain feelings of self-worth.

Although there are many different Dance Therapy methods, one of the most common is a circular formation because it creates a feeling of security and unity. A typical session begins with warm-up exercises, then progresses into arm, wrist, and finger movements set to appropriate music. These arm movements are derived from folk dances such as the Japanese fan dance. At the same time participants are encouraged to move the head, neck, and shoulders and to sway the body. Various props such as balls, fans, rhythm instruments, and scarves are used to give the participants an object they can manipulate or hold on to. The group may move around the room using simple steps like walking, jumping, hopping, sliding, or running. The session is ended by relaxing to slow, quiet movements. Many Dance Therapy methods use a "group hug" as their finale.

Dance therapists can be found throughout the United States, in Canada, Europe, South America, Asia, the Middle East, and Africa. Additional information on Dance Therapy can be obtained from the American Dance Therapy Association.

⚘ | DEEP COMPRESSION MASSAGE | ⚘

Deep Compression Massage is a specialized bodywork technique that utilizes a "pumping" action on the muscle. It is frequently used in sports massage. The technique involves alternate pushing into and releasing of the muscle by a massage therapist. Done in rapid succession, this in-and-out action works the muscle like a pump and turns it into a kind of "heart." Actually, all muscles act as a "heart" by moving blood when exercised.

Deep Compression Massage is used to rapidly pump fresh blood to tendons, ligaments, and muscle bellies (the large center portion of the muscle), and to remove adhesions.

The main benefit of Deep Compression Massage is accelerated healing in areas of the body which normally do not get enough circulation. It is very invigorating and works well on athletes and nonathletes who have a large buildup of lactic acid in their muscles. Many massage therapists are trained in this technique and use it when appropriate.

❧ | DEEP TISSUE MASSAGE | ❦

Deep Tissue Massage is a generic term for bodywork techniques that go into deep layers of muscle and connective tissue where aches, chronic pain, and fatigue are trapped.

Deep tissue work encompasses many different types of bodywork such as Cross-Fiber Friction work, Rolfing, Deep Tissue Sculpting, Hellerwork, Chua Ka, and others.

To be effective, this technique requires that the client's muscle be profoundly relaxed so the therapist can work on tissue right down to the bone. Starting at the skin and going deeper into the body, each layer of muscle must be relaxed in order to reach the next lower layer.

Although some practitioners try to force their way into the deep tissue, the deep layers cannot be reached this way. Using a great deal of pressure causes the body to fight back by tensing the muscles and making them impenetrable. When the muscles are properly relaxed, a client often will not perceive the work as feeling "deep."

Deep Tissue Massage usually concentrates on "clearing out" a specific area of the body such as the feet, legs, back, arms, neck, or shoulders rather than being a full body type of massage such as Swedish massage.

Benefits of deep tissue massage are numerous. It is used to remove chronic muscular pain, help with injury rehabilitation, and reduce inflammation-type pain caused by ailments such as arthritis and tendonitis.

By helping to remove accumulated lactic acid and other waste products from the muscles, deep tissue massage works to detoxify tissue. Lactic acid is a natural chemical by-product of muscular contractions. An accumulation of lactic acid deep within a muscle causes soreness and stiffness if it is not removed.

Although it can be used alone, some forms of deep tissue work are integrated with other massage techniques. Most massage therapists are able to perform some Deep Tissue Massage.

❧ | DEEP TISSUE SCULPTING | ❦

Deep Tissue Sculpting, also referred to as Muscle Sculpting, is a form of bodywork (Deep Tissue Massage) that is characterized by firm, constant compressions and strokes applied parallel to the muscle fibers.

It is a sensitive yet penetrating system of therapeutic touch that produces effective, lasting relief of chronic muscular tension and of soft tissue pain and dysfunction. It can also evoke emotional release.

Deep Tissue Sculpting was developed by Carole Osborne-Sheets. Born in New Orleans, Louisiana, in 1949, she graduated from Louisiana State University, New Orleans, in 1971, with a degree in secondary education. She then taught English and journalism to public high school students.

Osborne-Sheets's introduction to bodywork began informally in 1972. It started with what she calls "her love affair with the human anatomy." Fascinated by the anatomical structure of her lover, including his bones, she began to explore the depths of his muscles and all the bumps and curves on his skeleton. She discovered that when she applied pressure in a certain way, his skin and muscles seemingly melted and opened beneath her touch, and she could reach even greater depths into his body.

Her interest in anatomy continued and spread to the study of friends and family members. As her investigation of the body continued, she worked on herself and studied anatomy books to learn more about what she had been examining.

While exploring through the musculature for bones, Osborne-Sheets discovered that touch applied one way would cause the muscles to tighten up, yet applied another way would cause the musculature to seem to melt or dissolve under her touch.

She then discovered that emotions were released when the body was touched in certain ways. Recipients became profoundly relaxed and serene as a result of this work. She began to realize that perhaps this was some type of massage she was performing.

For several years prior, Gestalt and primal reeducation had been part of Osborne-Sheets's training at a center in New Orleans. It became a natural extension to begin blending her deep tissue work with the emotive work of the therapists. Although a high school teacher by day, she helped to facilitate primal release with her touch work in the evening.

In 1974 Osborne-Sheets learned that the Arica Institute in New Orleans was teaching a type of bodywork called Chua Ka, which was similar to what she was doing. The information presented on this centuries-old self-massage technique enhanced what she had already discovered on her own. With the help of classmate Barry Green she was able to pull together the various aspects of her work. This became the foundation for an approach to bodywork that Osborne-Sheets has used for the past eighteen years.

After moving to San Diego in 1976 to pursue her love of the body/mind therapies full time, she studied Tai Chi Chuan, learned Swedish massage and Esalen Style Massage, underwent Rolfing, and satisfied her interest in passive joint movement by training with Milton Trager, M.D.

In 1977 she co-founded with Barry Green the Institute of Psycho Structural Balancing or IPSB, later changed to the International Professional School of Bodywork. At that time the name *sculpting* was coined to label the related yet different systems of deep tissue work that had been synthesized from their various explorations.

Osborne-Sheets has since taught Deep Tissue Sculpting, integrative bodywork, and Bodywork for the Childbearing Year throughout the United States and in Europe.

Like other methods of deep tissue work, the techniques used in Deep Tissue Sculpting are intended to go beyond the skin level and get into the deeper structures of the musculoskeletal system, including connective tissue and muscles.

Connective tissue surrounds, penetrates, or covers every muscle in the body. It is composed of a semiliquid matrix, or ground substance, and two types of fibers.

When a practitioner or "sculptor" applies pressure or traction to a muscle, the fiber component in connective tissue initially takes the load. If pressure is released quickly it springs back. If pressure is maintained over a more sustained period of time, thirty to ninety seconds, the force is absorbed by the ground substance. It is this substance which becomes movable and makes a permanent change in the tissue. When the pressure is relieved, the tissue does not spring back completely.

To reach deeper layers, the sculptor uses her fingertips, knuckles, elbows, or forearms, the heels of her hands, or any bony body part as tools. Deep Tissue Sculpting is most effective when it is used in conjunction with other forms of bodywork.

With very few exceptions Deep Tissue Sculpting is performed without the use of oil. Exceptions include individuals with extremely dry skin and individuals with a lot of body hair. In the case of body hair, the oil is applied on the hair and not the skin.

Through balancing and releasing of the connective tissue, Deep Tissue Sculpting is able to relieve tension in chronically tight musculature caused by injury, emotional upsets, or repetitive movements such as those performed by an assembly line worker, an athlete "pumping iron," or a baseball pitcher.

It is also a particularly effective way to release enduring emotional tension held in the body, the result of chronic and traumatic emotional states caused by a single or repeated emotional trauma.

In addition to the technical procedures used, Deep Tissue Sculpting integrates an intuitive and/or artistic quality to working with the human body. This aspect of the work is necessary to access not only the physical, but the emotional, psychic, and spiritual response of the body as well.

While the practitioner is applying pressure, that part of the client's body is attuned to receive messages from the tissue. The muscle can reveal information about its tension, its resistance, and how it releases.

Like an artist, the deep tissue sculptor begins by holding a vision of an idealized body to work from. Then pressure is applied to areas of the body that are not within the parameters of the ideal configuration. Although the shoulder may be too high or the chest collapsed, pressure brings the body from its misaligned or disorganized state to one that is optimal.

Deep Tissue Sculpting is especially helpful for people with whiplash injury, scoliosis (lateral curvature of the spine), extreme lordosis (swayback), postural deviations, short and tight muscles from athletics, and muscular tension and shortening of connective tissue due to chronic emotional problems.

It is also used as an adjunct to psychotherapy. Psychotherapists often refer individuals under therapy to bodyworkers. Those with early childhood or later life traumas, and those with various addictions, benefit from touch therapy to release stored energy.

Deep Tissue Sculpting is taught at a number of massage schools throughout the country in either intensive or extended format. Level I consists of twenty-eight hours of instruction; Level II is thirty-six hours.

Carole Osborne-Sheets's book, *Deep Tissue Sculpting: A Technical and Artistic Manual for Therapeutic Bodywork Practitioners,* is written for bodywork professionals and not for the layperson. It is available from Integrative Bodywork Consultants.

For a referral to a practitioner of Deep Tissue Muscle Sculpting contact the International Professional School of Bodywork or Integrative Bodywork Consultants.

DMSO THERAPY

DMSO Therapy is the use of a chemical compound known as dimethyl sulfoxide, abbreviated DMSO, for a wide variety of therapeutic purposes.

The pharmaceutical grade of DMSO, when administered by a physician knowledgeable in its use, is a very effective and versatile compound which has been successfully adapted for use in the treatment of a number of health problems.

Depending on the condition being treated, physicians can administer DMSO in various strengths and amounts—orally, topically as a liquid or cream, or by injection either intramuscularly or intravenously.

Dimethyl sulfoxide was first synthesized in 1866 by a Russian chemist named Alexander Saytzeff. In addition to its medicinal uses, DMSO is an excellent solvent. It has the ability to remove paint and varnish and dissolve many different types of plastics. It is also used in the manufacture of synthetic fibers. DMSO does not affect natural materials such as cotton, wool, or leather.

Chemists' interest in DMSO was activated after World War II. In the late 1950s a chemist for Crown Zellerbach Corporation in Camas, Washington, a large paper manufacturer, was asked to find new commercial applications for a by-product of the company's wood pulp manufacturing operation. The by-product was dimethyl sulfoxide.

Zellerbach chemist Robert Herschler, while exploring agricultural uses for DMSO, noticed that some plant antibiotics and fungicides penetrated into the plant's circulatory system more quickly and deeply when mixed with DMSO than they did on their own. Also, Herschler noticed that when he got DMSO on his hands, a funny oysterlike taste developed in his mouth. Several other observations of DMSO's interesting properties led Herschler to think he was onto something.

When Herschler's superiors at Zellerback were not interested in his "discovery," he realized he needed someone to test DMSO in a clinical setting. Fortunately he met Stanley Jacob, M.D., an assistant professor of surgery at the University of Oregon Health Sciences Center.

In the 1960s Dr. Jacob began experimenting with DMSO's ability to carry substances into the body normally administered by injection, and its toxicity and side effects on laboratory animals. Since that time, thousands of studies appearing in numerous scientific publications, as well as abundant anecdotal evidence, have shown DMSO to be an amazing healing tool. Recently published research seems to show that DMSO delays or retards the growth of several types of cancer.

Although approved for medical use in over fifty countries throughout the world, the use of DMSO in the United States is under intense scrutiny by the FDA. Currently DMSO is approved by the FDA for only one medical application: the treatment of a rare bladder condition. All other therapeutic uses of DMSO are not approved by the FDA.

Currently, DMSO is used by a wide variety of people and age groups for a multitude of applications, from a young bodybuilder who is in excellent physical condition to an elderly arthritic who can barely walk.

The therapeutic benefits from DMSO use are numerous. It stops bacterial and fungal growth, relieves pain from a wide variety of causes, and reduces swelling and inflammation caused by arthritis, bursitis, tendonitis, and other musculoskeletal injuries. It "carries" other drugs into the body, avoiding the use of a hypodermic needle. It is a muscle relaxant. It softens scar tissue and soothes burns. It increases blood circulation in a local area by enlarging (dilating) the small blood vessels.

DMSO is manufactured in two grades: pharmaceutical and industrial solvent. Only the industrial solvent grade is currently available over the counter. Almost every health food store in the United States carries the industrial solvent grade of DMSO.

According to the vast amount of literature published, DMSO has been found to be a safe product. However, the application of 100 percent DMSO can sometimes cause skin irritation. A product commonly found in health food stores today contains 70 percent DMSO and 30 percent aloe vera, which prevents skin irritation.

For self-help use, it is most often applied topically to areas of pain and inflammation. When used in this manner, caution should be exercised because of DMSO's ability to pull other substances with it into the body. The skin must be absolutely clean when DMSO is applied, otherwise dirt, bacteria, and other harmful substances will be introduced into the body.

Two excellent books on the subject are *DMSO: The New Healing Power* by Morton Walker, D.P.M., and *DMSO: The Remarkable Story of a Pain Killing Drug* by Barry Tarshis.

❧ | DONG DIET | ❦

The Dong Diet is a nutritional plan used to treat arthritis which is based on a traditional low-fat, high-fiber Chinese diet consisting mainly of fresh vegetables, rice, fish, and small portions of chicken.

The Dong Diet was developed by Colin H. Dong, M.D., a graduate of the Stanford Medical School. At the age of thirty-five, after practicing medicine for seven years, Dr. Dong found himself overweight and suffering from crippling arthritis and a generalized dermatitis. For three years he ingested large amounts of aspirin and other related painkillers in order to withstand the agony of his disorder. The drugs produced severe side effects but no relief.

Dr. Dong's learned medical colleagues were baffled as to why his arthritis was becoming progressively worse. There was nothing further they could suggest to treat his joint pain or skin condition, and the last advice he received was to see a psychiatrist.

During three years of suffering, he read virtually every journal, scientific paper, and book on the subject of arthritis. All described the same type of treatment he had been given, treatment that had not worked on him. Written off by conventional medicine and faced with spending the remainder of his life in a wheelchair, Dr. Dong knew he must find a way to treat himself.

In something of a revelation, Dr. Dong remembered an old Chinese proverb that his father quoted: "Sickness enters through the mouth and catastrophe comes out the mouth." Dr. Dong recalled that almost every member of his family had some type of food allergy, and he had many. Also, he knew that allergies had been known and treated by traditional Chinese medicine for centuries.

He began to realize that in 1931, after he began to practice medicine, his diet had changed to the typical diet of most affluent Americans. This was very different from the one on which he had grown up: One of nine children, Dr. Dong had previously eaten a diet of beef, pork, chicken, fish, vegetables, and rice.

Dr. Dong decided to start himself on what he called a "poor man's diet" consisting of simple meats, vegetables, and rice. At first the results were not promising, but by eliminating different foods and medications his condition began to improve. Eventually he found that seafood, vegetables, and rice was the optimal combination.

Within a few weeks amazing changes took place. The sleepless nights of pain were gone. He was able to shave and play golf again as the stiffness and pain in his joints disappeared. His skin cleared and he went from 195 pounds to 150.

At the age of seventy-one, Dr. Dong played golf each morning and still treated thirty to forty patients daily while leading a full, active life.

Dr. Dong believed that arthritis is caused by an allergic reaction to various types of fresh foods, as well as processed and prepared foods which contain chemical preservatives, artificial flavor and color, and other additives.

Because of this philosophy, the following substances and foods are excluded from the diet: all chemical additives (particularly monosodium glutamate, or MSG); all preservatives; meats; fruits (including tomatoes); all dairy products; hot spices (including all varieties of pepper); alcoholic beverages (especially wine); nuts; chocolate products; any strong acid (like vinegar); and carbonated soft drinks.

Two excellent books by Colin H. Dong, M.D., *The Arthritic's Cookbook* and *New Hope for the Arthritic*, provide additional information on the Dong Diet.

ஜ | DRAMA THERAPY | ஜ

Drama Therapy is defined by the National Association for Drama Therapy as "the intentional use of drama/theater processes to achieve the therapeutic goals of symptom relief, emotional and physical integration, and personal growth."

Drama Therapy is an active approach to behavioral, emotional, and cognitive change that has been found to be effective with the severely disturbed and disabled. Yet it is equally applicable to the exploration of human potential in all people.

The National Association for Drama Therapy was incorporated in 1979 to establish and uphold high standards of professional competence among drama therapists. The association also develops national guidelines for master's and doctoral training programs in Drama Therapy and sets criteria for standards of registration for drama therapists.

In Drama Therapy clients have an opportunity to neutralize the intense emotions stemming from the unsettling events that have taken place in their lives. Drama Therapy helps to integrate them back into surroundings of family life, friends, and community.

The range of people benefiting from drama therapy includes those recovering from substance abuse, dysfunctional families, the developmentally disabled, prison inmates, AIDS patients, the homeless, psychiatric patients, children, adolescents, and the elderly.

Drama therapists are trained in theater arts, psychology, and Drama

Therapy. They provide evaluation and treatment with individuals, groups, and families. Drama Therapy is used in a variety of settings such as mental health facilities, hospitals, schools, prisons, community centers, and businesses, as well as in private practice.

Various methods are used in Drama Therapy. These include improvisational techniques such as role-playing, theater games, mime, puppetry, and mask work. Scripted dramatizations and theatrical productions are also used.

Registered drama therapists have fulfilled the requirements for registry and may use the appellation R.D.T. The eligibility requirements include a master's degree, five hundred hours of drama/theater experience, three hundred hours of Drama Therapy training, and one thousand hours of paid work experience as a drama therapist. Currently a Drama Therapy training program is available at the California Institute of Integral Studies in San Francisco and at New York University.

For more information regarding Drama Therapy contact the National Association for Drama Therapy.

🐚 | DREAM THERAPY | 🐚

Dream Therapy is the use of dreams and the dream state to accomplish physical and emotional healing. It involves both the interpretation of information obtained while dreaming and the active participation in the dream process through a technique called *lucid dreaming*. The various processes associated with dreams have been put under the generalized term of *dreamwork*.

Throughout history dreams and their interpretation have been of great interest to people because they provide a link between the mysterious inner world of the mind and the outer physical world of waking life.

Hippocrates practiced Dream Therapy, encouraged *dream incubation*, and taught about the therapeutic powers of dreams. In ancient Greece, more than three hundred dream temples were built to heal the sick.

Dream incubation was a practice in which people made a pilgrimage to a sacred temple in hopes of having a curative or prophetic dream while sleeping. There were elaborate preparations for the dream experience. The process lasted up to three weeks and included prayers, fasting, bathing, singing, and reciting poetry. The practice began in Egypt and was used for more than a thousand years in Greece.

Freud aroused interest in the importance of the dreaming mind. He stressed that dream interpretation by an expert psychoanalyst could be very healing. In Jungian analysis, therapy begins with free association and dream analysis. Great emphasis is placed on dream interpretation. Carl Jung said, "To be concerned with dreams is a form of self-realization."

Although psychotherapists use dream interpretation as part of their normal therapy, and there are practitioners in the healing arts who specialize in dream analysis consultation, dreamwork is mostly a self-help process.

Most dream interpretation is done by the individual having the dream, using one of the many books available on dream interpretation. Dreams may warn of oncoming health problems, help diagnose them, suggest treatment, accelerate the healing process, and contribute to lifelong health.

An individual with an injury, illness, or emotional problem can use lucid dreaming to heal himself. Lucid dreaming is a process in which the dreamer takes his conscious awareness (conscious mind) into the dream state to receive guidance or insight on a particular subject or problem. It is the unconscious awareness (subconscious mind) that provides answers and information in the form of symbols and pictures in the dream state.

During waking hours, our conscious awareness is the part of the mind that deals with memory, knowledge, and logic; it uses words, ideas, and thought to communicate. When the conscious awareness is taken into the dream state, there is a moment in the dream at which you are aware you are dreaming. By using a "script" prepared before going to sleep, you can influence the dream and make it turn out any way you want. For example you could say, "Help me heal" or visualize your skin free of the disease which now infests it.

Having the conscious awareness functioning while dreaming builds a bridge, so to speak, between the conscious and unconscious awareness and allows the two to work together. The conscious awareness is then able to interpret the pictures and symbols (answers from the unconscious awareness), and upon waking the dreamer will know why he had the dream and what the dream meant. The dreamer can then use this information to heal himself. Also, healing can take place within the dream and the individual can wake up and be fully healed without further effort.

There are many books available on the subject of dreamwork and dream interpretation. For a general overview of dreamwork, *Dreamtime and Dreamwork* by Stanley Krippner is very good. An excellent book that focuses on health and the healing aspect of dreaming is *The Healing Power of Dreams* by Patricia Garfield, Ph.D.

There are several organizations and publications specializing in the field of dreamwork. They are the Association for the Study of Dreams, Lucidity Association (Lucid Dreaming), and *Dream Network: A Quarterly Journal Exploring Dreams and Myths.*

🌊 | EGOSCUE METHOD | 🐚

The Egoscue Method is a treatment for musculoskeletal pain and a training technique to help athletes achieve peak levels of performance. It is based on the premise that the body needs motion to function properly and stay healthy. The Egoscue Method exercise program provides an individual with a means of receiving sufficient daily motion which is no longer supplied at work or at home in a modern industrialized society.

It is both a diagnostic and therapeutic technique that puts the responsibility for recovering from pain and physical dysfunction with the individual who is suffering. For those not in pain, the Egoscue Method can be used to increase energy levels, maximize physical and mental capabilities, and protect the individual from future dysfunction.

The Egoscue Method was developed by Pete Egoscue over a period of twenty years. It is derived from research and rigorous application. In the late 1960s, Egoscue was in a hospital recovering from a wound suffered in Vietnam. While immobilized, he began to realize that physical function is quickly lost under those conditions. Although it was a standard practice to rest an injured body part, Egoscue wondered if the recovery process did not contribute to the dysfunction.

Egoscue believes that people in the United States, Western Europe, Japan, and other parts of the industrialized world do not move enough. The current lifestyle in these countries does not provide the opportunity for sufficient movement to allow the body to maintain health and well-being. In a sense, we are suffering from "motion starvation." Through lack of motion, a person's body and overall health begin to deteriorate.

Previous generations, going back ten thousand years, depended on motion for their very survival. Even two generations ago, most people walked to the grocery store, and few families had two cars. That is not the case today. With technological advances and a myriad of so-called labor-saving devices, our daily movement is continuously being reduced.

Egoscue believes that the body needs motion to survive and be healthy, just as it needs shelter, companionship, food, and other biological necessities. Not supplying the body with its needs leads to deterioration and death. Conditions such as carpal tunnel syndrome, tennis elbow, low back pain, stiff neck, lack of energy, inability to perform as desired in a sport, and many other common problems are recognized by Egoscue as symptoms of dysfunction precipitated by lack of motion.

For the Egoscue Method to be successful, it is essential for an individual to realize that her pain and dysfunction are due to what she has done to herself, and not from some outside source. And it is her responsibility, not her doctor's, therapist's, or other health practitioner's, to correct the problem. According to Egoscue, once this mind-set takes, his method works every time.

In his clinics and in his new book, *The Egoscue Method of Healing Through Motion*, Pete Egoscue begins with an educational program to teach people how the muscles, bones, nerves, and other parts of the body function. With this knowledge, it is easier for an individual to understand how a variety of factors have led to pain and dysfunction in her own body.

Next comes the diagnosis. Function-dysfunction is divided into four categories, and every person fits into one of the four. Conditions I, II, and III relate to various dysfunctional symptoms. Condition IV, or D-LUX as he calls it, describes a person whose body geometry is perfect—a rare find. It is Egoscue's goal to get everyone into the D-LUX category.

Once it is known which category the individual falls into, an Egoscue Method workout is performed daily for about an hour to correct the dysfunction and alleviate muscle and joint pain. Each workout consists of a specific sequence of easy-to-do exercises, taken from a "menu" of twenty-two different techniques. These techniques are designed to restore lost functions by reintroducing the right types and amount of movement in the body.

Currently, Pete Egoscue operates clinics in San Diego and West Palm Beach where many world-famous athletes, including golfer Jack Nicklaus, and others have come for relief of their pain and dysfunction.

For additional information consult Pete Egoscue's book, *The Egoscue Method of Healing through Motion*, or contact his THE (Therapy, Health, Education) Clinic.

❧ | ELECTROTHERAPY | ☙

Electrotherapy is the use of electrical current for a variety of therapeutic purposes including pain relief, reduction of swelling, muscle relaxation, speeding up of the healing process, and stimulation of acupuncture points.

A device known as a transcutaneous electric nerve stimulator (TENS) dispenses minute amounts of pulsed electricity to stimulate specific areas of the body. Electrical stimulation can be used directly over the pain site or other related areas on the body, including acupuncture points. This can be accomplished with electrodes placed on the skin surface, or acupuncture needles penetrating the skin.

During the 1970s and 1980s, Robert O. Becker, M.D., did extensive work on the effects of electrical stimulation on the body; this work is detailed in his book, *The Body Electric.* Dr. Becker was able to stimulate the regrowth of severed limbs in salamanders and to speed the mending of broken bones through the use of electric current. Currently in Russia, electrical stimulation of broken bones to accelerate mending is a common practice in hospitals.

With repeated electrical stimulation (overexcitation), a muscle that is painfully contracted will become fatigued and finally release. Some of the latest research has shown that overexcitation can also relax a muscle by stimulating the "C-fibers" found deep within it. The C-fibers in turn trigger the body to release endorphins, thus reducing pain and relaxing the muscle.

As the pain subsides and the tensed muscle is relaxed, an increased blood flow is sent to the area. This brings fresh oxygen and nutrients to the muscle and accelerates the removal of waste products. At the same time swelling is reduced by moving fluid from within the tissue along the lymphatic system.

Repeated contraction with electrical stimulation can also be used to strengthen atrophied muscles. This is a very useful procedure in the rehabilitation of people recovering from a paralysis or who have been immobilized in a brace, cast, or hospital bed for long periods of time.

The healing rate for various injuries has been shown to be affected by the frequency and amplitude wave of the electric current used for stimulation. Acute injuries respond best to high frequency and high amplitude, while chronic injuries respond best to low frequency and low amplitude.

Today, electrical stimulation is used extensively by acupuncturists and in the field of physical therapy and rehabilitation.

A new use for electrical stimulation has found its way into the field of cosmetology. Certain acupuncture points are stimulated to strengthen the facial muscles, giving the face a tighter and more youthful look. Although this method of "electric face-lift" is less invasive than the traditional surgical method of face-lift, periodic maintenance treatments are required.

❧ | ENVIRONMENTAL MEDICINE | ❧

Environmental Medicine, sometimes referred to as Clinical Ecology, is the specialty in medicine in which doctors assist patients in uncovering the cause-and-effect relationship between their environment and their ill health, and help them to learn to avoid those inciting factors.

The term *allergy* was created to describe an abnormal response to substances that a person's system recognizes as foreign, yet which do not cause reactions in most people. Common substances that cause allergies, called *allergens* or *antigens*, include pollen, animal danders, molds, dust, foods, chemicals, drugs, air pollution, and perfumes.

Allergies can produce symptoms in almost every organ in the body, often masquerading as other diseases. They can affect the skin, eyes, ears, nose, throat, lungs, stomach, bladder, vagina, muscles, joints, and the entire nervous system, including the brain.

There are several ways to develop allergic reactions. Heredity seems to be a major factor. The more relatives a person has with allergies, the earlier in life that person is expected to experience allergic manifestations. It is possible to develop allergic sensitivity after a severe viral, bacterial, or fungal infection. Heavy exposure to industrial chemicals, pesticides, and other petrochemicals can lead to the development of allergic reactions. An increased load of stress, whether emotional or physical, positive or negative, can play a roll in allergies. Poor nutritional habits contribute to the development of allergies as well as other illnesses.

In many cases, an allergy exists latent in an individual for some time. It is believed by some that a latent allergy may be "triggered" by an allergen, and future contact with the allergen causes a reaction. When the severity and frequency of reactions increase, the individual may seek professional help.

As the allergy gradually becomes worse the individual's ability to adapt to these stresses finally runs out. At that point he is forced to seek medical attention to correct the debilitating condition.

To diagnose conditions, the physician takes a detailed environmentally oriented history and each complaint or symptom is traced chronologically to reveal any possible cause-and-effect relationships to environmental exposures. The history, along with an objective physical examination, leads to a provisional diagnosis which is used to direct the testing. Testing is used to determine those substances causing the symptoms, and which treatments will improve the condition.

Various testing procedures are used to measure an individual's reaction to the excitant (common foods and/or environmental chemicals). The simplest procedure takes place in a physician's office. This consists of placing concentrated solutions of the excitant under the tongue or injecting it under the skin and observing the reaction. More sophisticated testing involves hospitalization of the patient in a controlled environment, introducing excitants one at a time and recording the reactions to each.

Once the offending substances are identified, the individual's symptoms may be reduced or eliminated through various methods. Avoidance is the primary method. Immunization against a particular substance to control its adverse effects and increase the individual's tolerance to it is another. Environmental factors such as air, water, and building interiors can be controlled or mitigated by the use of air and water filters, negative ion generators, proper building materials, furnishings, and cleaning materials.

A rotary diversified diet can be used to see which foods cause a reaction. The individual is placed on a diet restricting most known food allergens. Foods are then returned to the diet singly or in groups, and reactions observed.

For additional information, consult the American Environmental Health Foundation and the Environmental Dental Association.

EXERCISE THERAPY

Exercise Therapy is the use of exercise to improve, correct, or alleviate a variety of physical problems or conditions. The benefits of exercise as therapy are overwhelmingly positive. Exercise can be separated into different types and categories which are utilized for different purposes.

Isometrics (exercise against unmoving resistance) involve muscle contraction with a minimum of other body motion. Weight lifting or the squeezing of a tennis ball are examples of isometric exercises. They are good for strengthening and building muscle.

Isotonics (dynamic exercise) involve body movement, including the arms and legs. Walking, jogging, and running are examples of isotonic exercise. These are continuous (sustained) exercises, which benefit the heart and circulation.

Low-impact aerobics (low-stress) are exercises that promote physical fitness using aerobic principles while avoiding physical risks such as knee and ankle injury, strained ligaments, tendon damage, and back pain associated with the more strenuous forms of exercise. They include walking, swimming, and bicycling.

High-impact aerobics are vigorous exercises that stress the body. They include jogging, running, and aerobic dancing.

Many doctors are now using Exercise Therapy as an alternative to many conventional treatment methods such as drugs and surgery. Under supervised conditions, exercise has been shown to alleviate or improve many physical conditions.

For example, exercise can be used in place of drug therapy to lower blood pressure. Exercise has been shown to help the mentally ill in some cases by helping to reduce or alleviate the need for antidepressive drugs. In obese individuals, exercise increases the metabolic rate, burns excess fat for effective weight control, and in some cases may prevent coronary bypass surgery. For the elderly, it is more desirable to increase brain function with exercise than with drugs. People who are chronically tense or nervous can be calmed and relaxed through exercise rather than through the use of tranquilizers.

Clinical studies carried out at Yale University during the 1980s tested the effect of stretching and exercise on a group of people with back problems, all of whom were diagnosed as requiring surgery to correct their condition. The group was divided in two. One half acted as the control and did not participate in an exercise program. The other half performed certain stretches and exercises for a specific period of time. At the end of the test, after examination it was determined that a significant percentage of the participants in the exercise program no longer required back surgery, while everyone in the control group still required surgery.

According to researchers even a modest exercise program helps prolong the quality and quantity of an individual's life. Also, exercise is both integral and complementary to many other programs, such as the well-known Pritikin Diet Program. Physical therapy and rehabilitation also benefit from exercise as it increases endurance, alleviates structural problems, and increases mobility and range of motion.

Exercise can also help prevent disease from attacking the body by increasing the release of growth hormones from the pituitary gland, which stimulates the immune system.

❧ | EYE-ROBICS | ❦

Eye-Robics is a method of improving visual deficiencies without the use of corrective lenses (glasses or contact lenses) or surgery. It is based on the Bates-Corbett Method of vision training.

Jerriann J. Taber, Ph.D., wore glasses for ten years before learning the Bates-Corbett Method. Dr. Taber was so pleased with regaining normal vision that she went on to become a teacher of the Bates-Corbett Method. In 1971 she founded the Vision Training Institute, and she has been teaching the art of seeing ever since. She is the author of a book titled *Eye-Robics*.

Eye-Robics is based on research and scientific discoveries made by an ophthalmologist named William H. Bates, M.D. (the Bates Method is described elsewhere in this book) and furthered by the efforts of Margaret Darst Corbett, who was personally trained by Dr. Bates in 1930.

In addition to using the Bates-Corbett vision-training techniques, Dr. Taber has adapted many self-growth techniques into her vision-improvement work. In vision training, all aspects of the whole person are experienced: mental, physical, emotional, and spiritual.

The basic premise of Eye-Robics is that tension in the mind causes imperfect sight. Relaxation of the mind and body are prime objectives in reversing the condition of imperfect sight. Different techniques are used to release mental and physical stress. Eye-Robics utilizes illustrated instructions, charts, and audio- and videocassettes to accomplish this.

Eye-Robics deals with the causes of vision problems, not the symptoms; most types of vision deficiencies can be improved. Eye-Robics teaches that through relaxation, the mind and body can be reeducated with good visual habits once again. The visual process is not a fixed state, as is commonly believed.

Eye muscles function better when they are in a relaxed state. By relaxing the six intrinsic eye muscles, the lens is better able to reshape itself. This allows for normal vision to be restored.

The Vision Training Institute offers a complete home training program in Eye-Robics vision improvement. It also offers a teacher training program in the Bates-Corbett Method of vision training. Students can become certified to teach the Bates-Corbett Method.

❧ | FASTING | ❧

Fasting, as a therapy, is the process of depriving the body of food (but not fluid) for a certain period of time. This allows the body an opportunity to cleanse itself and reestablish metabolic order.

There are many different types of fasts, including a water fast, a juice fast, and fasts that are limited to only one type of food, such as a fruit fast or rice fast. The duration of fasts also varies greatly, ranging from only one day to thirty days or longer under closely supervised conditions.

Fasting is the deliberate abstention from food, and is very different from starvation, which is to die or perish from lack of food or nourishment. The origin of the words, both Anglo-Saxon, are derived from different roots. "Starve" comes from the Old English word *steorfan*, which means "to die a lingering death from hunger," and "fast" is derived from the Gothic word *fastan* and the Old English word *faestan*, which mean "to go without food" or "to be strict."

Four of the six major religions of the world—Hinduism, Christianity, Islam, and Judaism—have distinct fasting traditions. Fasting was used for religious observance and for the spiritual effect derived from the cleansing process. The Bible relates many instances of fasting, with some editions mentioning it on seventy-five occasions. Many tribes of Native American Indians had ceremonies of renewal and rejuvenation in which fasting played a major part for the purification of mind and body.

Ancient Greek, Roman, Egyptian, and Chinese physicians have recommended fasting. During the past hundred years diet reformers have believed in the efficiency of fasting. Russian research claims that skin disorders such as eczema and psoriasis can be cured by fasting. Also, they say that fasting helps to restore the balance of hormones in the organism.

The desire of the body to fast seems to be inherent. When a person is sick she has little desire to eat, and fasting becomes a natural part of the healing process.

During normal times the body works to eliminate impurities that have been inhaled or ingested. The body must use a great deal of energy to process the food it is constantly consuming. When the body is under siege due to illness, energy is needed to fight the illness, and there is little energy left to clean out the digestive system.

Fasts have been used to improve overall health and as a therapy for specific health disorders. Some nonobese people fast on a regular basis to detoxify their bodies and give various parts of the body a chance to rest. Morbidly obese people have gone on medically supervised fasts for several months and lost hundreds of pounds in the process. Physiologically, in a prolonged fast the body consumes its own reserves of extra flesh, both fat and lean tissue (muscles, connective tissue, and organs).

A group known as "natural hygienists" believe in the holistic approach to health and healing. When they become ill they use fasting as the primary means of recuperation. The theory is that fasting allows the body to rest from most of its essential duties so that it can concentrate on healing itself.

Fasting has also been used to treat a multitude of diseases including rheumatoid arthritis, chronic headaches, stomach ulcers, bronchial asthma, diabetes, and schizophrenia. Research has shown that fasting also has some application in life extension.

Because fasting can be dangerous if done improperly, it should always be carried out under the supervision of a licensed health care practitioner.

FELDENKRAIS METHOD

The Feldenkrais Method is a powerful technique of body/mind integration that uses movement to enhance the communication between brain and body. Although it is not a therapy or healing technique, the lessons taught provide a way to improve a person's awareness, as well as physical and mental performance.

The lessons are taught with two different techniques, manipulative and group. The manipulative technique, called Functional Integration, is a hands-on, one-on-one, instructor-with-student arrangement. It is custom tailored to meet the needs of a certain individual and was the first of the two techniques to be developed. Awareness Through Movement is a group technique. It was created to produce the effects of the manipulative technique teachings to a group of people.

Although the Feldenkrais Method can help average persons of almost any age in their daily activities, it is particularly useful to professionals such as dancers and musicians who want to fine-tune their skills.

The Feldenkrais Method was developed by Moshe Feldenkrais (1904–84). Before he became immersed in the holistic health and New Age movements, Feldenkrais was an engineer with degrees in both electrical and mechanical engineering. The Russian-born Israeli received his doctorate in science from the Sorbonne in Paris and worked on the French atomic research program.

A judo master and excellent soccer player, he had always been interested in the body's mechanics. When a knee injury sustained while playing soccer began to flare up, he was led to apply his engineering-oriented mind to the mechanics of body and brain. In England during the 1940s he drew on the work of body/mind pioneer Frederick Mathias Alexander, originator of the Alexander Technique. This led to the development of the Feldenkrais Method.

Feldenkrais believed that ordinarily we learn just enough to function. For example, we learn to use our hands well enough to write and our legs well enough to walk, but our ability to function with a greater range of ease still remains undeveloped.

Movement only occurs when the brain sends a nerve impulse to a muscle and the muscle contracts in the correct pattern and time sequence. If muscle patterns never change (great numbers of them never do, especially after childhood), then the areas of the brain that control these patterns remain fixed.

The Feldenkrais Method uses over a thousand different exercises or movements to help the body program the brain, thus enhancing the whole body/mind system.

Lessons are usually done on a padded table with the student comfortably (fully) clothed. He lies on his back or in various other positions, sometimes with head and arms supported, to remove the effects of gravity normally experienced while standing.

The practitioner guides the student through a series of precise movements that alter habitual patterns and provide new learning directly to the neuromuscular system. Movements are light and performed as slowly, easily, and pleasantly as possible without any strain or pain whatsoever.

After a Feldenkrais session a student experiences improved posture, flexibility, and coordination, as well as relaxation and relief of muscular tension. Sessions normally last from thirty to fifty minutes.

Specialized training to become a Feldenkrais practitioner requires eight hundred hours of instruction, usually over a period of four years.

In 1977, Dr. Moshe Feldenkrais established the Feldenkrais Guild, the professional organization of practitioners of the Feldenkrais Method. A list of certified Feldenkrais practitioners is available from the guild. Additionally, numerous books, audio- and videotapes, and other information pertaining to the Feldenkrais Method are available from the guild.

🌱 | FIT FOR LIFE PROGRAM | 🌿

The Fit for Life Program is a way of eating that can be incorporated into a person's lifestyle as a way of life. It is a safe and balanced system based on natural physiological laws which apply to everyone, and on cycles of the human body. Fit for Life is truly a lifestyle, not a temporary pattern of behavior.

The Fit for Life Plan was developed by Harvey and Marilyn Diamond. Released from the air force in his early twenties, Harvey Diamond began to struggle with a weight problem. Nearly fifty pounds overweight, in an attempt to reduce he tried numerous types of diets and came to the conclusion that diets do not work.

While at a music festival one evening, Diamond overheard two healthy-looking individuals discussing their friend in Santa Barbara and his views on health and beauty. Very interested in what was said, he inquired about this person and was on his way to Santa Barbara, California, less than twenty-four hours later.

In Santa Barbara Harvey Diamond met this man who personified good health. Later, he was introduced to the concept of Natural Hygiene, a most remarkable approach to the care and upkeep of the human body. In 1970, within a month of his introduction to Natural Hygiene, Diamond had lost fifty pounds; he spent the next three and one-half years studying with this man. During this time, Diamond also read everything he could find on the subject of Natural Hygiene.

After leaving Santa Barbara, Diamond studied Natural Hygiene for ten years and did private consultations in Natural Hygiene. In 1981, he began a seminar program called the Diamond Method, which transformed the principles of Natural Hygiene into what became known as Fit for Life.

As Diamond explains, the word *hygiene* connotes cleanliness and the word *natural* implies a process unhampered by artificial forces. Therefore, "the basic foundation of Natural Hygiene is that the body is always striving for health, and that it achieves this by continuously cleansing itself of deleterious waste."

Although not a diet regimen, the Fit for Life Program provides a means for safe and permanent weight reduction. The key to the system is that it works with the body to free up energy, making energy readily available for other functions.

Digestion of food requires more energy than any other body function. The body needs energy to detoxify, and by eliminating this toxic waste, weight is lost in the process. With extra energy available the body automatically goes to work shedding any excess weight it is carrying. If weight loss is not a goal, then a significant boost in overall energy will be gained.

The unique part of this program is that in addition to stressing the importance of what foods are eaten, it also emphasizes the time of day and in what combinations they are eaten.

It has been found that certain combinations of foods digest more readily than others. In Fit for Life, proteins are not combined with starches because the body is not designed to digest more than one concentrated food at a time. Any food that is not a fruit or a vegetable is considered to be concentrated.

For example, fish with salad or vegetables would be a properly combined meal but fish with rice would not. A properly combined sandwich would be whole grain bread filled with tomatoes, avocados, sprouts, cucumber, and lettuce. But if turkey were added to that sandwich, it would not be properly combined.

The beauty of the Fit for Life Program is that if you get off the program for any reason, you just get back on it and results are immediately seen again.

In their excellent best-seller, *Fit for Life*, Harvey and Marilyn Diamond have synthesized the basic fundamentals of Natural Hygiene into a series of commonsense, easy-to-follow dietary principles.

The book includes numerous recipes and sample menus. When these guidelines are followed, the Fit for Life Program can facilitate the goal of eliminating obesity and alleviate the necessity for dieting.

Fit for Life was followed by *Fit for Life II—Living Health*, which goes beyond diet and teaches a total lifestyle.

For additional information on Natural Hygiene contact the American Natural Hygiene Society, the American Health Sciences Institute, or the International Association of Professional Natural Hygienists.

🦢 | GERIATRIC MASSAGE | 🐚

Geriatric Massage is the use of various bodywork and body/mind techniques on the elderly, typically those over sixty years old, for their therapeutic benefit. Although a fairly new specialty in the bodywork profession, it has been well received and is growing in popularity.

Massage for the elderly presents a special set of challenges because of the diversity found in this age group. While it is not difficult to identify a "typical" twenty-year-old, there is no typical seventy-year-old. The vast majority of the twenty-year-olds in the United States are in good health and free of conditions such as arthritis, osteoporosis, or rheumatism. The physical condition of seventy-year-olds, however, can range from those in training for their next marathon race to those individuals who are helpless, bedridden, and incontinent.

People over sixty years old, more than any other group in the population, can benefit from massage. Because of their extended number of years they have had more opportunity to subject their body to a wide variety of deleterious effects. Lack of nurturing, less than ideal nutrition, harsh climate, environmental pollution, accidents, traumas, emotional upsets, financial reverses, severe physical activity and/or occupation, and mental outlook all accumulate to take their toll on the body/mind.

Added to this are the built-in genetic factors that influence the body. The general slowdown of the body's built-in capacity for maintenance provides an explanation for the physical changes that can be observed in an elderly person. Many of these changes are expressed as poor blood circulation, joint stiffness, and hardening of the musculature.

The specialty of Geriatric Massage encompasses or overlaps at least marginally with several other disciplines including social gerontology, developmental anatomy and physiology, geriatrics, physiotherapy, and of course bodywork. Added to these are the human qualities of patience, intuition, gentleness, supportiveness, resourcefulness, and positive thinking.

Geriatric Massage resembles Sports Massage in many respects. Both address muscle problems that are the result of overexertion, injury, and general wear and tear. While athletes incur these muscle stresses in training and competition over a relatively short period of time, aged persons acquire them over a long life.

The elderly, because they typically do not move around as much as when they were younger, have reduced blood circulation, which slows down cell nourishment and cell detoxification. Massage increases the blood supply to the massaged area, thus nourishing and detoxifying cells. It also stimulates the lymphatic system and softens hardened muscle tissue. This results in a feeling of relaxation, improved joint movement, lowered blood pressure, and increased energy.

Health problems in the elderly that respond well to massage include myofibrositis (rheumatism), arthritis, hip and other joint problems, poor blood circulation, low back pain, neck and shoulder pain or stiffness, bad feet, walking problems, scoliosis (lateral curvature of the spine), and kyphosis (abnormal backward curvature of the spine).

Hospital patients, the seriously ill, and residents of nursing homes and extended care facilities are extremely responsive to even the briefest sessions of therapeutic massage and touch. Alone and isolated, they are denied physical contact, and oftentimes verbal contact as well.

The gentle touch of a massage therapist, along with verbal and nonverbal contact, not only works to improve physical conditions but serves to enhance quality of life for these people as well. Regular massage can often be the deciding factor in improving or at least maintaining the state of health in an older person.

Despite the tremendous growth of the massage and bodywork movement during the past twenty years, the elderly are the most underserved population group in America and also the neediest. By the year 2007, the first of the "baby boomers" will reach sixty years of age and the demand for Geriatric Massage will certainly increase.

❧ | GERSON THERAPY | ❧

The Gerson Therapy is an intensive medical treatment based on nutrition. It is a state-of-the-art, contemporary, holistic, and natural treatment which assists the body's own healing mechanism to combat chronic debilitating illness.

The Gerson Therapy was originated by Max Gerson, M.D. (1881–1959). Dr. Gerson graduated from Albert-Ludwigs Universitaet Medizinsche Fakultaet, Freiburg, Baden, Germany, in 1909. As a young doctor just out of medical school he suffered migraines usually three days a week, headaches so severe he would lie nauseated in a dark room totally unable to function.

Gerson sought an answer from medical school professors and teachers who were authorities on the subject. He was told that, according to all studies, there was nothing they could do for migraines. "When you are forty-five or fifty-five you'll feel better."

At this point Dr. Gerson realized that he would have to help himself, and so he began to read and study nutrition. At that time there was a relatively small amount of material available. His first experiment was with milk. He reasoned that since it is the first food babies can digest, if he took only milk it would be easy to digest and might help him. The milk diet did not work at all.

He then realized that in nature adult animals do not live on milk, and that milk is designed for fast growth and is suited to a baby's metabolism. Looking to man's closest ancestor in nature, the apes, Dr. Gerson noted that they lived on a diet of mainly fruits and nuts, along with greens and vegetables. Believing this was the right direction to proceed in, he put himself on a diet of apples. Within a very short period of time, he was free of migraines.

Dr. Gerson began his medical practice, in Germany, as an internal and nerve disease specialist. When a patient came to Dr. Gerson suffering with migraine headaches, Dr. Gerson suggested he try his personal diet. After a short time the man reported back that he was fine when adhering to the diet, and when not, the migraines returned.

A turning point came for Dr. Gerson when another migraine patient, to whom he had given his diet, reported back that not only had his migraines stopped but his lupus (skin tuberculosis) had cleared up. Dr. Gerson thought this impossible and that it must be attributable to something other than his diet, since there was no known cure for lupus.

Curious, Dr. Gerson tried his diet on lupus patients who did not have migraines, and they recovered also. From this experience Dr. Gerson concluded that with the right nutrition the body develops the ability to kill off the lupus. He applied his therapy to other types of tuberculosis and they also responded. In 1928 Dr. Gerson cured Dr. Albert Schweitzer's gravely ill wife of tuberculosis with his diet.

Soon Dr. Gerson's patients were recovering from all forms of tuberculosis and other complications such as arteriosclerosis, arthritis, and other diseases. They all cleared up with the same treatment. He realized that in this approach the basis of the treatment was to see the body as a total organism. And, when the body's ability to heal is restored, it will heal whatever is ailing it.

In 1936, fleeing the Nazis, Dr. Gerson and his family moved to New York City, and in 1938 he established a medical practice. Dr. Gerson went on to successfully treat hundreds of people, most of them with "terminal" or "incurable" cancer. At the age of seventy-five, Dr. Albert Schweitzer came to Dr. Gerson lacking energy and taking insulin for his diabetes. With Dr. Gerson's diet, Dr. Schweitzer was able to stop taking insulin and retain the energy to work and be active until the age of ninety-two.

Dr. Gerson considered degenerative diseases to be just that—degeneration of the body and its metabolism brought on by consuming toxic, degraded food, water, and air.

The objective of the Gerson Therapy is to regenerate the body to health instead of allowing or causing further degeneration toward death. It works closely with nature to help the sick body rid itself of disease through the supportive effects of simple foods, juices, and nontoxic medications.

The main features of the diet include sodium restriction, potassium supplementation, extreme fat restriction, periodic (temporary) protein restriction, high vitamin, mineral, and micronutrient intake, and high consumption of fluids. The medications used in the Gerson Therapy are classified as biologicals, materials of organic origin which are found in the body and supplied in therapeutic amounts.

The Gerson Therapy floods the body with nutrients from twenty pounds of fresh organic food daily. Most of it is pressed into thirteen glasses of fresh raw juices. Raw and cooked foods are also consumed. Another important part of the therapy is the detoxification of body tissues and blood by coffee enemas.

Gerson Therapy proponents believe that coffee enemas stimulate the enzyme systems of the gut wall and liver to promote excretion of toxic bile.

A wonderful quote from Dr. Max Gerson is, "Stay close to nature and its eternal laws will protect you."

From the 1940s, the American Medical Association has looked upon Dr. Gerson and his unorthodox treatment with disfavor. For years, the AMA contended that Dr. Gerson had failed or refused to acquaint the medical profession with details of his treatment even though Dr. Gerson had published more than fifty papers and three books on his diet treatment. Although many of his papers were submitted to various medical magazines for publication, they were rejected.

After Dr. Gerson's death in 1959, his treatments continued through the work of his daughter Charlotte and former aerospace engineer Norman

Fritz. To free their work of the influence caused by the decades-old boycott led by the American Medical Association, the Gerson Therapy Center of Mexico was opened in 1977.

Currently, the Gerson Therapy is available at the Centro Hospitalario Internacional del Pacifico, S.A., in Tijuana, Mexico. For further information contact the Gerson Institute.

❧ | HAKOMI METHOD OF BODY MIND THERAPY | ❧

The Hakomi Method of Body Mind Therapy, or Hakomi Method, is an efficient and powerful process for discovering and then studying mind/body patterns and core beliefs (self-limiting beliefs formed in childhood and stored in the subconscious) as they are experienced. It synthesizes aspects of Western psychotherapy, Eastern philosophy, and contemporary science into a unique process.

Hakomi is an ancient Hopi (American Indian) word meaning "How do you stand in relation to these many realms?" with a more modern translation of "Who are you?"

The Hakomi Method, developed in the late 1970s by Ron Kurtz, utilizes various philosophies, techniques, and approaches. Some of its origins stem from Buddhism and Taoism, and it also draws from such modern body-centered therapies as Reichian work, Bioenergetics, Gestalt, Psychomotor, Feldenkrais, Structural Bodywork, Ericksonian Hypnosis, Focusing, and Neurolinguistic Programming (NLP).

The main theory behind the Hakomi Method is that an individual has certain experiences (feelings, thoughts, and sensations) as a child that are powerful enough to form basic beliefs about herself and the world. Beliefs created in childhood then impose self-limitation on the adult. The Hakomi Method process often involves following these core beliefs back to the childhood events where lifetime habitual responses were created.

The objective of the Hakomi Method is to facilitate personal growth and transformation. Through various processes, people are able to discover, study, and revise limiting beliefs about themselves. Hakomi is offered through both individual sessions and workshops.

The Hakomi Method utilizes Hakomi Bodywork, a unique synthesis of bodywork and psychotherapy based on the recognition that body, mind, and spirit are one continuum of experience. Therapists work *through* the body, not *on* it. The body is viewed as a vast source of information that can be tapped into and used to elicit change, and not as an object to be repaired.

Much Hakomi therapy is done in a special state of consciousness, or deep knowing, called "mindfulness." Using this mindful awareness fosters open communication between the conscious and unconsciousness. In a state of mindfulness one not only has experiences but is able to observe the ongoing contents of the experiences without interfering.

Hakomi Bodywork includes both hands-on work (massage, deep-tissue work, structural work) and off-table work such as movement and body awareness. Both bodywork and psychotherapy are used simultaneously throughout the process to maintain a sense of relationship between the physical body and beliefs. Awareness of sensation is heightened, and associated memories, beliefs, and emotions emerge.

Hakomi bodywork can elicit a wide variety of experiences. Examining these experiences in the present sheds light on beliefs and the childhood events that shaped them. By reevaluating those parts of the individual's belief system that are painful and limiting, alternative choices and more satisfying options can be developed and incorporated into his daily life.

Hakomi Method Therapist Training and Hakomi Bodywork Training are taught at a number of locations in North America and Europe. Although classroom hours vary with training location, a typical therapist training format consists of a long weekend (three to four days) every four to six weeks over a period of eighteen to twenty-four months, with bodywork training being longer.

Additional information and a list of certified Hakomi therapists located throughout the United States may be obtained from the Hakomi Institute. The institute also has available the book by Ron Kurtz, *Body-Centered Psychotherapy: The Hakomi Method*, videotapes, and an *Introduction to Hakomi Bodywork* (which includes articles and tapes).

❧ | HANNA SOMATIC EDUCATION | ❧

Hanna Somatic Education, sometimes called Somatic Education, is the procedure for teaching voluntary conscious control of the neuromuscular system to individuals suffering muscular disorders of an involuntary, unconscious nature.

The process uses hands-on bodywork and a series of Somatic Exercises to relax chronically contracted muscles, restore voluntary control of the muscular system to the individual, relieve pain, and allow the body to move freely.

The Greek word *soma* has been used since the eighth century B.C. to mean "living body." A human being may be viewed in two ways: from the outside and from the inside. In conventional medicine or physiology, the person is seen from the outside, a third-person view, as a "body" with a certain size and shape. But, when an individual looks at herself from the inside, a first-person view, she is aware of internal feelings, movements, and intentions. This is a "soma."

Somatics is based on the work of Moshe Feldenkrais and Hans Selye, with the addition of the use of biofeedback principles. Feldenkrais, an Israeli physicist, developed a powerful technique of body/mind integration, known as Functional Integration, and combined it with Awareness Through Movement to enhance the communication between brain and body. Hans Selye, an endocrinologist and medical researcher, recognized that disease could be caused by stress.

The term "somatics" was coined by Thomas Hanna (1928–90). In 1970 he wrote a book, *Bodies in Revolt: A Primer in Somatic Thinking*, and then spent the next sixteen years developing his process through research and practical experience.

Born in Waco, Texas, the son of a pharmaceutical salesman, Hanna had a desire early in life to become a physician. By the time he went to college his interests had changed and in 1949 he graduated from Texas Christian University with degrees in philosophy and music. He then attended the University of Chicago and received a bachelor's degree in divinity and a Ph.D. in philosophy.

Unlike many who enter the health field to heal themselves, Hanna had always been healthy and athletic. While at Texas Christian University he played football and was the school middleweight boxing champion. Because of a strong interest in neurophysiology, Hanna was allowed to attend classes at the University of Florida Medical School, where he was a philosophy professor. This education in neurophysiology would later become the foundation for his somatics work.

In 1973 he moved to San Francisco, California, to become director of the Humanistic Psychology Institute. While there he arranged the first training session with Moshe Feldenkrais in the United States. Hanna became interested in Feldenkrais's work but did not adapt it in full. In 1975 he organized the Novato Institute for Somatic Research and Training.

From his study of neurophysiology Hanna realized that muscles chronically contracted due to constant stress and traumatic injury could not release because of the "closed-loop" principle in the body's sensory-motor system. In other words, when muscles are contracted from being constantly subjected to various types of stress reflexes and/or traumatic injuries for a prolonged period of time, they "forget" how to relax. Hanna termed this "sensory-motor amnesia."

In Somatic Education a practitioner, through bodywork and Somatic Exercises, puts new sensory information into the individual's sensory-motor feedback loop and muscles begin to relax. This is not a passive experience for the individual, as she actively participates and contributes to the process. Exercises are repeated at home to habituate the muscle to a new, easier pattern of movement.

It was Hanna's belief that so called "old age" and the attendant softening, weakening, and deterioration of the body that take place are due to decreased activity and are not inevitable. The "sensory-motor amnesia" that takes place slowly and insidiously within an individual can be reversed.

Before his untimely death in a car accident in 1990, Hanna wrote another book, *Somatics: Reawakening the Mind's Control of Movement, Flexibility, and Health,* in which he describes in detail his Somatic Exercise Program. It is available in bookstores and libraries. For additional information contact the Novato Institute for Somatic Research and Training.

❧ | HELLERWORK | ☙

Hellerwork is a holistic and preventive approach to health consisting of a series of eleven, ninety-minute sessions of deep tissue bodywork, movement reeducation, and therapeutic verbal dialogue.

Joseph Heller (not to be mistaken for the novelist), the founder of Hellerwork, was an aerospace engineer at the Jet Propulsion Laboratory in Pasadena, California, during the late 1960s. He analyzed the effects of stress and gravity on aerospace structures such as rockets.

Seeking relief from the stress of his very demanding occupation, Heller attended numerous workshops and encounter groups at Kairos, a center for human development in Los Angeles. Eventually Heller was offered the position of director at Kairos and enthusiastically accepted it.

It was through a workshop at Kairos that he met Ida Rolf, the developer of Structural Integration, more commonly known as Rolfing. Heller was impressed by Rolf's theories concerning body alignment, stress, and gravity, and the new Rolfing therapy that she was teaching. In 1972 Heller learned Rolfing and practiced it until 1975, when he was named the first director of the Rolf Institute in Boulder, Colorado.

After serving as director for three years, Heller departed from the Rolf Institute to found his own form of bodywork called Hellerwork. While a practicing Rolfer, he realized that restructuring the body alone was not enough to accomplish long-term change. The missing element in Rolfing, according to Heller, was teaching people how to use their bodies efficiently.

It made no sense to Heller to bestow on his clients a "new" body only to have them misuse it in all their old ways. To prevent this he incorporated a movement reeducation program into Hellerwork. It is based on exercises that teach stress-free methods of performing basic everyday movements such as standing up, sitting down, walking, and bending over to pick things up.

Hellerwork is designed to realign the body and release chronic tension and stress. In short it is a restoration program, using a body/mind approach, on the human physical structure.

It focuses on rebalancing the entire body by returning it to a more aligned, relaxed, and youthful state. Verbal dialogue is used to assist the client in becoming aware of emotional stress that may be related to physical tension.

The Deep Tissue Massage portion of Hellerwork focuses on fascia, the body's connective tissue, which envelops the muscles and joins them to the bones. By releasing chronic tension in the fascia, the major body segments—head, shoulders, chest, pelvis, and legs—are brought toward a vertical alignment.

According to Heller, there are three main causes of accumulated tension in the body: physical trauma, emotional trauma, and misuse. So, by releasing tension, buried memories of past physical and emotional traumas are unlocked.

The benefits of Hellerwork to the client include increased energy, vitality, and fitness, improved posture and body shape, and greater flexibility and ease of movement.

Hellerwork practitioner training is held throughout the world. Although formats vary, the same curriculum is used for each training. A list of Hellerwork practitioners is available from Hellerwork, Inc. A book titled *Bodywise* by Joseph Heller and William A. Henkin and an illustrated handbook describing the Hellerwork series is also available from Hellerwork, Inc.

❧ | HERBAL MEDICINE | ❧

Herbal Medicine, sometimes referred to as Herbalism or Botanical Medicine, is the use of herbs, in a wide variety of forms, for their therapeutic value. An herb is a plant or plant part valued for its medicinal, savory, or aromatic qualities. Herb plants produce and contain a variety of chemical substances that act upon the body.

Herbal Medicine was an integral part of the development of modern civilization. No other healing art has carried with it such a long, varied, and detailed history of usage. It is by far the oldest form of medicine practiced by mankind.

Necessity required primitive man to observe and appreciate the great diversity of plant life available to him. It provided food, clothing, shelter, and medicine. When pain, injury, or disease struck, besides animal products or mystical rites, he had little other choice but to turn to plants for relief.

Early medicine men treated the sick with prayer, ritual, and concoctions made from local herbs which may have been considered "magic potions." Countless plants were tested in the hope of finding one with magical powers. Much of the medicinal use of plants seems to have been based on a highly developed instinct which led the medicine man or healer of the tribe to the correct plant and its use.

Herbal treatments also developed empirically through observations of wild animals, and by trial and error. Over time, each group, tribe, or people added to their understanding of the therapeutic uses for plants indigenous to their local area.

The oldest known systems of medicine in the world are those from China, India, and ancient Egypt, which date back more than five thousand years. Information regarding the various uses of plants was recorded in books called "herbals." Much of today's knowledge of herbal medicine is based on these ancient volumes.

About 4000 B.C., the Sumerians inhabited an area in southern Mesopotamia around the Tigris and Euphrates Rivers. From the clay tablets, written in cuneiform, it is known that they used opium, thyme, mustard, licorice, and the chemical sulfur for medicines. Later, the Babylonians added garlic, cinnamon, coriander, saffron, and other herbs to the Sumerians' list of medicinal substances.

In 2800 B.C., the Emperor Shen-nung (c. 3737–2697 B.C.), a Chinese herbalist, recorded a list of 366 plant drugs in a *Pen Ts'ao* (an herbal). This is the oldest of the Chinese pharmacopoeias (books describing medicinal preparations). Additional information on herbal medicine was included in *The Yellow Emperor's Classic of Internal Medicine*, attributed to the Yellow Emperor Huang-ti (c. 2697–2595 B.C.). The *Materia Medica of Li-Shih-Chin*, a compendium which analyzes over one hundred plants and lists twelve thousand formulas and prescriptions, was translated into English and first published in 1596.

Ayurveda, the oldest medical system known to man, has been practiced in India for more than four thousand years. The Vedas, originally written in Sanskrit, recorded many references to healing plants. The *Rigveda*, an ancient Hindu scripture, lists more than one thousand medicinal plants. A comprehensive Indian herbal, *Chakra Samhita*, mentions more than five hundred herbal remedies.

Egyptian herbal medicine was developing concurrently with Chinese and Indian. Extensive information on herbal-based healing was found in the *Ebers Papyrus*, a document dating back to the sixteenth century B.C.. It contains a listing of some eight hundred medicinal preparations including aloe, anise, peppermint, fennel, castor oil, saffron, garlic, and many others. Ancient temple carvings at Karnak depict medicinal plants being brought back to Egypt from Syria by a royal expedition.

Hippocrates (460–377 B.C.), a Greek physician, was the first to move the healing profession away from superstition and magic and regard it as a science. In his writings, Hippocrates described the use of some four hundred healing plants used as purgatives, diuretics, ointments, liniments, and for numerous other applications. Some of the plants he recommended are still in use today, including sage, mint, mugwort, verbena, and others.

Roman medicine, which had its roots in Greek medicine, later served as the foundation for most European medicine. The two central figures in Roman herbal medicine were Galen (c. A.D. 130–200) and Dioscorides (first century A.D.). Dioscorides wrote a pharmaceutical guide, *De Materia Medica*, which deals with more than six hundred plants. The work of Dioscorides,

Galen, and Theophrastus (c. 371–287 B.C.) formed the basis of European herbalism until well into the sixteenth century.

From about A.D. 400–1500 the Catholic Church controlled almost all medical knowledge in Europe. During the Dark Ages (A.D. 641–1096), the herbal healing doctrines of Galen and Dioscorides were perpetuated when monasteries cultivated herb gardens for medicinal uses. At the same time, folk remedies and practical herbal know-how became the realm of the common people.

The Arab world rediscovered classic Greek medical works during the Dark Ages in Europe. They added plants such as camphor, saffron, and spinach to their existing pharmacopoeia. After the Crusades, Arabian knowledge of herbal medicine took root in Europe.

Starting with the reign of Elizabeth I of England (1551–1603), the Great Age of Herbals began in which many notable books were written. The massive *Theatrum Botanicum* by the English herbalist John Parkinson, covering 1,800 pages and detailing 3,800 plants, was published in 1640. This was followed by Nicholas Culpeper's classic work, *The Complete Herbal* (also called *The English Physician*), which contained detailed information on the medicinal properties of hundreds of herbs.

The plants and herbs brought to America by English colonists were an important part of their existence in the New World. Because some of these plants would not thrive in America, the colonists replaced them with native species which they discovered. At Monticello, Thomas Jefferson grew more than twenty-five different herbs in his "kitchen garden."

Although the use of herbal medicine declined in the United States during the twentieth century, due to advances in medical science and pharmaceutical chemistry, it is currently making a strong comeback. There are many reasons for this, including the holistic health movement, greater availability of herbal and health foods, and an increased desire of individuals to take charge of their own health. But the main reason for the resurgence of herbal medicine is the realization that over the millennia, there have been many botanical remedies that have worked consistently and effectively to treat a wide variety of physical and emotional problems.

Today, the use of herbal remedies is not an obscure method of treatment; approximately 75 percent of the world's population relies on it as their primary source of health care. Major pharmaceutical companies are currently conducting extensive research on plant materials gathered from the Amazon rain forests and numerous other locations throughout the world for their potential therapeutic value.

Substances derived from plants remain the basis for a large proportion of the commercial medications manufactured today which are used to treat heart disease, high blood pressure, pain, asthma, and other problems. Some of these plants have been used since antiquity for their same therapeutic value.

An example of this old/new use of an herb is ephedra, which has been used in Traditional Chinese Medicine for more than two thousand years to treat asthma and other respiratory problems. The active ingredient in ephedra, ephedrine, is currently used in commercial pharmaceutical preparations for relief of asthma symptoms and other respiratory problems by helping an individual to breathe more easily.

A more recent example is the foxglove plant. Discovered in 1775 by the English physician William Withering, the powdered leaf of this medicinal plant is more commonly known as the cardiac stimulant digitalis to the millions of heart patients it keeps alive.

Herbal Medicine can be broadly classified into various basic systems: Traditional Chinese Herbalism, which is part of Traditional Oriental Medicine, Ayurvedic Herbalism, which is derived from Ayurveda, and Western Herbalism, which originally came from Greece and Rome to Europe and then spread to North and South America.

Chinese and Ayurvedic Herbalism have developed into highly sophisticated systems of diagnosis and treatment over the centuries. Although Western Herbalism originally had such a system during Greco-Roman times, the present system did not continue to develop after the Middle Ages in Europe and is today primarily a system of folk medicine.

Central to the philosophy of Chinese Herbalism is the Taoists' dualistic concept of *yin* and *yang*. Yin is described as that which is dark, cold, moist, yielding, negative in polarity, and feminine, while yang is described as that which is light, warm, dry, dominant, positive in polarity, and masculine. Although yin and yang are opposite in nature, it is their ability to interact and balance that creates health.

The classification of foods and herbs in Chinese Herbalism is based on four categories: the Four Natures, the Five Flavors, the Four Directions, and the Organs and Meridians Affected.

The Four Natures consist of cold, cool, warm, and hot, which relate to the theory of yin and yang. For example, a cool/cold or yin herb would be used to treat a warm/hot yang disease by creating balance. Additionally there are herbs classified as neutrals which can be used to treat either yin or yang disease.

The Five Flavors consist of sour, bitter, sweet, spicy, and salty. Each of the flavors relates to a general physiological effect and is classified as either yin or yang in nature.

The Four Directions are rising, sinking, floating, or descending. They relate to how a substance reacts in the body. In this system the direction of yin is downward and yang is upward. Heavy or yin herbs are used to treat deep, more chronic diseases while the lighter or yang herbs treat more surface conditions such as inflammation or a cold.

The Organs and Meridians Affected is a relatively new classification in the Chinese system. Only a few hundred years old, it is not as highly developed as the other classifications. Chinese physiology is based on the interaction of the twelve vital organs, and this classification uses certain foods and herbs to affect specific organs.

Chinese Herbalism uses formulas of related groups of herbs to achieve its results rather than a specific herb for a specific ailment. The main principle of herbal formulation is based on four categories, with each one having a particular function in the formula. These include chief herbs, supporting herbs, assisting herbs, and conducting herbs. Herbal Medicine is a huge part of Traditional Oriental Medicine and is used in the treatment of virtually every type of ailment.

Ayurveda recognizes five basic elements: air, fire, water, earth, and ether. They manifest in the human body, condensed, as three basic elements: *vata* (air), *pitta* (fire), and *kapha* (water). Vata, pitta, and kapha, known as *tridoshas* (three humors), are the vital life forces that govern all bodily functions.

Ayurvedic healing is based on the knowledge of *prakruti*, or the human constitution of the individual person. Each constitution is a combination of all three doshas, vata, pitta, and kapha, with a predominant tendency toward one or more.

When the doshas are in balance they sustain the body, and when out of balance they serve to destroy it. Thus, health in the body consists of the correct balance of the creative and destructive forces of the doshas. For a more complete description of Ayurvedic medicine, see elsewhere in this book.

The classification of foods and herbs in Ayurvedic Herbalism, like Chinese Herbalism, is also based on four categories: energy (*virya*), taste (*rasa*), postdigestive effect (*vipaka*), and special potency (*prabhava*). Specific herbs are used to either increase or decrease vata, pitta, or kapha and put the body into balance.

Western Herbalism in Europe before the seventeenth century utilized the energetic classification of herbs associated with Galen and the Greco-Roman medicine previously described. Similar to Ayurveda, people were classified according to four biological humors: *sanguine* being hot/moist, *melancholic* being cold/dry, *phlegmatic* being cold/moist, and *choleric* being hot/dry.

The Native peoples of North America had extensive knowledge of medicinal plants. Through careful observation and trial and error, the Native Americans found medicines that were useful in treating a wide variety of ailments. American Indian Herbal Medicine was based on treating the symptom. They used one herb to treat one ailment rather than formulas of herbs as the Chinese use.

The American Indian pharmacopoeia included such well-known herbs as American ginseng, willow bark, sassafras, witch hazel, and many others. Willow bark was used by the Indians to treat headaches and rheumatism. Today, the active ingredient of willow bark, salicin, which was later synthesized into acetylsalicylic acid and commonly known as aspirin, is used millions of times daily throughout the world for the same purpose.

Natives of South America and Africa also have extensive knowledge of the medicinal value of native plants. The rain forests of South America are still among the most unexplored regions in the world for medicinal plants. Recently, two South American herbs, *pau d'arco* or *lapacho* from Argentina, and *suma* from Brazil, have become familiar to herbalists.

Pau d'arco has been shown to be effective in the treatment of inflammatory diseases, tumors, and candida yeast infections. Suma, much like *Angelica sinensis* in Chinese Herbalism, is used as a gentle tonic for women. Both herbs are known to increase immune defense.

It should be noted that different systems of botanical medicine may also use the same herb for completely different purposes. For example, in Chinese Herbalism the hawthorn berry is used for treating food stagnation, while in Western Herbalism it is used as a heart tonic for a variety of heart-related problems.

Also, within one system a certain herb may be of a major significance, while in the other system it is relegated to a minor role. An example of this would be the herb haritaki (*Terminalia chebula*); used only as an astringent in

Chinese Herbalism, in Ayurvedic Herbalism it is used for strengthening and purification, and is regarded as the most potent and sacred herb of the Himalayas.

Many herbs that are commonly used as condiments or spices also have valuable medicinal properties. In Chinese Herbalism a prime example is cinnamon. Popular as both a spice and a major medicinal herb, cinnamon is used therapeutically as a carminative to aid digestion and relieve vomiting. Another example is cayenne pepper. A popular spice in foods, medicinally it is used to aid the cardiovascular, respiratory, and digestive systems. Others in this spice/herb category include oregano, basil, nutmeg, and many more.

Currently, ginseng is the most popular herb of the world. It is widely used in Asia and is becoming increasingly popular in the United States and Europe. Native Chinese ginseng, in short supply after being harvested for thousands of years, has become very expensive. A large, wild ginseng root will command a price of twenty thousand to thirty thousand dollars in China today. Due to the high cost of the native species, American ginseng has now become very popular in China.

Herbs can be prepared in a variety of forms depending on their purpose. These include juice squeezed from herbs; mashing herbs into a paste; decoction, or extracting the active ingredient by boiling down the herb; a hot infusion (made like hot tea); a cold infusion (made like sun tea); herbs ground into a powder and used in that form or pressed into a pill; an herbal wine made by adding the herb to water and sugar and letting it ferment; a tincture, made by combining ground herbs with alcohol and used internally; a liniment, made like a tincture except it is used externally; salves and ointments made by adding herbs to a medium such as petroleum jelly; syrups in which herbs are added to a medium such as honey; and a poultice in which the herbs are applied directly to a wound or body part and held in place with a cloth.

Although herbs come naturally from plants, they must be treated with the same respect one would afford any prescription drug. It is necessary to use the correct herb in the appropriate quantity and at the appropriate time to achieve the desired results. Improper use of herbs can bring unwanted and sometimes dangerous results.

There are numerous self-help books on Herbalism available in libraries, bookstores, and health food stores, but it must be remembered that herbs are potent substances and should be used with caution. It is suggested that an individual consult a health care professional in a major healing modality such as Acupuncture, Naturopathic Medicine, or Ayurveda, or a qualified professional herbalist for guidance regarding the use of Herbal Medicine.

There are numerous general information books available on every aspect of Herbalism. Some interesting ones are *Planetary Herbology* by Michael Tierra, *Green Pharmacy* by Barbara Griggs, *A History of Plants* by Richard Le Strange, *Rodale's Illustrated Encyclopedia of Herbs*, and *Reader's Digest Magic and Medicine of Plants*.

Organizations that can provide additional information on Herbalism include the American Botanical Council, the Herb Research Foundation, the Herb Society of America, and the American Herb Association.

HOLISTIC MEDICINE

Holistic Medicine is a philosophy of medical care which recognizes the person as a whole, an integration of body, mind, and spirit, and emphasizes personal responsibility for lifestyle and wellness. It focuses on patient education and participation in the healing process.

Everything has an effect on an individual's health: all factors, gross and subtle, physical, emotional, mental, spiritual, and environmental. All are interconnected and affect one another. A symptom or illness can be seen as an indicator or warning that one or more aspects of a person's life are out of harmony and that a change is called for. Sometimes these early warning signs are very subtle and must be watched for.

Holistic Medicine is an approach to health care that differs from the "treatment only" perspective of conventional medicine. The holistic practitioner can serve as a guide to assist the patient in the process of self-evaluation that leads toward optimal integration of body, mind, emotion, and spirit.

A holistic practitioner fosters and maintains a partnership with the patient by using therapies that they both feel comfortable with. But the practitioner views the patient as being ultimately responsible for her own well-being.

Holistic Medicine is not limited to a particular specialty or ideology, but encompasses a wide range of modalities for diagnosis and treatment. Many ancient healing methods such as Traditional Chinese Medicine (Acupuncture and herbs) and Ayurveda, the Indian art and science of healing, utilize the principles of Holistic Medicine and more modern modalities such as Chiropractic and Homeopathy.

Additional information on Holistic Medicine and a list of holistic practitioners can be obtained from organizations such as the American Holistic Medical Association and the International Association of Holistic Health Practitioners.

❧ | HOLOTROPIC BREATHWORK | ❦

Holotropic Breathwork, sometimes called Holotropic Breathing, is a powerful technique of self-exploration based on ancient spiritual practices and modern consciousness research. This approach combines breathing, evocative music, and a specific form of bodywork. It includes and integrates the physical, psychological, and spiritual dimensions.

"Holotropic" comes from the Greek *holos* meaning "whole" and *trepin* meaning "to move in the direction of." It means literally "moving toward wholeness."

The Holotropic Breathwork process was developed in 1976 by Stanislav Grof, M.D., a psychiatrist with over thirty years' experience in psychotherapy research and nonordinary states of consciousness, and his wife, Christina. The Grofs do not call Holotropic Breathwork a therapy or spiritual technique, but prefer to refer to it as "an adventure of self-discovery."

Holotropic Breathwork is presented in a two-day workshop by facilitators certified by the Grofs. Many facilitators are in the mental-health field and use the process in their everyday work. Participants in the workshop lie flat on the floor in a dimly lit room. Facilitators coach the participants on how to breathe while stereo speakers fill the room with the sound of African drums. Participants alternate in the roles of experiencer and "sitters." Focused bodywork and mandala drawing are also important elements used in the holotropic process.

During the course of a session, two to four hours long, the participants try to access the four "levels" of experience that are available during breathing: sensory, biographical, perinatal, and transpersonal.

By accessing buried memories, an individual can relive his own birth experience or traumatic life events, free up "stuck" emotional viewpoints, or in some cases experience mystical states of awareness such as connecting to the universe.

The facilitator training program requires 150 hours of general experience in Holotropic Breathwork, 350 hours of training combining theory and experience, and a two-week certification seminar. The 350 hours of training, given over two years, consist of seven courses given in six-day modules.

The theory and practice of Holotropic Breathwork is described in detail in the books *Beyond the Brain: Birth, Death, and Transcendence* and *The Adventure in Self-Discovery* by Stanislav Grof.

Currently there are Holotropic Breathwork facilitators in the United States, Japan, Europe, and Australia. A list of facilitators can be obtained from Grof Transpersonal Training, Inc.

❧ | HOMEOPATHY | ❦

Homeopathy is a highly systematic therapy that uses small doses of specially prepared plants and minerals to powerfully stimulate the body's defense mechanisms and healing processes in order to cure illness.

The word *homeopathy* is taken from the Greek *homeos* meaning "similar" and *pathos* meaning "suffering." Thus, Homeopathy means "to treat with something that produces an effect similar to the suffering." This "law of similars," the concept of "like cures like" or "likes are cured by likes," is the basic principle of Homeopathy.

Homeopathic physicians consider disease from a different perspective than does modern conventional medicine. Disease is viewed as a result of a deeper disturbance or imbalance of the person as a whole, of which symptoms are simply the outward manifestation. Symptoms, whether mental, emotional, or physical, are expressions of this imbalance.

In Homeopathy, symptoms are not treated because they are only signs of the body's attempt to cure itself. Homeopathic treatment is based on the whole body and personality of the person, her totality and uniqueness, not solely on the specific condition or disease. In short, Homeopathy treats people, not diseases. In this respect Homeopathy is akin to the holistic school of medicine.

In conventional medicine, health is seen as the absence of disease. If nothing is wrong with a person, it is assumed he is healthy. Homeopathy views health as more than that. A truly healthy person is seen as one who is free of problems on all levels—physical, emotional, and mental.

In the fourth century B.C. Hippocrates first announced the essential homeopathic principle, which stated that if a remedy produces certain symptoms in a healthy person, it will cure a sick person of those same symptoms. Paracelsus, a well-known sixteenth-century physician and alchemist, referred to the law of similars in his writings and used it extensively in his practice. It was also utilized by many other cultures, including the Chinese, Greeks, Indians, Mayans, and Native Americans.

Samuel Christian Hahnemann (1755–1843), a German physician and the founder of Homeopathy, was born in Meissen, Saxony. He earned his medical degree in 1759, in Vienna, and practiced the conventional medicine of his day, but eventually grew disillusioned with the cures. These were the days when bloodletting, blistering, purges, leeches, sweating, and baths were the popular remedies for all ailments.

Through practical experimentation Hahnemann noticed that herbs given in a low dose tended to cure the same symptoms as they produced in a large poisoning dose.

Hahnemann's life changed after he obtained a copy of *Materia Medica* written by an Englishman named Cullen. It devoted several pages to a new Peruvian bark *(cinchona)*, used to cure the countess of Cinchon of a fever in Peru. He obtained some of the bark, took four drams of it daily, and contracted the fever. When he discontinued taking the bark the fever disappeared.

For the next six years Hahnemann systematically tested this observation on himself and fellow physicians. He found that any substance that can experimentally produce a specific set of symptoms when given to a healthy person can cure those same symptoms when given to a sick person.

In 1810 he wrote *The Organon of the Rational Art of Healing* in which he stated the laws and principles of a new system of healing he called Homeopathy. Although attacked by orthodox medical men, Hahnemann attracted a large following of thinking physicians to Vienna to learn about the new art, and a school of Homeopathy came into being. Currently, there are still four-year homeopathic medical schools in Europe.

Because he distrusted apothecaries of the day to make up his medicines correctly, Hahnemann chose to dispense his own medicines, an illegal practice in Germany at that time. In 1820, after being arrested in Leipzig, he was found guilty and forced to move. But through special permission granted by the royal house, he was allowed to practice again in Germany.

In 1831, when a cholera epidemic spread through Eastern Europe and thousands died, Hahnemann studied the symptoms and decided that camphor would cure the disease. His advice was accepted and the epidemic was put down—a great triumph for Hahnemann.

When cholera swept through Britain in 1840, it was found that nearly four times as many people survived when treated by Homeopathy versus those treated by orthodox methods.

Homeopathy was introduced to the United States in 1825 with the emigration of a Danish homeopath named Hans Gram. It became so popular that homeopaths organized the American Institute of Homeopathy in 1844. In 1846 another group formed an organization, called the American Medical Association (AMA), which was intent on slowing the rapid growth of Homeopathy.

After the AMA was formed, all of the physicians who used Homeopathy were expelled from its ranks. Throughout the late 1800s the AMA continued its witch-hunt of homeopaths and censured anyone in the medical profession who had even the remotest connection with the discipline. This persecution, combined with other factors such as economics, led to the decline of Homeopathy by the end of the nineteenth century. In 1900 there were more than twenty homeopathic colleges in the United States, but by 1923 only two remained. By 1950 they were either closed or no longer teaching Homeopathy.

In the 1970s Homeopathy reemerged as a viable health care field. Today, more and more people are rediscovering Homeopathy. Homeopathic medicines are used by many alternative health care professionals including acupuncturists, chiropractors, naturopaths, and many others. Additionally, some medical doctors and doctors of osteopathy are beginning to use homeopathic remedies in everyday medicine.

There are several companies that manufacture homeopathic remedies in the United States today. Homeopathic Medicine, or remedies, are made from over 1,500 natural plant, animal, and mineral products gathered from all parts of the world. These remedies are prepared in homeopathic pharmacies in accordance with the *Homeopathic Pharmacopoeia of the United States*, the official manufacturing manual recognized by the FDA.

Each substance is triturated (crushed, ground, or pulverized) by a slow, exhaustive method that results in an infinitesimal breakdown of the active ingredients, permitting ready diffusion and assimilation, thereby enhancing their therapeutic effectiveness.

For example, a known quantity of a plant substance, finely ground, is mixed with alcohol or water to obtain a solution. One drop of the solution is mixed with ninety-nine drops of alcohol or water (to achieve a ratio of 1:100); the mixture is then strongly shaken, a process known as *succussion*, and labeled as "1C." One drop of 1C is then mixed with one hundred drops of alcohol or water and the process is repeated to make a 2C. By the time 3C is reached, the dilution is one part in 1 million.

Through this special process of dilution and succussion not only is the potency increased, but because the remedies are so dilute, they cause no side effects and are perfectly safe. Homeopathic remedies act by stimulating the immune system and other restorative systems in the body.

Today, such notables as Her Majesty Queen Elizabeth II of England and rock music star Tina Turner are strong proponents of Homeopathy.

Organizations such as the National Center for Homeopathy, the International Foundation for Homeopathy, and Homeopathic Educational Services provide information about Homeopathy and promote its use in the United States.

❧ | HOSHINO THERAPY | ❦

Hoshino Therapy is a unique pressure-point system that integrates the art of hand massage with the science of Acupuncture. It is based on the detection of "aging" or loss of vitality in the soft tissues that results from the improper functioning of the biomechanical body.

Prevention evaluation is a distinctive feature of the therapy, which utilizes 250 pressure points to evaluate biomechanical functioning and to localize areas of wear and tear. The stimulation of selected points, using Hoshino's unique manual techniques, brings about the revitalization of soft tissue and the restoration of harmonious movement of the body parts. A program of special Hoshino exercises complements the therapy.

Hoshino Therapy was developed by Japanese acupuncturist Professor Tomezo Hoshino. He was born in 1910 in Atsugi, Japan (near Yokohama), into a family who for generations had been practitioners of Acupuncture and Traditional Oriental Medicine. At the age of sixteen, after being blinded in a motoring accident, he studied the traditional Japanese muscle massage called *hamma*. Eighteen months after the accident he bumped into a wall and was knocked unconscious. When he awoke, he was able to see again.

Hoshino then emigrated to Argentina and worked on a ranch. After six years, he developed neuralgia and returned to Japan, where he was cured by his uncle with treatments of Acupuncture and physiotherapy.

His uncle told Hoshino he had "special hands," and encouraged him to study Acupuncture. Hoshino began to study Acupuncture in 1935, received his diploma in 1939, and returned to Argentina.

In Buenos Aires he began searching for a method to cure arthrosis (any condition caused by a hardening of muscles, tendons, and ligaments). Since Acupuncture was not recognized in Argentina, he worked as a pedicurist. When he developed bursitis in his shoulder, Hoshino returned to Japan to be cured.

Seeking help from his former classmates at the Acupuncture institute, Hoshino found they were unable to cure him. He then went to a Japanese mountaintop resolving not to come down until he cured himself. After a month, using only the warmth and pressure from his own hands, he was able to reverse the condition in his shoulder. When he came down from the mountain he was free of pain and knew he had perfected a means to cure arthrosis.

Again he returned to Argentina and began to practice his new therapy with great success. In 1952 his therapy was recognized by the Argentine government as an official medical therapy.

In Hoshino Therapy, 250 vital points that relate to the body's bio-mechanical functioning are used. These selected Acupuncture points are located directly over the muscles, tendons, and ligaments. The combination of finger pressure applied to a specific vital point, and warmth from the therapist's hand work together to reverse the hardening of the soft tissues, thereby loosening the afflicted area.

Hoshino Therapy is used to treat such maladies as osteoarthritis, bursitis, tendonitis, nontraumatic disc disorders, and sciatica as well as nonspecific complaints such as headache, muscular pain, tension, fatigue, nausea, numbness, dizziness, and back pain.

Hoshino treatments are complemented by a program of four "Hoshino Exercises": the shoulder exercise, the knee exercise, the twisting exercise, and the chest exercise. They are designed for proper maintenance of the biomechanical body and help to prevent recurrence of symptoms after a series of Hoshino treatments.

For several years Professor Hoshino operated a research and treatment clinic in Boca Raton, Florida. Currently, all training of Hoshino therapists is done at the Center for Biotherapeutics/Hoshino Therapy Clinic.

The Hoshino Therapy advanced training program is open to health professionals and consists of a two-year program totaling four hundred hours of instruction. Tomezo Hoshino currently supervises the training of Hoshino therapists in the United States. Graduates of the program receive certificates.

❧ | HOXSEY TREATMENT | ❧

The Hoxsey Treatment is a program for the treatment of cancer utilizing a specially formulated herbal tonic combined with a diet of fresh foods that excludes salt, sugar, and alcohol. Certain other foods are also banned because they conflict with the tonic and neutralize its effect.

The tonic can be taken internally to treat internal cancers, or used as a salve or lotion and applied topically to treat external cancers.

Analysis has shown it to contain potassium iodine, licorice, red clover, burdock root, stillingia root, berberis root, poke root, cascara amarga, prickly ash bark, and buckthorn bark. Several of these well-known North American herbs are thought to have anticancer attributes.

In 1840 John Hoxsey noticed one of his horses, one that had developed cancer, selecting and eating certain herbs that grew around the farm. After a period of time he noticed the horse's cancer was cured.

John Hoxsey then set about to gather these same herbs and brew them together into a potion. He used the potion or tonic to treat and cure other cancerous animals.

The tonic's formula was passed down from father to son and when Harry M. Hoxsey, John Hoxsey's great-grandson, turned eighteen, he was given the formula.

In the 1920s, Harry M. Hoxsey, a charming self-taught healer, founded the Hoxsey Cancer Clinic in Dallas, Texas. The course of treatment at the clinic was limited to herbal mixtures.

In 1924 Hoxsey was allowed by the established medical profession to test his herbal method. Although the test proved successful, continued use of the treatment became contingent on Hoxsey's agreeing to stringent terms. Finding these terms intolerable, he refused.

Hoxsey then made further efforts to convince the medical establishment in this country of the legitimacy of his treatment. He asked the American Medical Association and the National Cancer Institute to test his treatment, but this never happened. He continued his work, curing people of cancer, in spite of threats and persecution. Numerous problems with the American Medical Association ensued and he was arrested several times for practicing medicine without a license.

In 1954 the *Journal of the American Medical Association* conducted an investigation of the Hoxsey Cancer Clinic of Dallas, Texas, from "behind their desk." The conclusion was that the tonic was merely a "cough medicine" because it contained potassium iodine, an expectorant included in some cough medicine formulas. The essence of the report, published in the June 12, 1954, issue of *JAMA*, stated in brief, said the Hoxsey tonic "is without any therapeutic merit in the treatment of cancer." In 1960, the Food and Drug Administration banned the sale of Hoxsey's remedy.

Although the Hoxsey Treatment has not been obtainable in the United States for over thirty years, it is still available at the Bio-Medical Center, an alternative medicine clinic in Tijuana, Mexico.

❧ | HYDROTHERAPY | ❦

Hydrotherapy is the use of water, hot or cold, fresh or mineral, for therapeutic or healing purposes. Hydrotherapy comes from the Greek words *hudor*, which means "water," and *therapeutikos*, which means "to take care of," or "to heal."

The use of water for healing is practically as old as mankind. It has existed as a healing therapy for thousands of years. As early as 4000 B.C. baths and remedies are mentioned in Sanskrit. The Egyptians, Babylonians, and Cretans made extensive use of water therapy and baths long before the Romans developed a fondness for them. The ruins of a Roman temple and a Bronze Age ax circa 1200 B.C. were discovered near the mineral springs at Lenk, in the Swiss Alps. The Greek physician Galen (c. A.D. 129–200) advocated the use of baths combined with massage and exercise to affect a cure.

The Spartans of Greece would plunge newborn babies into cold water to toughen them and immunize them against disease. The Chinese, Hindus, and Hebrews also used the water cure.

In Europe during the Middle Ages, bathing fell into disfavor for various reasons, which probably included the plague. In North America, some Native American tribes were using baths to cure disease. They used vapor baths in the form of sweat lodges followed by a plunge into a cold river or snow.

The well-known Turkish bath was developed in Constantinople during the fifteenth century. During the late eighteenth century John Wesley, founder of the Methodist Church, used cold-water bathing to cure a variety of diseases.

Since the mid-1800s water therapy has been very popular in Europe. An obscure German priest, Father Sebastian Kneipp (1821–1897), was searching for a remedy after contracting tuberculosis. He discovered a cold water treatment described in an eighteenth-century book by Johann Siegmund Hahn. After Father Kneipp plunged himself into the cold Danube River for a minute, two to three times a week for several weeks, he was cured.

Father Kneipp, regarded as the great "water doctor," later developed many different methods of water treatment, including hot and cold contrast baths, and cold water washes combined with warm wraps. Kneipp's treatments were less severe and shorter in duration than Hahn's.

In 1890, after more than thirty years of practical applications Father Kneipp published *My Water Cure*, in London. Around the turn of the century, several facilities utilizing the Kneipp water cure system were opened in the United States.

Dr. John Harvey Kellogg (1855–1946) did much to promote the use of Hydrotherapy in the United States. In 1876 he opened a sanitarium in Battle Creek, Michigan, to treat the ill with diet, Hydrotherapy, and other drugless therapies. By 1900 he had published a monumental 1,100-page work titled *Rational Hydrotherapy*.

Today therapies that utilize water in some beneficial way are so numerous that the list is almost endless. Drinking water is used in fasting and to help transport and eliminate waste products from the body. Swimming gives the therapeutic benefits of exercise without putting stress on the body. Soaking in warm water stimulates blood circulation, which increases oxygen to tissue and removes waste products. Warmth provided during an underwater massage or the buoyant support provided in underwater medical gymnastics is virtually unachievable by other means.

Naturally occurring springs are found in many parts of the United States such as those in Hot Springs, Arkansas, and Calistoga, California, and others can be found throughout the world. Springs where the water is hot and/or high in mineral content (sodium, calcium, potassium, magnesium, sulfur) are ideal for Hydrotherapy. In theory, minute amounts of the minerals present in the water will enter the system through the skin or mucous membrane to promote healing, resulting in a healthier overall state.

Benefits of Hydrotherapy are numerous. Water with high sulfur content is very helpful to arthritis sufferers and effectively treats skin problems such as eczema and psoriasis. Water's warmth promotes circulation and relaxation in spasmed muscles, while cold water decreases pain and reduces swelling. Moving the feet through a tub of cold water or taking a cold shower can be very invigorating and energizing.

Today, Hydrotherapy is becoming increasingly popular. Modern whirlpool spas, like the Jacuzzi, are common items in health clubs, spas, resorts, and many private residences throughout America.

Whirlpool spas are used by professional athletes after a game to reduce the effects of stresses placed on their bodies. People in every type of occupation find that sitting in a whirlpool helps them relax and relieve tension.

❧ | HYPERBARIC OXYGENATION THERAPY | ❦

Hyperbaric Oxygenation Therapy is a method of exposing an individual to 100 percent pure oxygen, under conditions of greater than normal atmospheric pressure, for therapeutic purposes.

Normal atmospheric air contains approximately 20 percent oxygen, with the remaining 80 percent made up of mostly nitrogen with some carbon dioxide, carbon monoxide, and various other gases in small amounts.

During Hyperbaric Oxygenation Therapy, an individual is sealed into a cylindrical enclosure called a hyperbaric chamber. Pure oxygen is introduced into the chamber to raise the barometric pressure inside to greater than normal atmospheric pressure.

The increased pressure, which completely surrounds the individual, forces pure oxygen into the body. The pressure inside the body is then equalized to the pressure within the chamber. This causes all body tissues to become flooded with more than the usual supply of oxygen.

Hyperbaric Oxygenation Therapy is used to treat disorders in which the oxygen supply to the body is deficient. If the heart, lungs, or blood vessels—due to injury or disease—are unable to maintain good circulation, an increase in oxygen can compensate for the reduction in circulation.

Hyperbaric Oxygenation has been found to be beneficial for all types of heart disease, circulatory problems, multiple sclerosis, gangrene, stroke, and many other conditions. Additionally it has been shown to slow down the aging process and help return natural color to graying hair. It is available at some alternative therapy clinics in Mexico. For additional information contact the American College of Hyperbaric Medicine.

❧ | HYPNOTHERAPY | ❦

Hypnotherapy is the use of hypnosis for therapeutic purposes. Although numerous investigations have been made to determine just exactly what hypnosis is, both theoretical and clinical, much disagreement exists.

A single theory on hypnosis that will fit in every respect does not exist at present. This is partly due to the difference between light and deep states of hypnosis. But hypnosis can be described as a somewhat altered state of consciousness and altered awareness, although the conscious mind is still present.

Although many people think of hypnosis as a fairly recent discovery, it has been practiced since ancient times. Hypnoticlike behavior has been reported from the dawn of history. Hypnotherapy in the form of waking and sleeping suggestion is among the oldest of the healing arts. Today, this type of behavior can be observed in the rites and ceremonies of many primitive cultures.

In ancient Egypt, priests used hypnotic incense and chanting to induce a state sometimes known as "temple sleep," during which curative suggestions were given to people suffering from a variety of ailments.

During the Golden Age of Greece, there were "sleep temples of the sick," where people were put into prolonged sleep induced by soft music, repeated phrases, and drugs.

Shamans, medicine men, and witch doctors used drums, objects of fixation, music, costumes, and ritual dance to induce trance states during which they would make waking suggestions of healing to the sick.

Medieval Christian religion made extensive use of rituals and ceremonies in which they used music, incense, selective illumination, and chanting in a church of overwhelming scale and magnificent architecture. Subjected to this awe-inspiring display, the peasants of the time were put into a hypnoticlike state and surrendered themselves to God.

It is generally agreed that modern hypnosis began with Franz Anton Mesmer (1734–1815), an Austrian physician. Mesmer revived the ancient healing art of hypnotic suggestion. His form of hypnotism, called *animal magnetism*, was based on his theory that the human body has a magnetic polarity with a force field. It became known as *mesmerism*, a term still used today.

Although Mesmer began to cure people with animal magnetism, he was ridiculed and persecuted by the orthodox medical world of Vienna. At that time there was no logical explanation, in scientific terms, for the results he was achieving. In 1778 Mesmer left Vienna for Paris, where he established a practice.

Mesmer was not well received by the medical world of Paris even though he accomplished miraculous cures. In response to the growing opposition to

Mesmer's work, a royal commission was established to investigate it. Unfortunately, the commission, failing to understand the psychotherapeutic basis of his work, deemed Mesmer a quack without allowing him to demonstrate the healing potential of his technique.

Because Mesmer's work had been so thoroughly discredited it was not until the 1840s that James Baird, a Scottish doctor, began to investigate the scientific value of mesmerism. It was Baird who coined the terms *hypnosis* and *hypnotism*. The medical use of hypnosis began with Baird, who used it widely in his medical practice.

In Vienna, Sigmund Freud (1856–1939) and Joseph Bauer (1842–1925) used hypnosis successfully in psychotherapy with patients they then classified as hysterical. Later Freud rejected hypnosis and substituted his method of free association and psychoanalysis.

At the end of World War I, British psychologist William McDougall (1871–1944) used hypnosis to treat soldiers suffering from "shell shock" induced by trench warfare.

Charles Hull (1884–1952), a professor at the University of Wisconsin, carried out detailed scientific studies on hypnotic phenomena and published the classic *Hypnosis and Suggestibility* in 1933.

After World War II and the Korean conflict, renewed interest in hypnosis came from psychiatrists who found it could achieve results more rapidly than the methods of psychotherapy they had been using.

In 1955 the British Medical Association reported hypnosis to be a valuable medical treatment. The American Medical Association followed suit three years later, in 1958, when an internal investigative committee reported favorably on it.

As noted earlier, the hypnotic state can be described as a somewhat altered state of consciousness. The relationship between the functioning of the conscious and subconscious minds during normal and hypnotic states is reversed. In the normal waking state, the conscious mind is in a dominant or primary role and the subconscious mind is in a secondary role. Under hypnosis, the conscious mind is in the secondary role, while the subconscious mind is in the primary or dominant role.

Hypnotherapy is a valuable therapeutic tool and not a parlor game. Ethical, professional hypnotherapists recommend that it only be used for serious and justifiable reasons. One should not be strongly influenced or compelled to submit to hypnosis, but should submit willingly.

Although some people cannot be hypnotized and the degree to which others can be hypnotized varies, most subjects are very susceptible to suggestions given them while in a hypnotic state. This capacity to accept hypnotic suggestion is a key to hypnotism's ability to effectively accomplish its goals.

Hypnotherapy has been used successfully to treat a wide variety of functional disorders such as blindness, paralysis, inability to speak or sing, personality disorders, alcoholism, addiction to nicotine, obesity, sexual problems, phobias such as fear of heights, water, flying in airplanes, driving over bridges, or enclosed spaces, and many others.

The practical applications of Hypnotherapy are vast. In the field of medicine it is used in anesthesiology, obstetrics, surgery, psychiatry, and other specialties. In dentistry it can be used to alleviate anxiety and reduce pain and discomfort. In psychotherapy, besides treating functional disorders it can be used for rehabilitation, relief of guilt, despair, venting of hurt, and more.

Anyone can be taught to hypnotize; the basics can be learned in a weekend seminar. Unfortunately, this does not necessarily make an individual qualified to practice hypnosis on a professional basis. It is prudent to know the background of a hypnotherapist with regard to education, experience, and professional competence.

Today many clinical hypnotherapists, psychologists, and psychiatrists use hypnotic regression to treat problems stemming from childhood traumas and past life experiences.

In 1980 the American Council of Hypnotist Examiners was founded to create a new level of specialized education and professional competency in the field of Hypnotherapy. The International Medical and Dental Hypnotherapy Association offers a referral service of certified hypnotherapists for the health care community and general public. There are many additional organizations listed in the resource section which can also provide information and referrals to trained professionals.

Virtually every library has a good selection of books on hypnosis and Hypnotherapy, and it is recommended that anyone considering using it for any type of healing become familiar with all aspects of it before receiving treatment.

Additional information may also be obtained by contacting any of the professional organizations listed in the resource section.

❧ | IMAGERY AND VISUALIZATION | ❦

Imagery and Visualization, also known as Creative Imagery, Guided Imagery, Mental Imagery, and Creative Visualization (the terms are used interchangeably) is the effective use of images or symbols to focus the mind on the workings of the body in order to cause real physiological changes.

Creative Imagery, in practice, is the conscious creation of positive thoughts and images, and the communication of them to the body to accomplish some particular goal or desired outcome. It can be utilized for the relief of pain, the curing of disease, or to affect behavioral change.

Imagery can take on many forms. It is a flow of thoughts you can see, hear, feel, smell, and taste. It is the interface language between mind and body.

Imagination, although associated with fantasy, the impractical, or day-dreaming, is an important part of the visualization process. It is the ability to create a mental picture in the mind of what is desired.

Imagery and Visualization have been recognized by all great cultures and traditions. These peoples understood that through Visualization human beings could transform the circumstances of their lives. Since the 1950s researchers and clinicians in the United States, Europe, Japan, and China have systematically explored the role Imagery plays in determining health and illness.

For over thirty years a large body of information regarding basic stress research, biofeedback instrumentation, clinical use of relaxation, and most recently from the field of psychoneuroimmunology, indicates that psychological factors can and do affect the physiology of the body. In other words, the mind/body connection does exist.

The exact mechanisms of Imagery are still a mystery. In the context of a healing tool, it is holistic in nature by recognizing the intimate relationship between mind and body. It is not a passive treatment. The individual requiring a cure or relief from an illness consciously participates in the healing process.

Although proven effective from a strictly physiological standpoint, Imagery can be employed in a broader scope of healing. While recovering from an illness, Imagery can provide insight into other areas of one's life that may require change to either complete the recovery or maintain it once completed. This may include changes in lifestyle, attitude, emotional state, or relationships.

Imagery can be used to treat a wide variety of physical maladies, from tension headaches to life-threatening disease. Conditions that are caused or aggravated by stress often respond very well to Imagery techniques.

Anecdotal evidence has shown that Imagery can effect profound changes in the body, such as curing cancer or putting it into remission, lowering blood pressure, and reducing or eliminating pain in all parts of the body.

Imagery has also had an impact on sports by increasing stamina and enhancing performance. An athlete can visualize the perfect golf swing or high dive.

Imagery is not a cure-all for every type of problem; other forms of treatment are often needed as well. Whatever type of treatment is used, however, from conventional medicine and surgery to more holistic approaches, Imagery is a helpful and effective supplement to other therapies.

Although there are practitioners who specialize in Imagery, the responsibility for and ultimate success of the technique rests with the individual practicing it. This makes it a wonderful self-help tool.

There are a number of books available on the subject. *Healing Yourself: A Step-by-Step Program for Better Health through Imagery* by Martin L. Rossman, M.D., is excellent. Another is *Psycheye: Self-Analytic Consciousness* by Akhter Ahsen, Ph.D.

Imagery audiotapes are available from the Academy for Guided Imagery and other sources. For additional information, contact any of the organizations listed in the resource section.

❧ | INFANT MASSAGE | ❧

Infant Massage is a program of stroking (massage) that can be used on babies aged three weeks to crawling. The interaction that takes place between the parents or caregiver and the child during stroking contains the basic elements of bonding. As the child grows, Infant Massage can be adapted to meet the needs of toddlers, older children, and the developmentally disabled.

In many cultures throughout the world, Infant Massage is an ancient tradition, but it has only recently been rediscovered in the West. In 1973 Vimala Schneider, while working at an orphanage in India, encountered the use of Infant Massage and became very interested in it. After returning to the United States she did extensive research and put together a curriculum for parent-infant classes. Subsequently she founded the International Association of Infant Massage Instructors.

It is common knowledge that loving, nurturing contact between caregiver and infant has a positive impact on the child's later development. Research continues to verify that loving, nurturing touch is necessary for the proper physical and psychological development of children. Infant Massage is a pleasant, easy method of providing this early positive contact.

Recently conducted studies by Tiffany Field, Ph.D., at the University of Miami showed that premature babies that received fifteen minutes of massage and movement three times a day showed a weight gain 47 percent higher than those receiving routine care. The infants massaged every day showed more progress than those not massaged, in both physical and neurological development.

Pediatrician Frederick Leboyer, well known for his first book, *Birth without Violence*, has been a strong advocate of Infant Massage. He relates the importance of touch for an infant because of the terrible contrast they suffer when exposed to the "outside" world after birth. They crave the sensations and sensory input they previously experienced and had been accustomed to in the womb.

According to Leboyer, "being touched and caressed, being massaged, is food for the infant. Food as necessary as minerals, vitamins, and proteins. Deprived of this food, the name of which is love, babies would rather die. And they often do."

The benefits of Infant Massage are numerous: it helps to strengthen and regulate the respiratory, circulatory, and gastrointestinal functions; helps the baby to relax and relieve the stresses which build up daily from the numerous new encounters with the world; enhances the loving communication between caregiver and baby; helps to tone muscles; and helps the caregiver to stay in touch with the infant's nonverbal cues.

Additional information on Infant Massage can be obtained from the International Association of Infant Massage Instructors and the International Loving Touch Foundation. Both organizations offer classes taught in four or five sessions. In these classes, mothers, fathers, and other caregivers are taught the benefits of nurturing touch, and step-by-step massage and relaxation techniques.

Infant Massage is also taught to bodyworkers as part of Bodywork for the Childbearing Year program developed in 1980 by Kate Jordan and Carole Osborne-Sheets. For details, see Bodywork for the Childbearing Year, elsewhere in this book.

Some excellent books on the subject are *Infant Massage: A Handbook for*

Loving Parents by Vimala Schneider-McClure, *Loving Hands: The Traditional Indian Art of Baby Massage* by Frederick Leboyer, and *Touching, the Human Significance of the Skin* by Ashley Montague.

IRIDOLOGY

Iridology is the study of the iris. The science of Iridology is a diagnostic technique which studies and analyzes the very delicate and intricate structures on the iris. Over 90 specific areas on each iris have been "mapped," making a total of over 180 zones available to reveal important information about conditions in the body.

In physiological terms the iris is the colored, opaque, contractile membrane portion of the eye which is perforated in the center by the pupil. Through contraction and dilation the iris regulates the amount of light entering the eye.

In the civilizations of Mesopotamia and the Indus Valley it was acknowledged that the first appearance of disease was often preceded by signs in the eye. It is well documented in Traditional Chinese Medicine that examining the eyes was part of the diagnostic procedure. Many years ago sclerology, the reading of one's health from the tiny blood vessels in the whites of the eyes, was developed by Native Americans in the southwestern United States.

In Europe during the late seventeenth century, doctors discovered a relationship between changes in the iris and certain disease states. In the early 1800s, near Budapest, Hungary, a young boy named Ignatz von Peczely tried to capture an owl in his garden. During the struggle, he broke the owl's leg. At that moment he looked into the owl's eye and noticed a black streak rising in the eye. After nursing the bird back to health, he released it, but it remained in the garden for several years. During this period of time von Peczely noticed the black streak had turned to white.

He later became a physician and while working on hospital wards observed the irises of accident victims and those of surgical patients before and after their operations. From the many observations of changes in the eye due to accident, illness, or surgery he was convinced that some type of reflex relationship existed between markings in the iris and the various parts of the body. Ignatz von Peczely published his text in Germany in 1881, complete with charts that correlated sections of the iris with the various organ systems of the body.

A short time after von Peczely's publication, a Swedish minister and homeopath, Nils Liljequist, discovered through observation changes in iris pigmentation due to toxic accumulations in the body. Given large quantities of quinine as a youth, Liljequist correlated the yellow-green discoloration of his eyes to the quinine. He published his findings in *Diagnosis from the Eye.*

Dr. Bernard Jensen pioneered the science of Iridology in the United States. He first published the internationally acclaimed *The Science and Practice of Iridology* in 1952. He also developed a comprehensive iris chart showing locations of the organs as they reflect in the iris. This chart remains the most accurate available today.

Dr. Jensen still teaches Iridology seminars and certifies iridologists. Additional information can be obtained from Bernard Jensen International in Escondido, California.·

The iris is very complex and contains several hundred thousand nerve endings. In Iridology theory it is generally believed that through these nerve filaments the iris is connected to every organ and nerve system in the body via the optic nerves, optic thalami, and the spinal cord.

In simplest terms, each specific area, or zone, on the iris acts as a readout gauge to reflect the dynamic changes occurring in the corresponding area of the body. For example, the area of the iris known as zone 6 is where the lymphatic system is gauged; a chain of small cloudlike spots resembling a string of pearls indicates that the lymphatic system has become overburdened with waste materials. No spots appear if the lymphatic system is healthy.

An Iridology chart represents a miniature human body with the head at the top, the feet at the bottom, and other areas of the body arranged in relation to each other. The left iris represents the left side of the body and right iris represents the right side of the body. Dual organs such as the kidneys are represented on each chart. By observing the color, texture, and density in all the different zones of the iris, the iridologist can get a very clear picture of the body's overall health. Interpretation of these color, texture, and density changes—or "spots" as they are called—uniquely reveals the condition inside the body.

Additional information may be obtained from Bernard Jensen International.

❦ | JAZZERCISE | ❧

Jazzercise is a complete program of body conditioning and fitness that combines the flow and rhythm of jazz dance with basic exercise principles.

The Jazzercise Workout is a carefully designed aerobic exercise program that can be used to achieve individual fitness goals. It can be used to increase cardiovascular fitness, muscle strength, flexibility, and muscle endurance, and to reduce body fat to produce a more fit and trim appearance.

Jazzercise is a safe, easy-to-follow, fun program of exercise for people of all ages. One specialty known as Jazzercise on the Lighter Side is for seniors aged fifty-five to ninety.

The creator of Jazzercise, Judi Sheppard Missett, literally grew up with dance. Born in San Diego, California, in 1944, her family soon moved to Iowa. When she was three her parents enrolled her in dance school, and from that point on, dance became her main challenge and focus in life.

As a freshman at Northwestern University in Evanston, Illinois, Sheppard landed a part in the school's major annual production. During the performance, she was spotted by a local agent and producer, which led to the establishment of her professional career.

During her junior and senior years at Northwestern, she continued her classes and danced professionally on a regular basis. Sheppard then graduated in theater and radio/television with an emphasis on dance. In 1966 she married Jack Missett.

In addition to her professional career, she devoted a great deal of time to teaching dance because she enjoyed it so much. Teaching grew frustrating to her, however, because of the large turnover in her classes. Curious as to why this was happening, she determined that her students only wanted to feel like dancers, to enjoy the movements and physical activity associated with dance; they did not want to train to become professionals.

Rethinking her teaching techniques, she created some simple dance routines based on jazz dance, which students could follow simply by watching her. During the hour class, students not only enjoyed the feeling of being dancers but benefited from the physical exercise they were receiving. Thus, Jazzercise was born in Chicago in 1969.

Judi Sheppard Missett moved to Southern California in 1972. Jazzercise began to grow in popularity as her students moved to different parts of the country. Today it is taught throughout the United States and in many foreign countries.

The Jazzercise Workout is divided into levels I, II, and III, with III being the most physically demanding. The program provides various methods to ascertain a person's "Jazzercise Fitness Level," which determines what level of intensity she should be using.

Each level consists of a warm-up/isolation segment, an aerobic segment, a muscle-toning segment, and a cooldown/flexibility segment.

In levels II and III the aerobic segment is more intense, while the muscle-toning segment covers more areas of the body than in level I. Each segment has a choice of different musical selections that accompany it. To produce the desired effect the selection must have the proper beat, rhythm, tempo, and continuity.

Today Jazzercise classes are available in virtually any city or town. A detailed explanation of Jazzercise can be found in Judi Sheppard Missett's book, *The Jazzercise Workout Book*.

❧ | JIN SHIN DO BODYMIND ACUPRESSURE | ❧

Jin Shin Do Bodymind Acupressure is a complete body/mind system of Acupressure which focuses on the deep release of muscular tension through gentle yet deep finger pressure, liberating both physical and emotional tensions.

Jin Shin Do means "the Way of the Compassionate Spirit" or "the Way of the Heart." It is an integrated system which combines traditional Japanese Acupressure techniques, Western psychology (Reich, Jung, etc.), and Taoist philosophy and breathing methods. Not only does Jin Shin Do address pain, it affects both physical and emotional tension within the body.

Jin Shin Do Bodymind Acupressure was developed by Iona Marsaa Teeguarden over a period of nearly twenty years. During this time she was involved with different types of professional therapeutic bodywork in the United States, Canada, and Europe. She studied with Acupressure/Acupuncture masters in both the United States and Japan.

Jin Shin Do is both a self-help technique and a professional therapeutic method. In its most basic form it is an easy-to-learn self-help tool. A unique thirty-point system, color-coded chart, and simple-to-use "release recipes" make it easy for beginners to help themselves, family, and friends.

In the hands of a skilled and sensitive practitioner, Jin Shin Do can be a

powerful healing and transformational tool that complements other therapeutic methods. During a Jin Shin Do session, which lasts about sixty to
ninety minutes, the client lies on a table and remains clothed.

Jin Shin Do therapy is effective in treating headaches, insomnia, back
pain, physical and emotional stress, eyestrain, tension and fatigue, and other
ailments. It is also effective in dealing with distressing emotional feelings
like hurt, anxiety, depression, guilt, and anger, and promotes a deep sense
of relaxation, increased awareness, and inner harmony.

To become a registered Jin Shin Do Acupressure practitioner requires the
following training: 125 hours of training from an authorized teacher plus
25 additional hours of counseling/process skills, 125 hours of Jin Shin Do
Acupressure practice, ten private sessions with an authorized practitioner-
teacher, a practical hands-on examination, and licensure/certification in a
health/helping profession.

A directory of authorized teachers and registered acupressurists is available from the Jin Shin Do Foundation for Bodymind Acupressure. For additional information, two books written by Iona Marsaa Teeguarden are
available: *The Acupressure Way of Health: Jin Shin Do* and *The Joy of Feeling:
Bodymind Acupressure.*

❧ | JIN SHIN JYUTSU | ☙

Jin Shin Jyutsu is the art of releasing tensions from within the body
which are the causes of various physical symptoms. It is considered an art as
opposed to a technique because a technique is a mechanical application,
whereas an art is a skillful creation.

The literal translation from Japanese is *Jin*: "Man of Knowing and Compassion," *Shin*: "Creator," and *Jyutsu*: "Art." The common translation is "Art of
the Creator through man of knowing and compassion."

According to ancient written records, which remain in the Archives of
the Imperial Palace in Japan, Jin Shin Jyutsu was widely known before the
birth of Guatama Buddha (the Indian philosopher and founder of Buddhism) or the birth of Moses (as recorded in the Bible).

Jin Shin Jyutsu came to Japan via Tibet and China. Based on ancient
knowledge of the body and creation, it was passed on orally from one generation to the next. Individual parts of the information, in written form,
were buried in different Shinto temples throughout Japan. It was said that if
a map of man were superimposed over a map of Japan, that each point on

the body would mark the location of a Shinto temple and in that temple could be found information for that particular body point.

This information disappeared and was virtually unknown in Japan until it was rediscovered in the early 1900s by a Japanese philosopher named Jiro Murai.

Murai had contracted an illness that was diagnosed as terminal. As custom dictated, he asked his family to take him to the mountains and leave him in solitude for seven days. Before leaving, a shaman (natural healer) showed him some hand techniques he could use on himself. While on the mountain he incurred chills and fever, and was in and out of consciousness. At the end of seven days Murai realized he had recovered, and vowed to learn this system that had healed him.

Through extensive study of the Bible, ancient Greek, Indian, and Chinese texts, and the *Kojiki* (the Japanese "Record of Ancient Things" dating back to A.D. 712), Murai unraveled the mystery. Combining the information he had learned with fifty years of experimentation, Murai concluded that Jin Shin Jyutsu was more than a philosophy of the body. He later studied the Chinese acupuncture points to add to his understanding.

Mary Ino Burmeister, a Japanese-American born in Seattle, Washington, wanted to be an interpreter for the United Nations. In the late 1940s she went to Japan to study the language. Through a casual meeting she met a man named Jiro Murai. His first words to her were, "How would you like to study with me to take a gift from Japan to America?" This began Burmeister's five years of study with Murai in Japan, which were followed by seven more years in the United States by correspondence.

After completing her studies with Murai, nearly twenty more years passed before she began to share her knowledge. Today Jin Shin Jyutsu practitioners can be found worldwide. Training seminars, for those wanting to become practitioners or those wanting to learn it for self-help, are held on a regular basis throughout the United States and in Europe.

Jin Shin Jyutsu works like Acupuncture by helping energy flow freely through the body. The vital life force energy, or *chi*, flows in meridians (energy channels or pathways) that travel throughout the body and on the surface of the skin. When one or more of these pathways becomes blocked, this damming effect can lead to discomfort or pain. Disease is viewed as a symptom of physical, mental, or emotional stress—created blockages in the body's energy pathways.

Vital life energy flows up the back and down the front of the body. The Jin Shin Jyutsu energy map of the body is somewhat similar to Acupuncture's meridian map, but has considerably fewer points. In Jin Shin Jyutsu, energy flow can become blocked in any of the twenty-six points called "safety energy locks," which are located throughout the body and in the organs themselves.

To clear these blockages, the practitioner places her hands on two different points (various combinations of the twenty-six) on the recipient's body and applies gentle pressure for one to five minutes.

Jin Shin Jyutsu utilizes the vital life energy flowing throughout the recipient's body, making use of what is flowing through the practitioner's hands, to recharge the recipient's energy in blocked areas.

This process does not take away energy from the practitioner since she is acting only as a conduit or channel through which energy flows. The practitioner's hands merely act as "jumper cables."

The recharged energy is then able to release the stress-caused blockages in the energy pathways. Harmony is restored to the system and the body, mind, and spirit are brought into balance.

Jin Shin Jyutsu does not diagnose, heal, or cure any illness, physical or emotional. It merely restores the free flow of energy, allowing the body to function at its optimum level.

Like traditional Acupuncture, Jin Shin Jyutsu also deals with the organ-emotion relationship. Weakness in a particular organ will make the individual more susceptible to the corresponding emotion. For example, weakness in the kidney and bladder would make an individual more likely to exhibit fear.

Mary Burmeister maintains that Jin Shin Jyutsu is an inborn art (ability) that anyone can learn without a great deal of training. Although it can be received from a practitioner, one of the major benefits is that it can be used as a self-healing tool. It can be practiced at almost any time as it works through clothing and can even penetrate a cast or brace.

Jin Shin Jyutsu, Inc. offers two-part seminars in the Jin Shin Jyutsu technique throughout the United States, and in Canada, South America, and Europe. Additionally, several self-help books on various aspects of Jin Shin Jyutsu and a chart of the twenty-six safety energy locks are available. For additional information and the name of a practitioner in your area contact Jin Shin Jyutsu, Inc.

❧ | LABAN MOVEMENT ANALYSIS | ☙

Laban Movement Analysis is a method for observing, describing, and interpreting the component parts or elements that make up every movement, from a simple conversational hand gesture to a complicated dance step.

Laban Movement Analysis was developed by Rudolf Laban (1879–1958), an Austro-Hungarian dancer, choreographer, philosopher, and teacher. Laban formalized a framework of basic principles for the understanding of movement structure and purpose.

The work in movement studies was further advanced by a student and colleague of Laban's, Irmgard Bartenieff (1900–81). She applied her Laban training to the field of physical therapy and developed her own system of body reeducation, which is called Bartenieff Fundamentals.

In addition to being a Labanotation expert, she was a pioneer in the development of dance therapy. Bartenieff originated a professional training program in Laban Movement Studies in 1965. In 1978 she founded the Laban/Bartenieff Institute of Movement Studies in New York City.

Laban Movement Analysis gives an increased awareness of what movement communicates and expresses. There are three primary elements of movement: (1) the body, (2) the space in which the body moves, and (3) the intention behind the movement. This triad of elements provides a valuable basis for understanding and analyzing movement in many different fields, including dance, theater, nonverbal communication, and therapy.

It can be effectively used by bodyworkers and physical therapists to analyze a client's movement patterns and suggest new possibilities, and by dance therapists and psychotherapists to understand a patient's nonverbal behavior and to support a diagnosis.

Today, a professional training program leading to a certificate in Laban Movement Studies as a certified movement analyst (C.M.A.) requires approximately five hundred hours of class instruction time with regular evaluation sessions and comprehensive movement, oral, and written examinations.

Currently there are more than five hundred certified movement analysts practicing in various fields. For additional information contact the Laban/Bartenieff Institute of Movement Studies. They can provide the name and address of a certified movement analyst in your area.

❧ | LIFE EXTENSION | ❧

Life Extension is the use of various drugs, therapies, nutrient supplements (vitamins, minerals, amino acids), and other ostensible health aids, and the modification of various lifestyle and environmental factors to increase an individual's life expectancy.

Although the basic idea of Life Extension has been around for many years, it received a great amount of notoriety in the late 1970s and early 1980s when Life Extension guru Durk Pearson appeared on several television shows, and then, with Sandy Shaw, wrote the classic *Life Extension: A Practical Scientific Approach* in 1982, followed by *The Life Extension Companion* in 1984.

Durk Pearson graduated from the Massachusetts Institute of Technology in 1965 with a degree in physics and enough extra class credits for degrees in biology and psychology as well. After graduation, he started a scientific consulting business in aerospace, energy, and Life Extension. Pearson's biomedical research was aimed at extending human longevity.

Sandy Shaw earned a degree in chemistry from the University of California, Los Angeles, in 1965. She has been a consultant to major food, nutrient, pharmaceutical, and cosmetic companies. Shaw spent many years researching the biochemical aging processes and how to control them.

The aging process, commonly thought of as something that is inevitable and happens with the passage of time, is really a naturally occurring progressive deterioration of various biochemical and cellular functions within the body.

Aging is not a single process; different systems within any individual body age at different rates. The rate of aging depends on how well the body repairs itself in relation to the damage that has occurred.

When damage to the different body systems outstrips its ability to repair itself, aging occurs. So, as an individual's physiological functions become progressively impaired, his chances for continued vitality and longevity are reduced.

The goal of Life Extension is not merely adding years to one's life, but more important, to improve the quality of life and to live in peak mental and physical condition for as long as possible. It would make little sense to add ten or twenty years to the life of a person who was already decrepit and marginally functioning.

Life Extension takes a conscious effort and is a lifetime activity. There are various degrees of Life Extension, depending on how much time, effort, money, resolve, and determination an individual has to accomplish his goal.

Although most Life Extension activities would be considered self-help in nature, it is recommended that a medical doctor knowledgeable in the field of Life Extension be consulted prior to starting, and while on a Life Extension program the doctor should monitor bodily functions and prescribe nutrients and/or drugs.

A program of Life Extension can be as simple as avoiding activities that are harmful such as smoking, drinking excessive amounts of alcohol, running or jogging in polluted air, and overeating to obesity. If an individual is unwilling to change his lifestyle and insists on putting harmful substances into his body, he can take inexpensive nutrients to counteract the deleterious effects of these substances.

In contrast to vitamins, minerals, and amino acids, Live Cell Therapy and Gerovital are more sophisticated Life Extension therapies that utilize expensive drugs and other therapies which are available only in Europe and Mexico.

In Live Cell Therapy, live cells are injected into the body. Pioneered in Switzerland by the late Paul Niehans, M.D., this therapy is used to regenerate weak and exhausted body systems and slow down the aging process.

Gerovital (GH_3) Therapy was developed in Romania by Dr. Ana Alsans. Given by injection, this drug is used for rejuvenation, longevity, and immune system enhancement.

Extensive research into the mechanism of aging is an ongoing process. The Life Extension Foundation in Hollywood, Florida, publishes a monthly report that provides up-to-date information in the field of Life Extension.

✍ | LIVE CELL THERAPY | ☙

Live Cell Therapy, also called Cellular Therapy or the "fresh-cell" method of Cellular Therapy, is the implantation of healthy cells, especially those taken from unborn animals, into human beings for a variety of therapeutic purposes including revitalization of the body and the treatment of degenerative diseases.

In the 1930s Paul Niehans, M.D., a noted Swiss surgeon and endocrinologist, developed a method of cellular revitalization he called Live Cell

Therapy and pioneered its use in treating patients for a myriad of degenerative diseases.

Live Cell Therapy can be used to help regenerate organs and organ systems that are weakened from aging and/or chronic disease. To be effective, Live Cell Therapy requires that the malfunctioning organ is still able to react to stimulation.

Another use of Live Cell Therapy is to strengthen the immune system. Cells from an unborn calf are normally used because the calf has not yet developed an immune system and therefore the cells will not be rejected by the patient's immune system as a foreign invader. This treatment has been used as an alternative cancer therapy of the immunotherapy variety.

Live Cell Therapy is based on the scientifically validated fact that specific fetal cells, when injected into a host, travel to the corresponding organ from which they were procured and revitalize the homologous cell activity. For example, fetal liver cells migrate to the host liver and stimulate regeneration.

Live Cell Therapy has long been popular among world leaders and Hollywood celebrities, including Winston Churchill, Konrad Adenauer, Charles de Gaulle, Dwight Eisenhower, Charlie Chaplin, Elizabeth Taylor, Bob Hope, and many others to prolong vitality and preserve youthful appearance.

A book titled *Live Cell Therapy* by endocrinologist Wolfram Kuhnau, M.D., is available for further reading (see resource guide).

Although Live Cell Therapy is currently unlicensed for use in the United States, the treatment is available at a number of alternative therapy clinics in Mexico and it is also available at some exclusive clinics in Switzerland.

❧ | LIVINGSTON TREATMENT | ❧

The Livingston Treatment is a specialized treatment based upon immunological enhancement to strengthen a patient's natural immune defense system to fight disease.

Included among these immunological enhancement therapies and techniques are vaccines, diet and nutrition, vitamins, psychological counseling, detoxification, use of antibiotics to overcome underlying infections, and traditional drug therapy—as long as it is consistent with enhancing the natural immune system.

The late Virginia Wuerthele-Caspe Livingston, M.D., was born in Meadville, Pennsylvania. After graduating from Vassar College, she received her M.D. from New York University. After holding various professorships and research positions she founded the Livingston Medical Clinic in San Diego, California, in 1971, with her late husband, Afton Munk Livingston.

Until her death in 1990, Dr. Virginia Livingston specialized in the research and clinical treatment of immune-deficient diseases such as cancer, arthritis, lupus, and scleroderma. This work laid the foundation for the present Livingston Foundation Medical Center's clinical program of immune system enhancement to fight these diseases.

Dr. Virginia Livingston believed that cancer is caused by a microbe she called *progenitor cryptocides*, which lives within the body of every individual. Disease is caused only when an individual's immune system is in a depressed or weakened condition.

Proper diet is an integral element of modern immunotherapy. Because the immune system cannot be sustained on a diet of foods devitalized by overprocessing, Dr. Livingston recommended a vegetarian diet of "live foods." Raw or lightly cooked vegetables provide the enzymes and vitamins essential to a healthy immune system. The diet eliminates all poultry because she believed it is contaminated with the *cryptocides* microbe.

Two excellent books by Dr. Virginia Livingston are available: *Food Alive: A Diet for Cancer and Chronic Disease*, published in 1977, describes her "live food" vegetarian diet, and *Conquest of Cancer*, published in 1984, details the medical techniques and remarkable results obtained through her treatments.

Today, the Livingston Foundation Medical Center provides immunological treatment programs based on the models developed by Dr. Virginia Livingston during her more than fifty years of research. For additional information on the Livingston Treatment contact the center.

✍ | LOMILOMI MASSAGE | ✍

Lomilomi Massage is an ancient massage technique from Hawaii. Culturally, it is *the* massage form of the indigenous Hawaiian people.

In the Hawaiian language, *lomilomi* basically means "rub rub." When used in a context of massage, however, Lomilomi refers to the technique of breaking up muscle spasms with a special movement of the fingers.

"Aunty" Margaret Machado defines Hawaiian Lomilomi as "the loving touch—a connection between heart, hand, and soul with the source of all life."

Although the history of Hawaiian Lomilomi is not well documented, it is known to be an ancient form of massage. Throughout Polynesia, a huge area of the southwest Pacific Ocean dotted with volcanic and coral islands, this honored healing art was passed from generation to generation within a family. Although each family's technique was somewhat different, some religious aspect of Lomilomi was common to most.

The skills needed to practice Lomilomi were also passed on to family successors by "kahunas" as part of their knowledge of healing methods and religious ceremonies. In old Hawaii, kahunas were similar to a medicine man or shaman in the Native American culture. They were trained as expert caretakers and transmitters of knowledge. Kahunas were a powerful group in Hawaii and other parts of Polynesia before the influence of Christian missionaries in the early nineteenth century.

Probably the first Hawaiian outside of the Kahuna family to share the secrets of Lomilomi Massage was Margaret Machado. Today, hers is the outstanding name associated with Lomilomi Massage. Familiarly known as "Aunty," Margaret Machado was born in Hawaii in 1916. After completing her high school education, she became a nurse. Eventually Machado opened a massage salon, and word of her healing abilities rapidly spread. This led her to develop charts that diagram Lomilomi Massage as she practices it. Later, she formally taught her methods.

Authentic Lomilomi Massage is therapeutic in value, and is characterized as being both relaxing and reviving. It uses a variety of massage strokes and pressure points such as those found in Reflexology or Shiatsu, except that the pressure point is held for a shorter length of time. A distinguishing feature of Lomilomi is that it incorporates both physical and spiritual aspects. Awareness of the relationship between God and man is of foremost importance.

Lomilomi is a direct massage technique that is applied to muscles in a state of acute or chronic tension. A unique feature of Lomilomi is the use of the forearm and elbow by the practitioner. In old Hawaii, a specially carved stick was used for deeper massage. A steam bath and shower after the massage are also considered an important part of the process in order to rid the body of toxins released during the massage.

Lomilomi can be used to treat a variety of musculoskeletal problems; the benefits, as in other massage techniques, are increased circulation of blood and lymph, which bring oxygen and nutrients to the affected area and remove waste products. It is also used in the Hawaiian culture as part of childbearing practices. Basic technique is a moving cross-fiber friction done with oils.

Currently, Aunty Margaret Machado teaches Lomilomi Massage at her school in Hawaii. For additional information contact the school.

❧ | LOOYENWORK | ❧

LooyenWork is a unique synthesis of painless deep tissue body therapy, movement reeducation, and environmental evaluation.

The LooyenWork technique is a hybrid. It utilizes essential parts of several well-established physical restructuring techniques including Postural Integration, the Feldenkrais Method, Aston-Patterning, Rolfing, and others. When these different elements are synthesized as LooyenWork, the results achieved are greater than if any single technique is separately applied.

Ted Looyen is the creator of LooyenWork. He was born in Holland and educated in Sydney, Australia. As a counselor and therapist with the Government Health Commission in Sydney, he became known for his ability to form immediate and profound connections with his clients.

In 1973 he began his career as a bodyworker in response to a severe back problem. Looyen received many different therapies in Australia and found that deep tissue work (Rolfing) produced the most effective results. He was not convinced, however, that the pain of deep tissue work was necessary, and set out to develop a noninvasive approach that could still effect profound structural changes.

Looyen studied a wide range of therapies including Postural Integration, the Feldenkrais Method, Aston-Patterning, and many more. Twelve years later, he had perfected a technique that accomplished all the positive effects of deep tissue work, but without the pain usually associated with it.

In 1986 Ted Looyen brought LooyenWork to the United States. Currently, his unique method of bodywork is known and practiced worldwide.

It is Looyen's belief that a bodyworker inflicting pain on a client is a repetition of the assault on the body that caused problems in the first place. Therefore, this approach to treatment would not produce optimum results, since the client would have to deal with the additional trauma that was inflicted by the bodyworker.

Ted Looyen always felt it was imperative that the approach to treatment be painless for change to occur. Traumatic painful experiences, whether emotional or physical, need gentle unraveling.

LooyenWork addresses the uniqueness of each individual. The practitioner does this by first identifying the individual's "core issue" through a sophisticated form of body reading. This core issue comprises the visible effects of emotional, psychological, and physical traumatic experience.

Once the core issue has been determined, the practitioner develops a session to treat the client's particular problem. Each session is different because every physical body has different problems. In LooyenWork, there is no standard number of treatments. Each session is complete in itself and different facets of the problem are worked on in subsequent sessions. There is no standard number of treatments.

The practitioner, using the fingertips in a gentle yet deep manner, releases connective tissue adhesions, lengthens chronically contracted muscles, and separates tendons. Although gentle to the client, these penetrating movements of the fingertips result in profound structural change.

In this process the client surrenders to and forms a healing partnership with the therapist. Understanding the body's resistance and fear patterns enables the practitioner to release accumulated holding patterns such as postural imbalances, and emotional and physical traumas.

Often a few sessions of LooyenWork, working with the core issue, are more effective in facilitating change than many years of traditional bodywork and psychotherapy. LooyenWork is often prescribed as an important adjunct to traditional medicine.

❧ | MACROBIOTIC SHIATSU | ❧

Macrobiotic Shiatsu is a preventive health care system which effectively combines dietary therapy and a natural healing art based on the principles of Traditional Chinese Medicine.

Shizuko Yamamoto, one of the world's leading macrobiotic counselors and Shiatsu practitioners, founded Macrobiotic Shiatsu. She also originated Barefoot Shiatsu, the application of which includes nutrition, exercise, and proper breathing. Yamamoto was trained in martial arts, natural healing, Yoga, and cooking arts.

The word *macrobiotics* comes from the Greek words *macro*, meaning "large or great," and *bios*, meaning "life." Macrobiotics is a way of living that respects the physical, biological, emotional, mental, ecological, and spiritual order of our daily lives. Eating and living within this natural order lead to happiness, health, and an appreciation for the simple things in life.

Shiatsu means "finger pressure" in Japanese. It is based on traditional Oriental medical practices. Shiatsu uses carefully judged pressure, properly applied to specific points on the body's surface with the fingers, knuckles, and hands. As a therapy it stimulates the body's natural curative powers and ability to recuperate from illness. In the practice of Barefoot Shiatsu, the feet are used as well as the hands.

Macrobiotic Shiatsu is holistic in nature. All aspects of an individual are considered, including physical, mental, and environmental factors in the individual's life as well as ancestral history. Its goal is to create balance within the individual.

As a preventive health care system, it stresses a lifestyle that is conducive to overall health and well-being. This is accomplished through proper diet and nutrition (eating a macrobiotic diet), abundant exercise, proper breathing, and a regulated sex life. It also requires other preventive measures such as making adjustments in diet and other routines during changes in seasons and weather. By adhering to these elements, optimum relative balance is maintained within and without the body.

Diagnosis is an important part of the Macrobiotic Shiatsu process. To assess the client's needs and determine the treatment necessary, Macrobiotic Shiatsu practitioners use a variety of diagnostic methods. They observe the face, body, posture (sitting and standing), and breathing patterns. They inquire into the client's health history, emotional state, and day-to-day routine. Many other signs visible on the body are also used. Through touch, the condition of the skin, muscles, and internal organs can be determined. Other techniques are used to determine the relationship between internal organs, energy, and diet.

To correct problems caused by imbalanced conditions the practitioner has remedies available in both Macrobiotics and Shiatsu; he may also use moxabustion (heating), tapping, and cupping.

The International Macrobiotic Shiatsu Society (IMSS) provides comprehensive education in Macrobiotic Shiatsu. Courses vary from a 15-hour seminar given over two days to a professional intensive residential program covering 360 hours of training.

For a more detailed description of Macrobiotic Shiatsu, a book titled *The Shiatsu Handbook* by Shizuko Yamamoto and Patrick McCarty, and a video titled *Barefoot Shiatsu* by Shizuko Yamamoto may be obtained from the IMSS, as can an International Practitioners Referral List and a newsletter.

❧ | MACROBIOTICS | ❦

Macrobiotics is a way of living that respects the physical, biological, emotional, mental, ecological, and spiritual order of our daily lives. Macrobiotic theory begins with the realization that there is a natural order to all things. Eating and living within this natural order leads to happiness, health, and an appreciation for the simple things in life. It is practicing the art of balance in all aspects of life.

Macrobiotics is not a specific diet, nutritional program, or the adhering to a set of dietary rules, but is more of an individual approach. The word *macrobiotics* comes from the Greek words *macro*, meaning "large or great," and *bios*, meaning "life."

Principles of the Macrobiotic diet go back several thousand years, when wise men in the Orient realized that food not only provides nourishment for the body but is also instrumental in creating health and happiness.

In the early 1900s, Japanese physician Sagen Ishizuka instituted the theory of nutrition and medicine based on the Oriental diet and Western science. The diet was very popular and he prescribed it for numerous patients daily. Ishizuka was born a weak child and in his early life suffered from disease.

Determined to improve his health, Ishizuka investigated diet and read thousands of books from both the East and West. From his lifelong study came two books, *Chemical Theory of Longevity* and *Biochemical Way to Health and Happiness*. After his death, Ishizuka's followers formed a Macrobiotic association, but due to lack of leadership it began to decline. Among these followers was George Ohsawa, twenty-two years old at the time, who took over the association and returned it to the successful status it once enjoyed.

George Ohsawa (1893–1966) devoted his entire life to educating people around the world about Oriental philosophy and its application. He was the first person to use the term *macrobiotics*. As a young man in Japan, he cured himself of tuberculosis with the diet. During his lifetime Ohsawa wrote roughly three hundred books.

In 1959 Ohsawa came to the United States from Japan and settled in New York City. Ohsawa began teaching there, and the first Macrobiotic summer camp in the United States was held at Southampton, Long Island, in July 1960. Later he moved to California and established the George Ohsawa Macrobiotic Foundation in Oroville.

The Macrobiotic dietary approach begins with a reorientation of everyday eating habits by selecting proper foods which will contribute to health and happiness. It recommends changing to a low-fat, low-protein, high-complex carbohydrate, and high-fiber diet.

Macrobiotic eating means gaining an understanding of how different foods affect each individual with regard to needs, preferences, and circumstances. What works one day may not work the next. Because we are in a constant state of change, diet can be modified by selecting foods most appropriate for meeting the current conditions or needs.

Although there are thousands of foods on earth, it is not within the natural order that all foods be for man's consumption. Macrobiotics makes a simple division between animal food and vegetal food, and chooses mainly vegetal.

Within the vegetal realm grains are most abundant on earth so they are the first choice in Macrobiotic cooking. Generally, man's foods, in order of importance, are grains, vegetables, salt, oil, nuts, fruits, and fish. An important part of Macrobiotic philosophy is that only locally grown produce that is normally in season at the time it is to be consumed be used. For example, if it is winter in New York you would not eat squash—normally grown there only in the summer—even though squash air freighted from South America is available.

Contrary to popular belief, Macrobiotic principles do not restrict the consumption of any particular food. Macrobiotic fare is more than just brown rice; it is based on a wide variety of unrefined grains, vegetables, soups, beans, and sea vegetables, as well as some meat, fruits, and nuts.

Typically, whole cereal grains comprise at least 50 percent by volume of every meal. These can include oats, barley, corn, millet, rye, wheat, and brown rice prepared in a variety of ways.

Soups made with vegetables, grains, seaweed, or beans and seasoned with tamari soy sauce or miso comprise about 5 to 10 percent of daily food intake.

A wide variety of vegetables, preferably local and organically grown, comprises approximately 20 to 30 percent of the diet. These vegetables include broccoli, green cabbage, Chinese cabbage, mustard greens, acorn squash, pumpkin, carrots, and many other perennials and seasonal varieties. They can be boiled, sautéed with oil, steamed, or eaten raw in small quantities.

Beans and sea vegetables comprise about 5 to 10 percent of the daily food intake. The preferred beans are chickpeas, adzuki beans, and lentils. Other types of beans may be used occasionally. Various sea vegetables and Irish moss can be prepared in soups, cooked with other dishes, or served as a side dish.

Certain foods if desired are for occasional use, usually one to three times a week, and should not constitute more than 5 to 10 percent of that day's total intake. These include white meat fish, fruits such as apples, berries, plums, peaches, and melons, and lightly roasted nuts and seeds such as peanuts, pecans, walnuts, and pumpkin or sunflower seeds.

Foods to avoid include meat, poultry, eggs, dairy products, animal fats, refined sugar, tropical and semitropical fruits, fruit juices, canned or frozen foods, coffee, tea, nightshade vegetables (potatoes, tomatoes, peppers, and eggplants), and others.

Preparation is an important part of Macrobiotic cooking as it can change the effect of food. For example, steaming or boiling food in more water with less salt will help to relax a person both physically and emotionally.

Vegetables are living foods and should be used whole to get total nutrition. They should not be peeled, nor should the leaves or roots be discarded. (There are some exceptions; for example, rhubarb leaves are poisonous.) Also, the direction and way in which vegetables are cut influence their yin and yang balance. The knife and cutting board should be cleaned after cutting each vegetable so that each may retain its own distinct qualities. Love, kindness, and generosity are basic ingredients in Macrobiotic cooking.

Eating Macrobiotically can range from very simple meals to an extensive number of dishes prepared with a variety of foods, depending on an individual's needs and circumstances. Another important aspect of Macrobiotic eating is chewing each mouthful of food thoroughly, from fifty to a hundred times. Also, through Macrobiotic eating an individual can gain insights into how different foods affect her health.

Although the Macrobiotic diet is not specifically a therapeutic nutritional program, it can have a definite impact on health. In his book *The Macrobiotic Approach to Cancer: Towards Preventing and Controlling Cancer with Diet and Lifestyle*, Michio Kushi details how the Macrobiotic diet and lifestyle have helped numerous individuals recover from illness, prevent disease, and find balance in life through peace of mind and better health.

Today, two of the most prominent names in the field of Macrobiotics are Michio and Aveline Kushi. Founders of the Kushi Institute, they have spent the past forty years teaching about the principles of Macrobiotic living. They teach how to attain and maintain health and a more peaceful world by adopting a more natural way of eating and living. The Kushis lecture at health conferences throughout the United States.

For additional information contact the Kushi Institute. The institute has available a wide variety of books on Macrobiotics and related subjects, cookbooks, audio- and videotapes, kitchenware, and Macrobiotic specialty foods. The Kushi Institute also conducts residential programs in cooking instruction, health seminars, and other programs.

Also, information can be obtained from the George Ohsawa Macrobiotic Foundation, including a complete line of books on Macrobiotics and other related subjects and a videotape on how to prepare Macrobiotic meals. The foundation publishes a bimonthly newsletter called *Macrobiotics Today*. Through the Vega Study Center they offer a variety of residential programs on cooking instruction and seminars on a variety of subjects.

❧ | MAGNETIC THERAPY | ❦

Magnetic Therapy, also known as Biomagnetic Therapy, is the application of specially designed magnets or magnetic fields to the human body for therapeutic purposes. It is a safe, noninvasive therapy.

The healing power of magnetism has been known to mankind for thousands of years. During the third century B.C., the Greek philosopher Aristotle was the first person in recorded history to speak about the therapeutic properties of natural magnets. Other ancient cultures including the Chinese, Arab, Egyptian, Indian, and Hebrew had knowledge of magnets and used them for healing purposes.

Around 200 B.C. a Greek physician and writer named Galen found that pain, caused by a variety of illnesses, could be relieved by applying natural magnets to different areas of the body. Lodestone shaped into amulets, bracelets, and other devices was used.

During the first century B.C. Chinese physicians recorded the effect that variations in the earth's magnetic field had on health and disease.

Around A.D. 1000 a Persian physician documented the use of magnets to relieve muscle spasms and treat gout, a disease marked by painful inflammation of the joints. In Europe during the Middle Ages physicians used powdered lodestone in potions and for topical application.

In the 1700s an Austrian physician named Franz Anton Mesmer wrote a dissertation on magnetism. Although he was severely ridiculed at the time, Mesmer's work has since proven to be a foundation for magnetic healing in the West. In 1843, I. Eydan studied the application of a magnetic field to the human body for therapeutic purposes. After World War II, Russian army doctors used magnets to reduce pain after the amputation of limbs.

By 1958 extensive work on Magnetic Therapy was being done in Japan. In 1959 Kyoichi Nakagawa, M.D., one of the world's foremost authorities on the therapeutic effects of magnetism on the human body, reported on a group of symptomatic conditions that responded favorably to Magnetic Therapy when other methods failed.

A recent study conducted by the Massachusetts Institute of Technology proved conclusively that biomagnetic products used on the body increase the flow of blood, which contributes to the healing process.

The therapeutic magnets used today are quite different in appearance from the standard bar or horseshoe magnet made from iron. Most therapeutic magnets are manufactured in Japan and Europe, where extensive research on the subject has been done.

Modern biomagnets are made from different materials and have a permanent magnetic charge. Two basic styles of biomagnets are the small, hard ferrite type, and the flat, flexible, rubberlike pad type.

Ferrite magnets are incorporated into a variety of devices such as mattress pads, pillowlike head supports, supports for the joints (wrist, elbow, and knee), vests, and jewelry such as necklaces and bracelets.

Flexible pad magnets are available in a variety of shapes and sizes that may be attached directly to an injury or pain site on the body. They can also be molded into various shapes such as insoles for shoes.

Today millions of people around the world reap the benefit of Magnetic Therapy by sleeping on magnetic futons or mattress pads, using magnetic shoe insoles which stimulate the Reflexology points on the sole of the foot as they walk, and using the many other biomagnetic products available.

Magnets themselves are not responsible for healing, but rather stimulate the body's innate capacity to heal itself. The magnetic field produced by therapeutic magnets affects living cells by creating an optimal environment in which they can exist at their best and most efficient level of functioning.

Many physical conditions, both injury and disease, are marked by impeded blood flow in the body. An ample supply of oxygenated, nutrient-rich blood is absolutely essential to the healing process. When a magnet is applied to the human body, magnetic waves pass through the tissue and a principle in physics known as the "Hall effect" works to stimulate blood flow.

Charged particles (positive and negative ions) in the bloodstream are attracted to the corresponding positive and negative poles of the therapeutic magnet, which is placed on or near the site being treated. These magnetic polarities create ionic currents and patterns which act to dilate the blood vessels and increase blood flow to the affected area.

Magnetic fields are more effective than electric current in increasing blood flow because the wavelengths emitted by magnets penetrate the skin more easily and flow into the body through fat, nerves, and bones. Electrical stimulation only penetrates to a depth of approximately ten millimeters.

In recent years magnetic field therapy has been found to aid in the recovery of both acute and chronic conditions. In the Soviet Union, doctors regularly used magnets to speed wound healing after surgery, to improve circulation, and to strengthen and mend bones.

Acute conditions include sprains, strains, broken bones, and soft tissue trauma (cuts and burns). Additionally, results have shown that when Magnetic Therapy is used, the quality of healing is better (less scar tissue) and occurs at a more rapid rate.

Chronic conditions such as degenerative joint disease, certain forms of arthritis, and diabetic ulcers have been reduced or reversed with Magnetic Therapy.

In Japan, the Ministry of Welfare (equivalent to the U.S. Food and Drug Administration) has already approved the use of biomagnetic products for the treatment of injuries.

In Japanese Acupuncture, magnets are used in conjunction with needles on specific Acupuncture points. A magnet can be incorporated into the head of a small, tacklike needle. These specialized needles are worn for a specific length of time.

Although the state of California has outlawed the use of magnets by licensed health care practitioners for healing purposes, they are still available for self-help use.

Food and Drug Administration approval of magnetic healing devices is probably a long time off. However, many magnetic devices proven and accepted in Japan and other parts of the world are currently available in the United States for self-help use. One Japanese company that manufactures a wide range of self-help biomagnetic products that are available in the United States is Nikken. Consult the resource section for additional sources.

Two recent books on the subject, *The Body Magnetic* and *Getting Started in Magnetic Healing* by Dr. Buryl Payne, provide excellent information. Dr. Payne is a physicist-psychologist, and the inventor of the first biofeedback instrument.

❧ | MAHARISHI AYUR-VEDA | ❧

Maharishi Ayur-Veda is an adaptation of the four-thousand- to six-thousand-year-old Indian holistic health system known as Ayurvedic medicine, which utilizes herbal remedies, diet, massage, and Hatha Yoga to promote healing.

Ayurvedic medicine, or Ayurveda, is a complete health care system which emphasizes prevention of disease as well as promotion of health and longevity. Ayurveda is more than just a healing system, it is the science and art of appropriate living.

During centuries of foreign rule in India, Ayurvedic institutions declined in India, and much Ayurvedic knowledge became misunderstood or lost. Recently Maharishi Mahesh Yogi, founder of the Transcendental Meditation (TM) program, in collaboration with several leading Ayurvedic physicians and scholars revived this ancient tradition and introduced it to the West.

Maharishi Ayur-Veda, the modern reformulation of this traditional health care system, is based on classical Ayurvedic texts and includes Transcendental Meditation as an integral part. It holds that the primary force in the cause of disease is imbalance resulting from the disruption of homeostasis or the immune system.

Because it has never separated body from mind, Maharishi Ayur-Veda places importance on mental, emotional, and behavioral factors, which are seen as critical in the development of these imbalances.

There are four comprehensive approaches to treatment: consciousness, physiology, behavior, and environment. Each of these approaches encompasses several types of therapies. All Maharishi Ayur-Veda treatments are based upon a person's body type or physiological constitution as determined by an Ayurvedic physician.

Treatment programs for most common diseases, including high blood pressure, insomnia, arthritis, weight problems, anxiety, headaches, and digestive disturbances, are offered at Maharishi Ayur-Veda medical or health centers located throughout the United States. Programs for disease prevention and rejuvenation of the body are also offered at the centers.

The Maharishi Ayur-Veda Association of America offers a Physician Training Program for physicians wanting to incorporate Maharishi Ayur-Veda methods into their regular practice. The names of practitioners who have completed this course may be obtained from the Maharishi Ayur-Veda medical center in Fairfield, Iowa.

Currently there are seven Maharishi Ayur-Veda medical centers throughout the United States and more than one hundred clinics world-wide. For more information contact any of the Maharishi Ayur-Veda medical centers.

Maharishi Ayur-Veda is well described and documented in two excellent books written by Deepak Chopra, M.D.: *Quantum Healing: Exploring the Frontiers of Body-Mind Medicine* and *Perfect Health*.

🐚 | MANUAL LYMPHATIC DRAINAGE | 🐚

Manual Lymphatic Drainage, or Lymphatic Drainage, is a gentle, noninvasive, rhythmical European massage technique designed to accelerate the movement of lymphatic fluid in the human body.

The technique was developed in France during the 1930s by Dr. Emil Vodder and his wife, Estrid, through clinical experience. While working on the French Riviera as masseurs, the Danish couple noticed that their English clients suffered from chronic colds, sinusitis, and similar respiratory problems.

Dr. Vodder noticed that all these clients had swollen lymph nodes in their necks and wondered if the blockage in the lymph nodes could be the underlying cause of the nose and throat infections. He found that by manually applying a precise amount of pressure on the skin of the neck, and lightly massaging it in a specific pattern and way, the infections and swelling disappeared.

The Vodders moved to Paris and for six years continued their research on this technique. By 1936 they were ready to present their findings at a health and beauty congress. At the outbreak of the war in Europe, they returned to their native Denmark and founded the Manual Lymphatic Drainage Institute in Copenhagen to train therapists.

Emil and Estrid Vodder eventually named Gunther and Hildegard Wittlinger as their designated successors. In 1972 the Wittlingers established the Dr. Vodder School in Walchsee, Austria. Health professionals from around the world travel to Austria for their four-week intensive training class.

Gradually, Manual Lymphatic Drainage gained a strong foothold in Europe, mostly in Germany, Austria, France, and the Scandinavian countries. In 1982 it was introduced to North America and is now widely practiced and taught in the United States, Canada, and Mexico.

The lymph system's function is to carry off wastes, toxins, bacteria, viruses, excess water, etc., from the body's connective tissue. Blockage in the lymph system or damage to lymph nodes results in swelling (edema), congestion, and eventual physical problems and abnormalities.

Manual Lymphatic Drainage is used to treat a wide variety of conditions, including acne, burns, edema, inflammation, arthritis, and sinusitis. Because it stimulates a natural cleaning system to help the body rid itself of accumulated toxins and poisons, it brings tissue to a healthier state.

The length and frequency of treatments vary depending on the condition being treated and its severity, but they are usually thirty to sixty minutes long. During this time the therapist uses precise, gentle, rhythmical movements on the client while she is lying on a massage table.

Strokes are always done in the direction of the muscle fiber because that is the direction in which the vessels run; the objective is to try and push the fluid and waste products along.

There are four basic manipulation techniques used in Manual Lymphatic Drainage that are not usually known to massage therapists. They are stationary circles, pumping, scooping, and rotary. These techniques are applied in a specific way, following the lymph pathways exactly unless there is a blockage. Normally only the skin is moved, as 40 percent of the body's lymph lies within superficial layers.

Many massage schools are now training practitioners in Manual Lymphatic Drainage. It is included in the thousand-hour holistic health practitioner curriculum. Local massage schools can be contacted for the names and locations of graduates.

Courses in the Vodder Method of Manual Lymphatic Drainage are taught throughout the United States. The basic course is five days. To be certified as a Manual Lymphatic Drainage Therapist by the Vodder School in Austria requires completion of four different courses.

Detailed information on the Vodder Method of Manual Lymphatic Drainage can be found in the three-volume *Introduction to Dr. Vodder's Manual Lymphatic Drainage*. All three volumes are published by Karl F. Haug Publishers, Heidelberg, Germany, and are available through Medicina Biologica in Portland, Oregon.

❧ | MASSAGE THERAPY | ☙

Massage Therapy, as defined by the American Massage Therapy Association, is "the manipulation of soft tissue for therapeutic purposes and may include, but is not limited to, effleurage, petrissage, tapotement, compression, vibration, friction, nerve strokes, and other Swedish movements, either by hand or with mechanical or electrical apparatus for the purpose of body massage. This may include the use of oil, salt glows, hot and cold packs, and other recognized forms of Massage Therapy."

The use of massage is widespread and well documented throughout history. The use of touch to soothe or gain some degree of relief from pain is a universal human experience.

Stroking and kneading of the neck, chest, back, and limbs were used in ancient civilizations to relieve pain and suffering. Massage was used by the Chinese, Egyptians, Hindus, Greeks, Romans, and Persians.

Written records go back several thousand years. The earliest are found in *The Yellow Emperor's Classic of Internal Medicine*, attributed to Huang-ti, the Yellow Emperor, who died in 2598 B.C. In Homer's *Odyssey*, massage is mentioned as a welcome relief to exhausted heroes.

In the fifth century B.C. Hippocrates wrote, "The physician must be experienced in many things, but most assuredly in rubbing."

During the third century B.C. the Greek physician and writer Galen wrote four treatises on active and passive massage. Plutarch, an ancient Greek biographer, described the use of massage by Julius Caesar, who praised it highly.

The walls of the temple at Borobudur, India, built in A.D. 800, contain a relief depicting Buddha receiving a massage treatment.

Indigenous peoples of Africa, North America, and the South Pacific islands all employed massage in their cultures.

The therapeutic massage in use today has evolved from both the East and West. Eastern contributions came from China, India, and Japan, while those of the West can be traced to Per Hendrik Ling in Sweden at the beginning of the nineteenth century. Ling developed a system that became known as Swedish Massage.

During the late nineteenth and early twentieth centuries, European doctors used massage techniques to treat a variety of chronic diseases. Until the 1980s, the term "massage" in the United States usually referred to Swedish Massage.

Although not a household name, the father of Massage Therapy in the United States was Cornelius E. De Puy, M.D. Graduating from medical school in 1814, De Puy published the first journal article on the subject in 1817. Unfortunately he died at the age of twenty-nine before he had a chance to further develop Massage Therapy in the medicine of the day.

Massage Therapy, as the term is used today, is nonspecific and encompasses many different techniques used for a variety of purposes. It could be said that all massage is therapeutic.

Filling cavities, cleaning teeth, or extracting teeth are all forms of dentistry, but each of these specialties treats specific problems. This is also true for therapeutic massage. Currently there are literally dozens of different massage techniques in use. A well-trained, knowledgeable massage therapist will use different techniques to accomplish different goals.

Currently the national examination given to massage practitioners by the American Massage Therapy Association is for certification in therapeutic massage and bodywork. Although the terms *massage* and *bodywork* are used interchangeably to cover everything in this field, bodywork more often refers to manipulative techniques such as Rolfing (Structural Integration), Hellerwork, or others, and movement-based techniques such as the Feldenkrais Method, the Alexander Technique, and others.

Since the end of World War II, many new discoveries and innovations in massage and bodywork have been brought forth. Some people in the field have developed new techniques by combining or synthesizing two or more known techniques, and others have taken a well-known technique and added special insight of their own to create a new and more effective technique.

With the greater awareness in physical fitness, and the increased pursuit of athletics by both professionals and amateurs, the field of sports massage was developed to meet the needs of this group.

The physical, mental, and emotional benefits of Massage Therapy are well documented. In general, most massage techniques accomplish the following: increased circulation of blood and lymphatic fluid, which brings additional quantities of oxygen and nutrients to tissue; removal and elimination of the waste products of metabolism and other toxic substances from the body; relaxation and reduction of stress with attendant decrease in pain; and movement of blood back to the heart in those individuals unable to exercise due to a debilitating disease or injury.

New information continually confirms the therapeutic value of touch in every age group and occupation. From infants to geriatric patients, corporate presidents to construction workers, all may benefit from therapeutic massage.

The United States seems to be lagging behind Europe in the use of massage as a medical therapy. Chiropractors and osteopaths commonly use "soft tissue manipulation" (massage) for certain musculoskeletal problems. In some countries in Europe, a medical doctor will prescribe therapeutic massage rather than drugs when appropriate, and it may even be covered by the individual's health insurance. However, it is not the customary practice of an M.D. in the United States to write a prescription for five therapeutic massages for an individual suffering from stress. A bottle of tranquilizers would be the more likely choice.

Many different massage and bodywork techniques are discussed in this book under the name of the specific technique or modality.

Today, there are massage therapists located even in small cities. Massage schools are good sources of referrals in cities where they are located. For additional information on therapeutic massage contact the American Massage Therapy Association or the Associated Bodywork and Massage Professionals.

MCDOUGALL DIET

The McDougall Diet is a vegan diet (strict vegetarian diet which includes only food of plant origin). It is low in fat, high in fiber and complex carbohydrates, has zero cholesterol, and is low in sugar and salt.

As a child and a young adult, John A. McDougall ate a typical American diet rich in bacon, eggs, milk, and hot dogs. At the age of eighteen he suffered a stroke, and he required stomach surgery by the time he reached twenty-six years old.

Dr. McDougall earned his medical degree from Michigan State University and received his postgraduate training at the University of Hawaii. For three years he practiced medicine in Hawaii, where he became interested in the effect of diet. Dr. McDougall began to realize that allopathic medicine was limited in treating his chronic disease patients.

While in Hawaii, many of his patients were first-generation Orientals who ate a traditional diet of rice and vegetables and showed an obvious absence of diseases typical to Western culture. In contrast, their children ate a typical American diet, were often overweight, and had typical American diseases such as high blood pressure, coronary disease, and diabetes.

Having learned in medical school that chronic disease is passed on genetically from one generation to the next, Dr. McDougall was amazed by his discovery. He searched the available medical literature for studies on diet and disease. From his research Dr. McDougall found that many diseased people who changed to a diet of simple foods became well.

The McDougall Diet is not a fad, but is based on the traditional foods people have eaten for thousands of years. It is basically the same diet throughout the world, except the main complex carbohydrates change with different cultures and geographic locations. For example, corn is used in North and Central America and rice in Asia.

Foods allowed on this diet include whole grains, whole grain flour and pasta, legumes, winter squashes, and root vegetables. Small amounts of fresh vegetables and fruits are used to supplement the main complex carbohydrate dishes.

Absolutely no fats (cholesterol) are permitted in the diet. Dr. McDougall agrees with Nathan Pritikin that cholesterol is responsible for hardening of the arteries and the heart diseases that result from it.

Dr. McDougall feels the body produces sufficient cholesterol by itself and when excess is introduced into the body, it settles in the lining of the arteries, which "prepares the soil" for atherosclerosis.

He also feels that if a diet rich in fats is replaced with a healthy, grain-based diet before irreparable damage to the heart and major blood vessels occur, reversal of the plaque deposits in the arteries is possible.

Although the McDougall Diet is primarily a self-help tool that can be used by an individual at home, it is also part of the McDougall Program currently offered at the St. Helena Health Center located in California's Napa Valley wine country. An intensive twelve-day residential program, personally supervised by Dr. McDougall, is designed to promote improved health through exercise, stress reduction, and diet.

Three books on the prevention and treatment of disease, *The McDougall Plan*, *McDougall's Medicine*, and *The McDougall Program: Twelve Days to*

Dynamic Health, published by Dr. McDougall, provide additional information on the McDougall Diet.

For additional information on the McDougall Program at the St. Helena Health Center, contact the center.

❧ | MEDITATION | ❧

Meditation "is the intentional directing of attention to the clear aspect of one's own inner nature" according to Roy Eugene Davis, a recognized expert in the practice of Meditation. Although this definition is correct, Meditation is not a single practice nor can it be easily defined in precise terms.

The use of Meditation for healing is not new. Meditative techniques are the product of diverse cultures and peoples around the world. The value of Meditation to alleviate suffering and promote healing has been known and practiced for thousands of years.

There are many different types of Meditation practiced today which are based on different principles. They can be roughly classified into four categories depending on whether they are based on the body or mind and whether they employ control or letting-go mechanisms as a means of achieving a meditative state.

The first category of Meditation, based on body control, is incorporated into certain types of Yoga to unite body and mind. This type of Meditation is concerned with the body assuming a certain posture. The spine is kept straight and the body remains still and immobile. This lowers the metabolic level and reduces stress.

The second category of Meditation, based on control of the mind, utilizes concentration, contemplation, and visualization to achieve the meditative state.

Concentration involves focusing the consciousness on a single simple object, such as a black circle. Contemplation uses the continuous repetition of a word or syllable. Visualization uses a scene complicated enough to require focus and attention by the meditator.

Many cultures use mind control in their Meditation and some have a religious connotation. Examples include the repeated intonation of vowel sounds, the chanting of Buddhist monks, the repetition of prayers such as the Hail Mary, and the war chants of Native Americans.

The third category of Meditation is based on the "letting-go" of the body. One technique involves the deliberate relaxation of muscular tension.

Other letting-go techniques encourage moving of the body freely and spontaneously as the urge is felt. This technique can be used with biofeedback.

Yet another technique involves immobility as the meditator consciously attempts no action. An example would be sitting still and doing nothing.

The fourth category of meditation is based on the letting-go of the mind. The mind remains passive and open to whatever enters it in the here and now. By leaving the mind open, the individual is able to receive insight into a particular problem or the answer to a question concerning his health.

Research has shown that Meditation can contribute to an individual's psychological and physiological well-being. This is accomplished as Meditation brings the brainwave pattern into an alpha state, which is a level of consciousness that promotes the healing state.

There is scientific evidence that Meditation can reduce blood pressure and relieve pain and stress. When used in combination with biofeedback, Meditation enhances the effectiveness of biofeedback.

Meditation is a self-help practice. There are numerous books on Meditation available in libraries and bookstores. Also, audiocassettes that teach Meditation techniques or provide guided meditations are available. Many metaphysical bookstores offer classes in Meditation techniques.

✍ | MOVEMENT THERAPY | ✍

Movement Therapy is an educational process that assists an individual in improving his movement functioning.

The movement therapist uses hands-on repatterning and verbal instruction to teach clients and students to recognize and improve problem movement patterns and stress-related emotional conditions. These difficulties restrict the functional aspects of their lives, and may contribute to chronic disorders.

Clients and students of Movement Therapy may include individuals recovering from an injury or accident, those suffering from a degenerative neurological disorder such as multiple sclerosis or immune suppression, and those with chronic pain.

While working with a client or student, an International Movement Therapy Association (IMTA) registered movement therapist may utilize several different approaches. These include physiological repatterning, movement analysis and performance, psychological/emotional expression, and health maintenance and improvement.

In physiological repatterning, a movement therapist appraises the cognitive-motor function problems caused by poor usage and awareness of such body systems as the perceptual, neurological, and musculoskeletal. She also studies how these systems interrelate to the environment and environmental tasks. The therapist then employs corrective measures to improve the problems.

Through movement analysis and performance, a movement therapist explores an individual's quality of movement in relation to specific tasks and functions he performs. The objective is to optimize his movement potential for efficiency and expressiveness within the spatial environment which he occupies.

Through psychological/emotional expression, a movement therapist can observe and explore the client's or student's nonverbal way of interacting with himself, other persons, groups, and the environment.

For health maintenance and improvement, a movement therapist designs exercise programs for individuals and groups to reduce stress, improve immune functioning, and improve overall health and quality of life. Generally, exercises are noncardiovascular intensive and based on total body organization in relationship to the individual's movement functioning.

During either a private or a group session, an IMTA registered movement therapist uses a wide variety of instructional methods. These include but are not limited to the use of verbal instructions, hypnosis, and imagery, the use of deep muscle and connective tissue manipulation, and the mobilization of body systems to reeducate specific body parts. An important part of this work involves active participation by the client-student.

The benefits of Movement Therapy are not limited to those suffering from a specific illness or physical problem. It can be utilized by those who wish to improve their self-awareness and quality of life. Others may wish to achieve optimal physical, cognitive, and emotional performance in daily work-related activities or in sports.

To become an IMTA registered movement therapist requires over five hundred hours of in-class, hands-on instruction, two hundred hours of postgraduate experience in teaching or private practice, and other conditions.

Graduates of training programs such as the Feldenkrais Training program, the Alexander Teacher Training program, and many others have fulfilled the educational requirements to become IMTA registered movement therapists.

❧ | MUCUSLESS DIET | ☙

The Mucusless Diet and Mucusless Diet Healing System are therapeutic methods to regain and maintain good health by eliminating accumulated waste matter, mucus, and toxins from the body, then preventing them from being reintroduced. Once the body is thoroughly cleaned, regeneration is promoted.

The Mucusless Diet consists of eating a wide variety of raw and cooked fruits, starchless vegetables, and raw or cooked mostly leafy-green vegetables. The Mucusless Diet Healing System combines short or long fasts with gradually changing menus of foods that do not produce mucus in the body.

Professor Arnold Ehret (1866–1922), born in Baden, Germany, developed the Mucusless Diet Healing System. While attending college, he suffered a severe attack of bronchial catarrh (buildup of mucus in the system) brought on by farm work, long walks to school, and the standard diet of the day. At the age of twenty-one, Ehret graduated as a professor of drawing for high school and college.

Ehret taught drawing at college until he was drafted for military service. After nine months he was released due to a heart problem and resumed his teaching position. By the age of thirty-one he was suffering from Bright's disease, a kidney condition marked by mucus or pus and albumin in the urine, and pain in the kidneys. After numerous attempts at recuperation and several years of treatment by no fewer than twenty-four physicians, Ehret was pronounced incurable.

After hearing about naturopathy, he received three treatments, which provided some relief but not a cure. He tried many other natural cure methods known in Europe, and, although he was not really sick, he was not well either. After the meat, eggs, and milk diet doctors placed him on caused the condition to worsen, Ehret decided to try and find his own answer. He went to Berlin and tried vegetarianism, with poor results.

The following winter Ehret went to Algiers in northern Africa. The combination of mild weather and abundance of fresh fruits improved his condition. He tried short fasts to cleanse his system. His health, both physical and mental, was better than he had ever known. The increased endurance allowed him to make an eight-hundred-mile bicycle trip from Algiers to Tunis. This was after doctors had told him he was near death.

After years of research, experimentation convinced Ehret that eating fruit, which produced no mucus in the body, and fasting was nature's way to regain and maintain superior health. He gained knowledge of how the body cleansed itself of the impurities from eating the wrong food, and how eating the right food could regenerate, repair, and strengthen the body.

Although the ideas of eating fruit and fasting were already known to naturopathy, Ehret developed his knowledge into a workable program he called the Mucusless Diet Healing System. He opened a "Fruit and Fasting" sanitarium in Switzerland, treating thousands of patients.

In 1915 he came to the United States to inspect the fruit raised here, especially in California. When World War I began, he was forced to stay in the United States. Ehret found others here who were involved in the same type of work and discoveries, and began to advocate the benefits of these methods that had proved so successful in Europe.

In 1922 Professor Arnold Ehret, while still in the prime of life and enjoying a superior state of health, had an unfortunate accident in Los Angeles, California. On a wet, foggy night he slipped on a stretch of oil-soaked pavement and fell backward, striking his head on the ground, which caused a skull fracture. He was taken to an emergency hospital and pronounced dead upon arrival.

It was Professor Ehret's teaching that every disease, regardless of name, was actually constipation, and that the uneliminated feces in the large intestine was the cause of continual poisoning of the bloodstream and other body systems. He believed that every sick person had a more or less mucus-clogged system resulting from the body's reaction to undigested and uneliminated food accumulated from a lifetime of eating unnatural food substances. His basic philosophy was that "nature alone is the primary healer."

Detailed explanation of the diet and healing system can be found in Professor Ehret's book, *Mucusless Diet Healing System*, which is available at most health food stores, bookstores, and libraries.

MUSIC THERAPY

Music Therapy is the use of music to accomplish a therapeutic objective. Music is used to restore, maintain, or improve an individual's physical and mental health. Music Therapy can take the form of either playing an instrument or listening to music.

The value of music as a healing tool was known by Pythagoras in the sixth century B.C. He regarded music and diet as the principal means of purifying the body and soul and maintaining the health and harmony of the whole organism.

For several thousand years, the cultures of aboriginal peoples around the world have used music and dance as part of their healing arts.

Beginning in the 1960s, clinical evidence, documented in medical literature, has shown that Music Therapy provides real improvement for a variety of conditions. A Dutch obstetrician found Music Therapy effective for certain situations during childbirth. When the mother became emotionally upset or jittery, or experienced excessive pain, he found that a serene and tranquil style of classical music was an effective substitute for a sedative. To overcome the feeling of fatigue from labor, music with a rhythmic beat was used.

In the early 1970s, composer Steven Halpern began what is known as "New Age music," a unique style that is designed to relax the listener by aligning and attuning her body, mind, and spirit. This style of music, which has no recognizable harmony, melody, or rhythm, is excellent for Meditation, Yoga, or massage work. It is also used as background music in holistically oriented restaurants, health care centers, and commercial establishments throughout the country.

It is known that music creates an emotional reaction—a fact utilized in both the motion picture and advertising industries. The musical score of a movie, or background music in television and radio commercials, is carefully chosen to effect a particular mood or reaction.

Certain kinds of music can lower the heart rate and blood pressure in humans. Studies have shown that music has a profound effect on plants also. Plants exposed to classical music thrived while those exposed to rock music did not fare well at all.

Today, music therapists treat individuals of all ages, in a variety of settings. These include hospitals, clinics, day care facilities, schools, community mental health centers, substance abuse centers, nursing homes, hospices, rehabilitation centers, and private practice. Both group and individual music experiences are utilized in therapy.

Music therapists work with a wide variety of mental and physical problems. Major areas include developmental disabilities, mental illness, geriatric problems (e.g., Alzheimer's disease), behavior disorders, learning disabilities, deprived and/or disadvantaged conditions, substance abuse, and physical disabilities such as brain injuries, orthopedic handicaps, sensory impairment, and other health and/or medical impairments.

Because Music Therapy is nonverbal, it provides a safe and acceptable means of communication for the emotionally ill and others. The musical experience provides the arena for the exploration of feelings and therapeutic issues such as self-esteem or personal insight. Music Therapy can be helpful to the individual in releasing emotions and feelings that have been held in check for long periods of time. This in turn can bring about desirable changes in behavior.

Currently, there are more than fifty colleges and universities throughout the United States that provide a four-year curriculum in Music Therapy. Some institutions also offer master's and doctoral programs. An organization known as the Certification Board for Music Therapists administers national Music Therapy examinations and certifies music therapists.

There are numerous books available on Music Therapy. A complete list is available from the National Association for Music Therapy. Both the American Association for Music Therapy and the National Association for Music Therapy can provide referrals to Certified Music Therapists.

❧ | MYOFASCIAL RELEASE THERAPY | ❧

Myofascial Release Therapy is a whole-body hands-on approach to the evaluation and treatment of the human structure. The technique is used by therapists to relieve soft tissue (muscle) from the abnormal grip of tight fascia (connective tissue).

The prefix *myo* comes from the Greek meaning "muscle." Myofascial Release is the literal release of the fascia in the body. Generally, it is a mild and gentle form of stretching that has a profound effect upon body tissues. It is used to relieve pain and improve physical functioning.

The fascial system is a densely woven sheet of connective tissue that lines and covers nearly every muscle, bone, nerve, artery, and vein, as well as all of the internal organs, including the heart, lungs, brain, and spinal cord.

It is not just a system of separate coverings, but is actually one structure that extends from the top of the head to the tip of the toes; it plays an important role in the support of the body. Fascia is composed of two types of fibers: collagenous fibers, which are tough and have little ability to stretch, and elastic fibers, which are stretchable.

In the normal healthy state, fascia is relaxed and has the ability to move without restriction. When the body experiences inflammation, disease, or physical trauma such as whiplash, surgery, or habitually poor posture, the effect on the fascia is cumulative over time.

Eventually the fascia loses some of its pliability; it becomes thicker and hardens. As fascia tightens it becomes a source of tension throughout the body. This tension can effectively "bind up" muscles and cause pain and/or restricted range of motion, which limits the body's ability to move freely.

Fascia can also become inflamed, causing severe pain. This is a relatively new syndrome in orthopedics, called fibromyositis.

Because fascia permeates all regions of the body and is interconnected, tension in the fascia can "travel" from its original source to adjacent and distant parts of the body. This same effect occurs with inflammation in the fascia.

For example, chronic low back pain may eventually create pain in the neck and head due to a gradual tightening of the fascia and muscles.

Until fairly recently the importance of the fascial system was virtually ignored. However, the importance of the role of the fascial system in pain and dysfunction has now been documented at Michigan State University's biomechanical research laboratory.

Therapists use different types of Myofascial Release techniques depending upon the area of the body found to have restricted fascia. Key to the success of Myofascial Release treatments is keeping the pressure and stretch extremely mild.

Muscle tissue responds to a relatively firm stretch, but that is not the case with fascia. However, it has been shown that under a small amount of pressure (applied by a therapist's hands) fascia will soften and begin to release when the pressure is sustained over time.

The Myofascial Release approach is used to treat neck and back pain, headaches, recurring sports injuries, scoliosis, and other problems.

The Myofascial Release Treatment Center in Paoli, Pennsylvania, offers seminars in Myofascial Release throughout the United States. They also have available a list of graduates of their Myofascial Release Seminars.

✍ | NAPRAPATHY | ✍

Naprapathy is a gentle system of treatment that uses manipulations of the soft connective tissue—ligaments, muscles, and tendons—to release tension and restore the normal flow of energy in the body. Its origin is rooted in Osteopathy and Chiropractic.

Naprapathy was developed by a young chiropractor, Oakley Smith. In 1907 he founded the National College of Naprapathy in Chicago, Illinois, which is still in existence today. In addition to his manipulative system, Smith developed unique charts and symbols which are used to record specific information on the patient's condition as well as the types of treatment she receives.

Naprapathic practitioners believe the body has an innate capability to function properly; however, when the soft connective tissue becomes contracted and rigid, it can interfere with the normal functioning of nervous and circulatory systems. This is due to a cumulative effect from such factors as improper posture, injuries of all types, poor nutrition, and mental/emotional conflict.

Through hand palpation and sensitive touch, the practitioner explores the soft connective tissue. Testing for resistance with gentle thrusts, he tries to locate areas in the body that have become contracted and rigid. Also, the practitioner will note any areas that are tender or painful to the touch.

Once these problem areas have been established, the practitioner begins repetitive, rhythmic, manipulative thrusts, called "directos," to gently stretch the painful and contracted areas of soft connective tissue. Once the tension in the contracted tissue is released, the impaired nerve functioning and congested blood circulation are restored to a more normal condition.

Manipulative sessions usually last about thirty minutes. Although the practitioner may work on other parts of the body, normally his attention is directed at the ligaments encasing the spinal column, where, because of its close proximity, connective tissue can affect the functioning of spinal nerves. In addition to manipulation, the major component of Naprapathy, practitioners also utilize diet and nutrition, exercise, and postural improvement to aid in improved functioning of the nervous and circulatory systems.

For additional information on Naprapathy contact the American Naprapathic Association, or for information regarding educational opportunities contact the National College of Naprapathy.

❧ | NATURAL HYGIENE | ❧

Natural Hygiene, also referred to as Life Science, is a health system whereby we live in accord with our biological or natural makeup. It teaches us how to live in harmony with nature by learning to eat a proper natural diet and maintain a lifestyle that promotes a happier, healthier existence.

By eating a wholesome diet of delicious natural foods, an individual can develop a healthy body and heal herself naturally.

The concept of Natural Hygiene is over 150 years old. It began as Hygiene in 1820 with the work of Dr. Isaac Jennings of Fairfield, Connecticut. Later, through the work of Dr. Jennings and Dr. Sylvester Graham, Hygiene was slowly elaborated as a philosophy of life.

During the 1850s and 1860s a brilliant man named Dr. Russell Thacker Trall did much of the original research and contemplation that led to the further development of Hygiene.

After Louis Pasteur developed the germ theory in the late 1890s, Hygiene slid from the forefront and lost support as a health movement. Although it did not completely die out, it continued to decline in spite of the championing efforts of many people.

In the late 1920s Dr. Herbert M. Shelton came on the scene as a giant in the movement. He wrote the classic book on Natural Hygiene diet, *The Science and Fine Art of Food and Nutrition.* The fundamental principles of Natural Hygiene are well detailed in the many books by Dr. Shelton.

In 1948 the American Natural Hygiene Society was founded. The word Natural was added to Hygiene to make it a distinct entity and to remove the misconception attached to the common definition of hygiene.

In the 1970s the term Life Science was used by T. C. Fry to denote Natural Hygiene. In October 1982, Dr. Henry E. Stevenson, T. C. Fry, and ten students launched a new educational effort in Yorktown, Texas. They began teaching Natural Hygiene for professional purposes.

In 1985 Harvey and Marilyn Diamond published *Fit for Life* and shared the ideas of Natural Hygiene with millions around the world. *Fit for Life* was followed by *Fit for Life II—Living Health*, which goes beyond diet and teaches a total lifestyle.

Supporters of Natural Hygiene or Life Science believe that the human body is a fully self-sufficient organism. It is self-directing, self-constructing, self-preserving, and self-healing. When its basic needs are met it is capable of maintaining itself in superb functioning order completely free of disease.

As Harvey Diamond explains it, the word *hygiene* connotes cleanliness and the word *natural* implies a process unhampered by artificial forces. Therefore, "the basic foundation of Natural Hygiene is that the body is always striving for health and that it achieves this by continuously cleansing itself of deleterious waste." Diamond's program, Fit for Life, works with the body to free up energy and make it readily available for other functions.

Digestion of food requires more energy than any other body function. The body needs energy to detoxify, and by eliminating this toxic waste, weight is lost in the process. With extra energy available the body automatically goes to work shedding any excess weight it is carrying. If weight loss is not a goal, then a significant boost in overall energy will be gained.

An individual can derive many benefits from practicing Natural Hygiene. There is anecdotal evidence that Natural Hygiene can improve or cure some chronic and acute ailments. Fasting is utilized along with a proper dietary program.

For additional information contact Natural Hygiene, Inc. Also, available from the International Association of Professional Natural Hygienists is a professional referral list. This is a registry of licensed medical doctors, chiropractors, osteopaths, and naturopaths who are certified to provide Natural Hygiene care and consultation.

❧ | NATUROPATHIC MEDICINE | ❧

Naturopathic Medicine, or naturopathy, is a complete health care system that utilizes a wide variety of natural healing therapies.

The term *naturopathy* was first used in the late 1800s by German homeopath John H. Scheel to denote a form of health care that utilized natural methods to treat the whole person.

Naturopathy was introduced into the United States by Benedict Lust in the late nineteenth century. Lust came to America to teach and practice the Hydrotherapy techniques and other therapies popularized in Europe by the great "water doctor," Father Sebastian Kneipp.

In 1900 a group of Kneipp practitioners decided to broaden the scope of their practice in order to incorporate all of the natural healing methods available at that time. From this meeting naturopathy emerged as a separate discipline. At that time it included botanical medicines, Homeopathy, nutritional therapy, medical electricity (now called bioelectric therapy or electrotherapy), psychology, and the new manipulative therapies.

The American School of Naturopathy, founded in New York City by Benedict Lust, graduated its first class in 1902. In 1909, California was the first state to enact a law regulating the practice of Naturopathic Medicine. The profession grew and spread rapidly across the country. During that time more than twenty naturopathic medical colleges were graduating naturopathic physicians who were licensed in a majority of the states.

Naturopathic medical conventions in the 1920s attracted more than ten thousand practitioners. During the 1940s and 1950s the discipline experienced a decline with the rise and popularity of pharmaceutical drugs, technological medicine, and the idea that drugs could eliminate all disease.

Since the late 1970s Naturopathic Medicine has experienced a resurgence as health-conscious people have begun to seek out alternatives to conventional medicine.

To treat disease and restore health, today's Naturopathic Medicine draws from the sciences of clinical nutrition, Herbal Medicine, Homeopathy, Exercise Therapy, counseling, Acupuncture, natural childbirth, Hydrotherapy, and physical medicine (manipulation of muscles, bones, and spine, and physiotherapy).

In states where they are licensed, naturopathic physicians provide primary care and perform physical examinations, laboratory testing, gynecological exams, nutritional and dietary assessments, metabolic analyses, allergy testing, X-ray examinations, and other diagnostic tests.

To receive a degree of doctor of naturopathy (N.D.) requires four years of graduate-level study in the medical sciences along with training in naturopathic therapeutics.

Presently there are two naturopathic medical colleges in the United States. John Bastyr University in Seattle, Washington, and the National College of Naturopathic Medicine in Portland, Oregon, are four-year postgraduate schools with admission requirements comparable to those of conventional medical schools.

Currently seven states—Washington, Oregon, Arizona, Montana, Alaska, and Hawaii—grant licenses to naturopathic physicians. Utah and Florida have "sunset laws" which recognize licenses previously granted to practitioners of "drugless therapy." Other states either have no regulations or have very specific practicing regulations.

The following principles are the foundation that naturopathic medical practice is built on.

The Healing Power of Nature: Nature acts powerfully through healing mechanisms in the body and mind to maintain and restore health. Naturopathic physicians work to restore and support these inherent healing systems when they have broken down, by using methods, medicines, and techniques that are in harmony with the natural process.

First Do No Harm: Naturopathic physicians prefer noninvasive treatments which minimize the risks of harmful side effects. They are trained to know which patients they can treat safely, and which ones they need to refer to other health care practitioners.

Find the Cause: Every illness has an underlying cause, often in aspects of the lifestyle, diet, or habits of the individual. A naturopathic physician is trained to find and remove the underlying cause of a disease.

Treat the Whole Person: Health or disease comes from a complex interaction of physical, emotional, dietary, genetic, environmental, lifestyle, and other factors. Naturopathic physicians treat the whole person, taking these factors into account.

Preventive Medicine: The naturopathic approach to health care can prevent minor illness from developing into more serious or chronic degenerative diseases. Patients are taught the principles with which to live a healthy life; by following these principles they can prevent major illness. It requires the patient to take an active role in the healing process.

The natural healing methods of Naturopathic Medicine treat a wide variety of health problems. They are used to treat everyday acute illnesses such as colds, flu, sore throat, bronchitis, and digestive problems. Naturopathic Medicine can also treat chronic degenerative diseases such as arthritis, other autoimmune diseases, and cancer. It also treats chronic structural problems.

Currently, the American Association of Naturopathic Physicians (AANP) is the unifying organization for Naturopathic Medicine. Contact the AANP to obtain the name of a naturopathic physician in your area.

NETWORK CHIROPRACTIC

Network Chiropractic is a new approach to Chiropractic, a health care system that deals with the relationship between the spinal column and the nervous system, and which maintains that there must be an unobstructed flow of nerve impulses from the brain through the spinal nerves and out to every part of the body for a person to experience harmony, vitality, and good health (see Chiropractic elsewhere in this book).

Network Chiropractic is not a new Chiropractic technique, but a "network" of the different methods commonly used by chiropractors. The primary difference between Network Chiropractic and standard Chiropractic is the sequence in which the adjustments are implemented. Through gentle touch, Network Chiropractic facilitates the release of physical and emotional trauma, which aids in an individual's personal growth and transformational process.

A graduate of New York College of Chiropractic, Donald Epstein, D.C., developed Network Chiropractic in 1979 in an attempt to unify the various methods in use by the Chiropractic profession. While first developing the work, Dr. Epstein was "shocked and frightened" when, after holding light pressure on a certain vertebra for a few seconds, some of his patients evoked screams, cries, laughter, and other emotions as they relived past physical and emotional traumas.

After many years of maintaining a private practice in the New York City area, Dr. Epstein now travels around the world devoting his full attention to the advancement of Network Chiropractic through teaching, lecturing, and research.

In Network Chiropractic, it is believed that an individual's physical, mental, emotional, and spiritual aspects are interrelated; rather than curing specific problems, it is oriented toward healing the body, mind, and spirit.

When the body is healthy and functioning optimally, life energy flows unobstructed through the body. Due to tension caused by physical and emotional trauma, chemical stress (e.g., environmental pollution), and subluxations (misalignment of the vertebrae), the flow of energy is reduced, causing interference in the transmission of nerve impulses from the brain to organs and other tissues of the body.

The Network Chiropractic process begins with light, sustained pressure applied to the spinal tissue, where the vertebrae attach to the thin covering of the spinal cord. Through gentle touches and taps, tension held in the brain and spinal cord is released. In some patients this release of trapped energy produces dramatic reactions such as screams, dialogue, laughter, assuming strange positions, etc., as they reexperience the traumas. Other patients release quietly and without incident.

If there is still a lack of recovery from physical or structural trauma after the release has occurred, the network chiropractor can then use any of the more conventional structural thrust adjustments to complete the process.

Individuals from all walks of life, including many celebrities and entertainers, find Network Chiropractic to be a life-changing experience producing both physical and emotional improvements. Through Network Chiropractic, many people find that they have a greater connection to their innate intelligence, helping them to make personal choices.

Currently, there are approximately three hundred network chiropractors in the United States who use this method exclusively in their practice. For additional information or the name of a network chiropractor in your area contact the Association for Network Chiropractic.

ᘓ | NEURO/CELLULAR REPATTERNING | ᘖ

Neuro/Cellular Repatterning is a process that integrates spiritual psychology with body/mind therapy to release negative cellular memory. It works on the physical, mental, emotional, and spiritual levels to help release emotional and physical dysfunctions.

For twenty-five years, Arthur H. Martin had been looking for a cure to his own physical problems. Conventional medical doctors told him his spine was deteriorating and he would wind up in a wheelchair. Unfortunately, they could determine no specific cause for his physical problem.

Studying and wandering through all of the alternatives to allopathic (conventional) medicine, Martin still was not able to find a single person who understood his problems or could alleviate his pain.

Trained as a psychologist, Martin thought that the discipline might have the answer. But from his training, he realized that conventional psychology seemed satisfied with blaming the problem on someone or on some unknown factor.

In his later training with Paul Solomon, psychology was approached from a holistic spiritual aspect. This was quite different from his original training. Although this did answer some of his questions regarding personal dialogue with his own body and the insights it could provide, it did not heal his body.

In 1978, a workshop with Ronald Beasley gave Martin the fundamentals of how the body stores cellular memory, and the basics of removing those memories. With this new knowledge he had the tools to integrate spiritual psychology with body/mind therapy for use as the basis for his counseling.

Physical dysfunctions reveal themselves in obvious ways, but their causes remained unknown. Martin became aware that his belief system contained suppressed emotional programs (negative emotional experiences from childhood) that were causing his physical problems. Until John Bradshaw introduced the concept of the dysfunctional family and inner child, few people were aware of this syndrome.

Before 1988, the process was called Cellular Repatterning. Martin then discovered his technique could erase patterns the neurological system used to keep muscles in trauma from past negative emotional experiences.

Each cell has a memory, a perfect image of how to regenerate itself. When the dysfunctional negative overlay of emotional energy is removed, it will regenerate itself perfectly. The blueprint will rebuild a perfect body. All cellular structures will regenerate this way.

It is believed that if the causes or reasons for dysfunction can be discovered, they can be released, which leads to healing in a short period of time.

Neuro/Cellular Repatterning is a new field of practice that uses love and forgiveness as the basic healing modality. Practitioners believe that these are the only modalities that will cause healing. Practitioners who utilize it are not "healers" or "therapists" but teachers helping an individual learn to love herself and to receive love.

Today, Neuro/Cellular Repatterning utilizes biofeedback instruments in a nonconventional way. As appropriate questions are posed, the instrument validates responses from the individual's subconscious. Blocked traumatic events that have occurred during the individual's life are located.

Childhood reality is reconstructed as it was. To change dysfunctional behavior patterns, the irrational, illogical, self-defeating programs locked into the cellular memory of the body/mind from childhood must be released.

During a Neuro/Cellular Repatterning treatment, the release of stored trauma is registered graphically on the instrument. Through this release, the individual is freed from denial/delusion to receive the basic needs of all people: self-love and "alrightness." Without these two basic human needs it is very difficult to achieve self-worth, self-esteem, acceptance, and approval.

Currently, Art Martin presents Neuro/Cellular Repatterning workshops on the West Coast several times a year. He has written two books on healing and recovery, *Recovering Yourself* and *Your Body Tells the Truth*. Contact the Wellness Institute for Personal Transformation for more information.

🙂 | NO-NIGHTSHADE DIET | 🙂

The No-Nightshade Diet is a nutritional program used to treat arthritis and other autoimmune diseases.

As the name implies, no plants from the nightshade family may be consumed. This family includes white potatoes, eggplants, all types of peppers (red and green chili, jalapeño, red and green bell peppers, etc.), and tobacco. Black and white pepper may be used for seasoning.

Norman Childers, Ph.D., a victim of arthritis, suffered from severe joint pain and stiffness. Motivated to some type of self-help action, he began to examine his own diet. After careful scrutiny he realized that within a short time of eating tomatoes in any form, his muscles became sore and his joints painful.

As a university professor of horticulture, he was very aware of the toxic nature of plants in the nightshade family (genus *Solanum*, family Solanaceae). Childers then proceeded to test the effect of each nightshade food on himself and found they all worsened his arthritic symptoms. He decided to exclude them all from his diet and within a few months the pain and stiffness he had suffered were gone.

Because the Arthritis Foundation showed little interest in his findings, Childers recruited volunteers through magazine advertisements to help in testing the No-Nightshade Diet.

Over the years he has collected data from several hundred individuals using the diet. From this information he has concluded that completely eliminating nightshade foods from their diet was beneficial to individuals sensitive (allergic) to them.

By adhering to the diet, the dysfunction caused by muscle pain, joint pain, and stiffness could be cured, reduced, or prevented.

It has been estimated that approximately 10 percent of the population is sensitive to edible foods in the nightshade family.

The No-Nightshade Diet is an easy-to-follow self-help measure. For those who consume a lot of prepared foods or eat in restaurants often, caution should be taken. Many varieties of peppers are used in ethnic cuisines for seasoning, and potato starch is commonly used as a thickener in commercially prepared foods.

❧ | ORTHO-BIONOMY | ❧

Ortho-Bionomy is an educational process designed to teach people how to be more at ease with their bodies—physically and energetically. It uses a noninvasive, gentle touch to deal with acute and chronic pain, emotional release, and structural balancing.

It is a technique/philosophy that integrates the body, mind, and spirit and connects with the Taoist way of thinking with respect to getting the most accomplished by doing the least. Ortho-Bionomy shares similarities with Osteopathic Functional Technique, CranioSacral Therapy, Aston-Patterning, and the Feldenkrais Method.

The term Ortho-Bionomy comes from the Greek roots *ortho*, which means "straight" or "genuine," and *bionomy*, the science that deals with natural laws. It loosely translates as "a balanced application of the laws of life" or "correct interpretation of the laws of life."

In simplest terms it means to respect the innate wisdom of the body; do not go against the healing process and do not force it back where you think it should go. In Ortho-Bionomy the concept of the body's capacity to self-correct and self-heal is fundamental.

Ortho-Bionomy was developed by British osteopath Arthur Lincoln Pauls, D.O., F.C.O. A black belt in judo, Pauls both practiced and taught the martial art. He had a sharp awareness of the relationship between energy and movement and understood the need for a movement or process to complete itself (such as the follow-through of swinging a bat or tennis racket).

Pauls' longtime interest in therapeutic bodywork to relieve pain and tension caused by martial arts injuries led him to study Osteopathy. Although he liked the results achieved through its practice, Pauls was not content with the manipulations that forced bones and joints back into place.

While a student, Pauls discovered an article, "Spontaneous Release by Positioning," written by the American osteopath Lawrence Jones, D.O., who after ten years of experimentation found that when patients were made comfortable in very specific ways—when they were put into positions their bodies appeared to be trying to achieve—release of muscle spasm would spontaneously occur.

Based on his understanding and experience, Pauls was in agreement with Jones's principles and techniques. He then developed a dramatically different system of healing based on stimulation of the body's own self-corrective reflexes. Dr. Pauls pursued this idea and began to develop his own system of techniques which he could teach to others. He called this work Ortho-Bionomy.

Ortho-Bionomy has been called the "Homeopathy of Bodywork" because it seeks to accentuate the existing condition in order to achieve a healing result. Like Homeopathy, it follows the line of least resistance.

In Ortho-Bionomy, practitioners use a unique educational approach of gentle positioning and movement of the body to restore balance and comfort. This helps an individual to rediscover comfort and to release the pain and patterns that have maintained them. The basic physical technique is the discovery of the preferred posture, one which is most comfortable for the body, not an idealized posture.

While held in a position of comfort, the body's innate (self-correcting) healing reflex is initiated; tense muscles and ligaments relax, stress and emotional tension are released, natural alignment and balance are restored, and a deep sense of inner harmony is achieved.

Sessions employ conversation and movements such as walking, sitting, standing, and reaching to discover new patterns of self-awareness and structural balance. Patterns of misuse are replaced with long-lasting flexibility and ease. It is compatible with any form of exercise, health care, or personal growth.

Ortho-Bionomy provides effective help for arthritis, whiplash, sports injury, rheumatic ailments, muscle pain, and emotional stress, and aids people with occupations which require habitually imbalanced posture or muscle strain. It restores range of motion and increases relaxation and circulation in different parts of the body.

It is the philosophy of Ortho-Bionomy that the body heals itself, and practitioners only show the individual how to move in his own ideal direction.

Many health care professionals such as massage therapists, physical therapists, naturopaths, chiropractors, etc., incorporate Ortho-Bionomy into their practice. A list of registered Ortho-Bionomy practitioners is available from the Society of Ortho-Bionomy International.

❧ | ORTHOMOLECULAR THERAPY | ❧

Orthomolecular Therapy is the treatment of disease by varying the concentration of substances (nutrients—vitamins, minerals, amino acids, enzymes, and others) normally present in the human body for good health.

Ortho comes from the Greek word for "correct" and *molecular* pertains to molecules, which are the smallest physical unit of an element or compound (substance).

Although Orthomolecular Therapy has been linked to so-called megadoses of vitamins, its real intention is to provide the body with substances it needs to create the correct molecular concentrations or conditions necessary for optimum health. Large or megadoses of a substance are only necessary in some cases and only when appropriate. In others it may mean taking only moderate or small amounts of the substance to correct the deficiency or problem condition in the body.

Early in the 1950s there were few alternatives available to treat schizophrenia other than large doses of sedatives or convulsive therapy, which used drugs or electricity. Violent schizophrenics were restrained with straitjackets.

Two psychiatrists, Drs. Abram Hoffer and Humphrey Osmond, were challenged by the need to relieve the suffering caused by schizophrenic illness.

Before his work with Hoffer, Osmond and a co-worker formulated ideas and did some work on the biochemical nature of the illness.

Hoffer and Osmond developed the theory that schizophrenics suffer from a biochemical condition. They believed schizophrenics abnormally metabolize adrenaline into a chemical called adrenochrome, which produces schizophrenic symptoms.

They then theorized that large doses of niacin (vitamin B_3) would help schizophrenics. This was based on a clue derived from their knowledge of pellagra, a protein-deficiency disease that causes schizophrenic symptoms that is successfully treated with vitamin B_3.

An experiment was conducted by giving schizophrenic patients large doses of niacin (or the amide form niacinamide) and similarly large doses of vitamin C. The results were encouraging and later supported by larger studies.

At that time anything in large quantities was termed *mega*, and thus megavitamin therapy was born and named. This also marked the beginning of what was to become Orthomolecular Medicine and in particular Orthomolecular Psychiatry.

In 1968 Nobel Prize–winning chemist Linus Pauling, in an article titled "Orthomolecular Psychiatry," coined the word *orthomolecular* to denote the use of naturally occurring substances, particularly nutrients, in maintaining health and treating disease.

During that early period, megadose niacin therapy for schizophrenia and the dietary treatment of hypoglycemia were the major emphases in the orthomolecular movement.

The biochemical/orthomolecular approach to good health is based on the understanding that each person is different and has different nutritional needs. This is due to genetically established metabolism, environmental factors, stress, and biochemistry.

Orthomolecular Psychiatry and Medicine treat unique imbalances in an individual's biochemistry which relate to problems such as depression, aging, alcoholism, substance abuse, allergies, hypoglycemia, hyperactivity, and learning disabilities in children, degenerative diseases such as arthritis, schizophrenia, AIDS, and cancer.

The Huxley Institute for Biosocial Research, established in 1971, is a nonprofit, tax-exempt charitable organization which advocates the biochemical/orthomolecular approach to good health. An extensive amount of educational material (books, audiotapes, and article reprints) dealing with the subject of Orthomolecular Medicine is available from them. They also have two quarterly publications, *Getting Better* and *The Journal of Orthomolecular Medicine.*

Today there are many qualified physicians who take the orthomolecular approach to diagnosis and utilize treatments based on diet, nutrition, vitamins, and nutrients. Additional information is available from the Academy of Orthomolecular Medicine.

ॐ | OSTEOPATHY | ॐ

Osteopathy, or Osteopathic Medicine, emphasizes the relationship of the body structure to organic function. It is a complete health care system that combines manipulative care with conventional allopathic medicine. Osteopathic Medicine focuses upon treatment of the individual, not just the disease.

The term *osteopathy* is derived from the Greek roots *osteon*, meaning "bone," and *pathos*, meaning "feeling."

Osteopathic Medicine was developed in 1874 by Andrew Taylor Still, M.D. Born in the state of Virginia in 1828, the son of a Scots mother and English-German father, he served as a surgeon in the Union army during the Civil War.

Dr. Still was dissatisfied with the effectiveness of nineteenth-century medicine and with the use of drugs and curative agents. He had always been a student of nature and insisted that the body was a perfect machine which would function smoothly if allowed to do so.

Dr. Still maintained that all diseases have a cause-and-effect relationship.

A doctor sees the effects of a disease and must find the causes in order to restore the patient's health.

He became interested in the skeleton and the relation of tissues to the bony framework. This led to his belief that a body's functions are determined by its structure. If the structure is out of alignment, other parts of the body will not perform efficiently.

For several years Dr. Still carried on his work as a bonesetter, eventually opening a practice in Kirksville, Missouri. In 1887 he began teaching his four sons the art and in 1892 founded the American School of Osteopathy.

Dr. Still pioneered the concept of "wellness" by helping patients develop a lifestyle that promotes health and prevents disease. This was accomplished through principles of exercise, and proper diet and nutrition. This philosophy has been a cornerstone of the osteopathic profession for more than a century.

Today, osteopathic physicians, or D.O.'s (doctors of osteopathy), undergo similar training as doctors of medicine, or M.D.'s. Osteopathic Medicine comprises a four-year graduate-level curriculum of medical training, a one-year internship, and an optional two-year to six-year residency program in the medical specialty of choice.

The osteopathic physician adheres to the Hippocratic ideal of medicine with a holistic approach to the body/mind and whole person. D.O.'s consider the patient's mental and emotional status as well as his musculoskeletal system. That is, they deal directly with both the internal and external conditions that caused the disease.

D.O.'s prefer treatments which stimulate an individual's natural abilities to maintain or return to a state of optimum health. However, they can prescribe drugs, perform surgery, and utilize all of the currently recognized diagnostic and therapeutic methods known to the practice of modern medicine to maintain and restore the health of their patients.

Osteopathic Medicine places special emphasis on the musculoskeletal system, which reflects and influences the condition of all other body organs and systems. D.O.'s offer a hands-on approach to the diagnosis and treatment of selected ailments involving bones, muscles, tendons, tissues, and the spinal column through the use of palpation, manipulation, and physical therapy.

To treat these problems, a variety of procedures are used. Soft-tissue manipulation or soft-tissue mobilization are osteopathic terms for what is actually massage. A lymphatic massage technique is also used to promote circulation of fluid in the lymphatic system.

Two other osteopathic bodywork modalities are Strain-Counterstrain Therapy and CranioSacral Therapy, described in detail elsewhere in this book.

Strain-Counterstrain Therapy, developed by Lawrence Jones, D.O., is a neuromuscular technique that involves identification of trigger points and use of a hands-on technique to relieve pain caused by trigger points.

CranioSacral Therapy, discovered by John E. Upledger, D.O., treats imbalances in the CranioSacral System, a physiological system in the human body, using a technique of gentle, noninvasive manipulation.

Currently there are fifteen osteopathic medical colleges located throughout the United States. It is estimated that by the year 2000 there will be forty-five thousand osteopathic physicians practicing in the United States.

Two organizations represent the field of Osteopathic Medicine. They are the American Osteopathic Association and the American Academy of Osteopathy. The latter can provide a listing of member physicians in your area. For additional information contact either group.

✑ | OXIDATIVE THERAPY | ✎

Oxidative Therapy is a type of therapy that supplies oxygen to the body for its potential therapeutic benefit.

Currently, the two most widely known types of Oxidative Therapy are Hydrogen Peroxide Therapy and Ozone Therapy. These are separately described elsewhere in this book.

Oxidation is a naturally occurring process in the body which is essential to life. In nature, examples of oxidation include rust on ferrous metals (slow oxidation), and fire (rapid oxidation).

In the course of normal metabolism in the body, chemically reactive entities known as "free radicals" are produced. Free radicals are also formed by exposure to radiation and harmful chemicals, by the breakdown of ingested substances such as fried foods and animal fats, and by other means.

Because they are a major source of cell damage, some researchers believe free radicals lead to aging, cardiovascular disease, and cancer. Antioxidants such as vitamin E can be taken to help reduce the formation of free radicals.

Oxidation is used by the body as a first line of defense against bacteria, virus, yeast, and parasites. Currently, Oxidative Therapy is used to treat a variety of ailments and degenerative diseases. It is an "underground" treatment for AIDS.

The theory behind the use of oxidative treatments for cancer is linked to research in the 1950s by Nobel Prize–winning scientist Otto Warburg. In a 1956 article in *Science* magazine Warburg showed that cancer cells are anaerobic (live without oxygen) and will die in the presence of a high oxygen concentration.

A more recently posed theory explaining the effectiveness of oxidative treatment in various diseases involves the free radical theory of cellular damage. It is thought that the oxidative agent acts as a scavenger in the body, attacking and removing the dangerous and destructive free radicals before they can cause harm.

Additional information about Oxidative Therapies can be found in the book *Oxygen Therapies* by Ed McCabe, available at most health food stores. Also refer to the list of professional organizations in the resource section.

ꔪ | OZONE THERAPY | ꕥ

Ozone Therapy is the use of ozone gas for therapeutic purposes. It is classified as an Oxidative Therapy, which in simplest terms is a therapy that supplies oxygen to the body for its potential therapeutic benefit (see above).

The use of Ozone Therapy is not new. It has been used in Germany since the early 1900s, and thousands of European physicians have utilized it as a medical treatment for more than fifty years. Drs. R. Rilling and R. Viebahn, co-authors of *The Use of Ozone in Medicine*, published in Germany, cite numerous scientific papers that show the effect of ozone in cancer treatment.

Ozone is simply three atoms of oxygen, or triatomic oxygen (O_3). Normal atmospheric oxygen is O_2. In nature ozone is produced when oxygen is exposed to the sun's ultraviolet (UV) rays. It is also produced by lightning. The chemical formula for converting oxygen into ozone is $3O_2$ + UV energy = $2O_3$.

Ozone is bluish in color with a pungent odor. When inhaled, it is an irritant. It is not as stable as normal oxygen. When ozone breaks down as shown in the following reaction ($O_3 \rightarrow O_2 + O_1$), O_1 is released. The O_1 molecule will attack a wide variety of organic molecules.

Because the O_1 kills viruses, bacteria, and fungis, ozone gas has many commercial applications such as sterilization of disposable medical equipment and purification of drinking water.

In humans, O_1 from ozone gas is used to kill bacteria, viruses, yeast, and parasites in the body. It is also used to treat a variety of ailments and degenerative diseases, including cancer and AIDS. Because the FDA has failed to give permission to use Ozone Therapy on AIDS patients, it has become an "underground" treatment in the AIDS community.

Ozone Therapy in humans requires the use of a medically pure grade of ozone, which is produced by a device called an ozone generator. It involves using the correct concentrations of ozone along with proper medical procedure. Ozone is administered by injection under the skin, into the muscle, or by intravenous infusion or enema.

Although numerous clinical reports and animal studies exist, Ozone Therapy is not available in the United States. Presently Ozone Therapy is available only in Europe and Mexico. The well-known Gerson Clinic in Tijuana, Mexico, began using it in 1983 to complement their metabolic program.

Additional information about Ozone Therapy can be found in the book *Oxygen Therapies* by Ed McCabe, available at most health food stores or from the International Ozone Association.

PARASYMPATHETIC MASSAGE

Parasympathetic Massage is a bodywork technique used to stimulate the body's parasympathetic nervous system to help relieve pain and heal the body.

The autonomic nervous system is concerned with regulating body activities automatically or unconsciously. It is divided into two systems, the sympathetic and parasympathetic, which at times work in conjunction with one another and at other times oppose one another.

The sympathetic system deals with energy, action, and survival, often called the "fight or flight" syndrome. During "fight or flight" the adrenal glands are stimulated, increasing blood pressure, heart rate, and blood sugar levels. Blood is diverted from the digestive organs and other normal body functions to support the increased activities of the brain, heart, and skeletal muscles. During this time the body burns all its available resources and produces a great deal of metabolic waste in the process.

When the body is at rest and not threatened, the parasympathetic is able to engage and dominate. It then begins to perform "housekeeping" functions by causing blood to flow from the surface to the internal organs. Digestion and other major body functions such as those of the kidneys, bladder, and large intestine begin to work normally, replenishing the body and increasing elimination of wastes.

Stress stimulates the sympathetic system. Unfortunately, the rigors of modern life keep many people in the sympathetic mode more than is healthy, sometimes to the point where they cannot turn it off. Parasympathetic Massage is used to artificially "turn off" the sympathetic mode.

Parasympathetic Massage is a hybrid technique somewhere between Esalen Style Massage and Manual Lymphatic Drainage that utilizes light, soothing strokes in a clinical manner. It produces a soothing quality in the body, which helps to turn off the sympathetic nervous system, and encourages the parasympathetic system to dominate.

The Esalen Style Massage, with its gentle, nurturing approach, works to relax the body while the Manual Lymphatic Drainage helps to increase the body's healing capacity by cleansing wastes from the body. With this technique, the bodyworker is mechanically flushing waste products through the tissues so the body does not have to work as hard.

The key to all bodywork is using the correct procedure or technique at the optimal time to accomplish what is necessary. For certain situations, Parasympathetic Massage is useful and beneficial. It can be used alone or in combination with other massage techniques.

Parasympathetic Massage technique is taught to massage therapists as part of the thousand-hour holistic health practitioner curriculum. Most massage schools should be able to refer an individual to practitioners with this training.

❧ | PAST LIVES THERAPY | ❧

Past Lives Therapy operates on the assumption that a person can trace the problems he is experiencing in the present lifetime, whether mental, emotional, or physical, to roots in his past lives.

By recreating various scenes from past lives, an individual is better able to understand how these past events relate to certain problems he is experiencing in the present.

Past Lives Therapy serves as a technique for undoing the harmful effects these past incidents have on the present. Through these insights an individual can learn to live his present life more easily and deal with the reality of the here and now. As in many other therapies, Past Lives Therapy assumes the existence of the unconscious mind and establishes the important connection between body and mind.

Although the principle of reincarnation is used as a tool in Past Lives Therapy, it is not essential for the individual to believe in it for the process to be successful.

The idea of past lives and reincarnation has been in existence for thousands of years. Among the ancient Greeks, Pythagoras led an influential religious cult supporting the doctrine of reincarnation. Also the cabala, a collection of Jewish mystical lore, acknowledges the idea of past lives.

Eastern cultures readily accept the idea of reincarnation. Over one billion Hindus, Buddhists, and Jains throughout the world consider reincarnation a fact of life which is deeply rooted in their religious philosophy.

Many people in the West still tend to think of reincarnation in terms of the occult or as bizarre. Past Lives Therapy, however, has had a following in the United States and Europe for over twenty-five years and is continually gaining acceptance.

Past Lives Therapy can be used on both adults and children. It is particularly effective for children because early discovery of past-life traumas can help to prevent emotional and physical problems.

Past Lives Therapists believe that physical pain experienced in past lives is linked to present-day problems. For the therapy to be effective, an individual must relive all of the details surrounding a past life incident fully and completely. This includes the pain and emotional trauma as it occurred moment by moment.

An individual can only detach himself from the past-life trauma, and the associated problems it is causing in the present life, by feeling the emotion of the original incident. With the help of a Past Lives Therapist, the incident can be released after the individual reexperiences it.

The idea of making an individual relive an incident to "detach" himself from his fear of it is not a new concept. Freudian therapy attempts to uncover hidden trauma experienced very early in life.

Today, some psychotherapists are using Past Lives Therapy as an adjunct to conventional psychotherapy; it is sometimes referred to as Regression Therapy.

The key to Past Lives Therapy is accessing the unconscious or subconscious mind. This can be done through either hypnosis or guided meditations.

In hypnosis, the subject is put under a hypnotic trance and taken back in time. This can trigger the recollection of traumatic events from past lives.

Although there are many different types of guided meditations used in Past Lives Therapy, the following is an example of one. The individual is put into a comfortable, relaxed position (usually lying down). With appropriate words and musical background, he is led into a dark tunnel with a light at the end. As he walks down the tunnel, he asks his unconscious to lead him to a past life that will shed light on problems he is having in the present life. As he emerges into the light, he is in another time and space and begins to see events of that past life.

There are many excellent books available on Past Lives Therapy in bookstores and libraries. One by Morris Netherton and Nancy Shiffrin titled *Past Lives Therapy* gives a good overview of the subject.

A very interesting book by Florida psychiatrist Brian L. Weiss, M.D., titled *Many Lives, Many Masters*, details a case history of a twenty-seven-year-old female who suffered from fears and phobias. With no sign of relief after eighteen months of conventional therapy, Dr. Weiss put her under hypnosis. She began to recall traumatic incidents of dying in several past lives, which seemed to explain and relieve her symptoms.

The Association for Past-Life Research and Therapies can provide referrals to member past life therapists in your area. The association also has a large selection of books, videos, and audiotapes available.

❧ | PFRIMMER TECHNIQUE | ☙

The Pfrimmer Technique is a type of deep muscle therapy that utilizes a specific series of cross-fiber tissue movements applied to the muscles by a fully trained Pfrimmer deep muscle therapist. The technique is designed to cause corrective changes in the muscle tissue at the cellular level.

The Pfrimmer Technique, called the original "deep muscle therapy," is based exclusively on over thirty years of research and practical application of Therese C. Pfrimmer, a registered masseuse and physiotherapist from Ontario, Canada. She discovered the technique in the 1940s after being paralyzed from the waist down. Application of the technique she discovered led to the reversal of her paralysis.

Due to injury, fatigue, lactic acid buildup, stress, trauma, etc., the normal flow of body fluids (blood and lymph) is disrupted. Deprived of oxygenated blood and free-flowing lymphatic fluid, the involved layers of muscle fibers begin to weaken, harden, and adhere to surrounding fibers, causing congestion and muscle malfunction.

There are several objectives to Pfrimmer Deep Muscle Therapy. It releases adherent and fibrous conditions existing in the deeper layers of muscle tissue, including the fascia, thus softening the hardened muscle fibers. It restores the free flow of lymph and fresh oxygenated blood, with its natural healing powers, to the whole body. It aids and improves freer joint movement. It assists glandular secretions supplied to muscles when required. And it helps to remove waste products and toxins from the muscles.

Common conditions that have benefited from Pfrimmer Deep Muscle Therapy include arthritis, headache, neuralgia, multiple sclerosis, muscular dystrophy, poor circulation, sciatica, sports injuries, trauma, occupational stress, fibrositis, and many others.

A two-week graduate course in Pfrimmer Deep Muscle Therapy is available to doctors, nurses, physical therapists, and massage therapists at the Alexandria School of Scientific Therapeutics and the Pennsylvania School of Muscle Therapy. For additional information contact the Alexandria School.

❧ | PHYSICAL THERAPY | ❧

Physical Therapy is a hands-on health care profession which has been called "the cornerstone of rehabilitation" because of its role in helping people recover from the effects of injury, surgery, or disease.

Physical Therapy has a long and colorful history. The use of heat as a therapeutic agent can be traced back to the Egyptians, who built temples to the sun god Ra, and worshiped the sun's healing power. In Peru the Incas used the sun to improve their health. A Chinese practitioner, Kong-Fu, wrote a book in 3000 B.C. on the value of massage and exercise.

The Romans used application of hot wax to relieve pain and were the first to use Hydrotherapy. Underwater exercise in warm springs was used to treat paralysis from war wounds and the pains of the aging civilian population. Both Greeks and Romans used vessels filled with hot water, sand, or coals for the localized application of heat.

While Europe was in the Dark Ages, medicine continued in Arab-dominated areas. Two Middle Eastern authors reported on the therapeutic and hygienic effects of exercise. In the sixteenth and seventeenth centuries several major British works praised the value of massage and exercise in the treatment of disease. In the middle of the nineteenth century German and French doctors wrote of the effectiveness of massage for circulation and overall health.

Sweden's Per Hendrik Ling (1776–1839), known as the "Father of European Physical Culture," demonstrated that exercises performed correctly could remedy bodily defects and disease. He established the Central Institute of Massage and Corrective Exercises in Stockholm in 1813. He also built the first swimming pool in Europe.

Although a large number of physical therapists work in hospitals, today more than 60 percent of them can be found in private Physical Therapy offices, community health centers, corporate or industrial health centers, sports facilities, research institutions, rehabilitation centers, nursing homes, pediatric centers and schools, colleges, and universities.

Individuals normally visit a physical therapist for a specific purpose with a prescription from their physician. The physical therapist is qualified to use different types of tests to determine the extent of the malfunction or damage to soft tissue and bony structures in the patient.

The physical therapist may employ a wide variety of sophisticated equipment, one of which can show the difference in muscle strength and range of motion between affected and unaffected limbs. A different piece of equipment is used in the case of postural problems or a condition that involves the skeleton and how it relates to soft tissue problems. Electroneuromyography, an electrical test procedure that evaluates the condition of nerves and muscles, can also be used by the physical therapist as a source of invaluable information.

Physical therapists also conduct hands-on and visual examination of patients, testing such things as joint movement and range of motion; they palpate bony structures to determine postural deviations, and examine soft tissue structures for abnormal conditions.

After the physical therapist has analyzed the results of various mechanical, electrical, and hands-on tests, a working diagnosis is arrived at. A treatment program is then implemented to address the problem.

This regimen of therapy may include a program of corrective exercises,

Electrotherapy (electrical stimulation), Hydrotherapy, traction, heat, ultrasound, Cryotherapy (ice), manipulation, or Massage Therapy, depending on the person's particular problem.

The goal of Physical Therapy is to assist the person's body in healing itself as rapidly as possible. Treatments are intended to assist individuals in their recovery process by helping them to increase strength, reduce swelling, relieve pain, and restore normal range of motion and function. They also help individuals to relearn normal daily activities such as walking, dressing, or bathing.

In the case of injury, therapist and patient also strive for stabilization and prevention of further injury or reinjury in the future. Physical therapists do this by teaching people the importance of fitness and showing them how to avoid injury to their bodies at work or play.

Physical Therapy is a licensed profession. After graduating from an accredited educational program, physical therapist candidates must pass a state-administered national exam. Other requirements for Physical Therapy practice vary from state to state.

For additional information contact the American Physical and Physio Therapy Association.

POETRY THERAPY

Poetry Therapy is the therapeutic use of poetry for the treatment and healing of emotional disorders or the facilitation of psychological growth. The process involves the individuals' creation of their own poetry or response to poems written by others, after reading or listening to them.

Closely allied to Poetry Therapy is Bibliotherapy (from the word *bibliography*). Bibliotherapy, which expands the scope of Poetry Therapy, is a term sometimes used to describe the wide range of materials available for therapy. Simplified, it is the use of various types of literature for the purpose of healing.

The Biblio/Poetry Therapy approach involves the use of metaphor and imagery derived from published poems and lyrics, other literary forms such as short fiction, plays, novels, stories, myths, and fables, audiovisual aids, and other material considered bibliotherapeutic.

Poetry Therapy is not a creation of the late twentieth century, as one might think. Its origins date back to prehistory, when Stone Age shamans used rhythmic spells and urgent appeals to communicate with the unconscious.

The relationship between poetry, insight, and healing goes back to ancient Greece. Apollo, god of medicine, prophecy, and poetry, was one of the principal deities on Mount Olympus. Presentations at the Aesclepius Temple theaters were attended for the explicit purpose of psychological healing. In 330 B.C. Aristotle expounded on the power of literature to stir up emotions and purge unhealthy feelings.

In his autobiography, John Stuart Mill (1806–73), son of Scottish historian and philosopher James Mill (1773–1836), described how he healed himself with poetry. In the mid 1800s the Reverend John Keble expounded on the virtues of poetry. He believed that poetry "is a safety valve which can prevent mental disease."

At the beginning of this century, it is obvious that Sigmund Freud realized the worth of poetry when he said, "Not I, but the poet, discovered the unconscious."

The work of a poet named Eli Greifer laid the foundation for the practice of modern Poetry Therapy. Originally educated as an attorney, Greifer later turned to poetry. Beginning in 1928 he opened several poetry clubs and galleries in New York's Greenwich Village. While making a living as a pharmacist, Greifer offered his clientele unique "prescriptions" in the form of poems. For therapy, he would advise his clients to recite poetry. Poems, selected to be uplifting and supportive of the ego-self, were to be repeated until they became a part of the individual's subconscious. This same principle is applied today in the repetition of positive affirmations.

The reading and writing of poetry became a "saving grace" for a segment of the inmate population in German concentration camps during World War II. Amidst brutal treatment and the atrocities of war, poetry helped this group of people maintain their sanity and sense of humanity.

One of the first major works on Poetry Therapy, entitled *The Healing Power of Poetry*, was written by psychiatrist Dr. Smiley Blanton in the 1940s.

By 1958 Eli Greifer was working in the mental hygiene clinic at Brooklyn's Cumberland Hospital. There he met a psychiatrist named Dr. Jack J. Leedy. Through a collaborative effort they established the first formal Poetry Therapy group in the United States. Soon, other groups were established around the country.

During the 1960s professional poets were attracted to the therapy groups, which added credibility to the emerging field. Dr. Leedy began working with drug abusers in New York City and later went on to compile and edit two major works in the field of Poetry Therapy.

In 1968 Dr. Leedy and Morris Morrison, Ph.D., jointly started the Association of Poetry Therapists. A few years later the name was changed to the National Association for Poetry Therapy.

Poetry is a unique and powerful form of communication. A poem can inspire, stimulate, evoke positive and negative emotions, or change our perspective on a given situation. Through metaphor and imagery a poem can convey feelings in a way no other medium can. It is precisely these qualities that enable Poetry Therapy to be an effective healing tool.

Poems used in a typical Poetry Therapy group session are chosen for specific qualities. They usually have strong emotional appeal; contain striking original metaphors; are relatively easy to comprehend; move along to rhythms that provide momentum; and are short enough to hold attention. The subtle nature of poetry is always one of its most important features.

By allowing an individual to bring up profound feelings in a safe and supportive atmosphere and express or release these feelings in a socially acceptable manner, Poetry Therapy provides a powerful approach to healing. For individuals in therapy who write their own poetry, the goal is not to make them into poets but to give them an appropriate and meaningful avenue of expression.

A wide variety of populations have successfully responded to Poetry Therapy, including geriatric patients suffering from Alzheimer's, strokes, and heart disease, the mentally retarded, the emotionally disturbed, schizophrenic patients, substance abusers, the eating disordered, veterans, depressed and suicidal patients, and those suffering with physical illness and disabilities.

In the elderly, especially those suffering from memory disorders, poems may rekindle memories and awake dormant pleasurable feelings which can add to the quality of life.

Poetry Therapy is usually not considered a stand-alone therapy. It is most effective when used in conjunction with other treatment techniques or as part of a comprehensive treatment program.

Before an individual can become certified in the area of Poetry Therapy, she is required to take specialized training. This usually includes the study of therapeutic processes, supervised work in a clinical setting, and instruction dealing with the proper selection of literature.

For additional information contact the National Association for Poetry Therapy. An extensive bibliography list is available from the association. Two classics are *Poetry As Healer: Mending the Troubled Mind*, edited by Jack J. Leedy, M.D., and *Poetry in the Therapeutic Experience*, edited by Arthur Lerner, Ph.D.

✍ | POLARITY THERAPY | ✍

Polarity Therapy is a natural system that seeks to balance the body's life energy. This complete, holistic method of health care combines diet, exercise, practitioner touch, and self-awareness to provide a simple, comprehensive method for health maintenance.

The principles of Polarity Therapy were developed by Randolph Stone, D.C., D.O., N.D. (1890–1982). Born in Austria, he emigrated to the United States in 1903 and settled in Chicago.

From an early age Dr. Stone studied all the available systems of natural healing in addition to Western science. He received doctoral degrees in Chiropractic, Osteopathy, and Naturopathy.

Dr. Stone did extensive reading in Western occult tradition and became involved with the profound questions of health and illness. He wanted to know why some people were inclined toward certain types of disease and what factors were involved in avoiding illness and maintaining optimal wellness.

After extensive travel to study the traditional healing systems of other cultures, Dr. Stone became especially interested in the Eastern healing methods. From China and Japan came Acupuncture, Herbal Medicine, and Shiatsu. The Hermetic and cabalistic systems came from the Middle East. And from India came the principles of Ayurveda and Yoga.

Using the knowledge he acquired from these different sources, in addition to his own inspiration and insights, Dr. Stone blended aspects of East and West to create a new and unique system called Polarity Therapy.

In 1948 he outlined the basic principles of his new system in a privately published book titled *Energy: The Vital Principle in the Healing Art*. Over the years he continued to develop the principles of Polarity Therapy and taught it to other health practitioners while maintaining a private practice.

In 1973 Dr. Stone retired and appointed Pierre Pannetier, his student for ten years, to succeed him. Pannetier was born in Kampot, Cambodia, in 1914. After assuming the leadership duties of the Polarity Therapy movement, he traveled extensively throughout the United States and Canada disseminating information and teaching Polarity Therapy seminars. He died in 1984, just two years after Dr. Stone.

The Polarity Therapy system of energy balancing asserts that energy fields and currents exist everywhere in nature, and that the free flow and balance of this energy in the human body is the underlying foundation of good health.

This life force or energy referred to in Polarity Therapy has similar concepts in other cultures. In China and Japan it is called *chi*; in India it is called *prana*; it is "bioplasmic" energy in Russian psychic research; and Wilhelm Reich called it "orgone" energy.

In Polarity Therapy, energy is either positive (+), negative (−), or neutral (0). Energy is not considered good or bad; what matters is whether it is blocked or free flowing in the body.

Dr. Stone taught that body, mind, emotions, and spirit are all interdependent, and each person is responsible for his own health. In Polarity Therapy the practitioner and client work together in a healing relationship to address problems caused by energy blockages in the body/mind.

As previously stated, Polarity Therapy utilizes four interrelated therapeutic methods: bodywork, diet, exercise, and self-awareness.

In Polarity bodywork the practitioner's hands are used for a variety of touching movements or contacts on the client's body. This is nonmanipulative bodywork in the sense that it does not work on muscles, connective tissue, or bones.

The practitioner (giver) places his hands on two designated points (energy centers), one charged positive and the other charged negative, on the client's (receiver's) body. The giver's hands are also charged, the left being positive and the right being negative. The giver places his positively charged hand on the receiver's negative body point and his negatively charged hand on the receiver's positively charged body point.

The giver's hands do not impart energy, they merely redirect the flow of the receiver's own energy. The receiver then recharges himself with his own freed energy.

When energy is balanced between positive and negative poles (points or locations in the body), the "neutral" principle is manifested. In this neutral state energy between two points is balanced and recharged, allowing the free flow to be reestablished. This results in harmony and is experienced by the individual as health and well-being.

A short-term diet is used for internal cleansing or purification, and a long-term diet for maintenance that leads to optimal well-being.

Exercise utilizes Polarity Yoga in a series of simple self-help techniques that create relaxation and balance.

In the self-awareness portion of Polarity, an individual learns to understand the source of his tension and discovers ways to sustain his health.

All of the major works of Dr. Randolph Stone are collected in three volumes: the two-volume *Polarity Therapy* and *Health Building: The Conscious Art of Living Well.*

For a list of Polarity Therapy practitioners in your area or for more information, contact the American Polarity Therapy Association, where also available is a large selection of books, videos, audiocassettes, and charts.

❧ | POSTURAL INTEGRATION | ❦

Postural Integration is a complete system of bodywork for releasing the blocks and tensions which have accumulated in the body/mind. It works simultaneously with the physical, mental, and emotional aspects of the whole person. These include tissue, breathing, postures, movements, positions, thoughts, and feelings.

Postural Integration was developed by Jack W. Painter, Ph.D., after many years of self-exploration in the fields of massage, Acupuncture, Gestalt, Reichian Therapy, and Rolfing.

Born in 1933, Dr. Painter was raised in eastern Tennessee and graduated from Emory University in Atlanta, Georgia. He also studied in Germany, France, and Poland.

Between 1962 and 1971 he was a professor at the University of Miami. During this time he researched Acupuncture, zazen, Yoga, Connective Tissue Manipulation, and Reichian and Gestalt bodywork.

Dr. Painter holds a Massage Therapy degree from Lindsey Hopkins Technical Education Center in Miami, and is an associate of the Wilhelm Reich Institute in Mexico. He was one of Ida Rolf's students.

In Postural Integration, different techniques are synthesized into a single process that is both powerful and loving. It utilizes a type of bodywork to move deep blocked layers of fascia and reorganize the muscular system. At the same time the process opens and releases most stubborn emotions and thoughts that are held within.

Fascia is the connective tissue which gives shape to the body and holds it together. The fascial system is a densely woven sheet of connective tissue that surrounds, penetrates, lines, or covers nearly every muscle, bone, nerve, artery, and vein as well as all the internal organs, including the heart, lungs, brain, and spinal cord.

The fascia is not just a system of separate coverings, but is actually one structure that extends from the top of the head to the tip of the toes, which plays an important role in the support of the body. Fascia is composed of two types of fibers: collagenous fibers, which are tough and have little ability to stretch, and elastic fibers, which are stretchable.

In the normal healthy state, fascia is relaxed and has the ability to move without restriction. When the body experiences habitually poor posture, disease, physical trauma, repeated patterns of self-use (such as in a job), surgery, emotional distress, and other factors, the effect on the fascia is cumulative over time. Eventually, as the fascia loses some of its pliability, it thickens and hardens. This leads to stiffness, restricted motion, pain, and an overall loss of freedom of movement in the body.

Fortunately, connective tissue has a physical structure that is like gelatin. It becomes amorphous (having no definite shape) when energy is applied to it. While in the amorphous state, it can be reformed into any position or shape desired. Then, as the energy is removed, the fascia solidifies and retains the new shape.

During a typical session the Postural Integration practitioner uses her hands, fingers, and forearms to smooth and redistribute bunched and disorganized layers of fascia. This allows overstretched muscles to contract and overcontracted muscles to relax.

Muscle tone is then restored to a balanced state. The skeleton, without manipulation, returns to an upright position, which distributes body weight more evenly. This creates a new flexible alignment which allows energy to flow freely throughout the body.

While the practitioner is performing bodywork the client is simultaneously encouraged to breathe more freely, to express blocked emotions and thoughts, and to explore new physical movements. The practitioner may enter into a dialogue with the client to clarify the client's feelings and ideas.

The practitioner is responsible for knowing how much pressure to use on the client at any given time. Pressure that is too light will evoke nothing new, and pressure that is too severe will cause tense muscles to become even more rigid.

The extraordinary power of Postural Integration to effect positive change is based on the willingness of the client and practitioner to work with the client on many levels. The client's body, mind, and emotions are addressed at the same time, giving a physical, emotional, and cognitive unity to the process.

Postural Integration is a process of ten separate seventy-five-minute sessions, although some individuals may require more. During the first seven sessions, the legs, pelvis, torso, arms, and head are each thoroughly and deeply released. Then in the final three sessions all of the parts are carefully brought back into a harmonious relation with one another.

Dr. Painter is the author of two books, *Deep Bodywork and Personal Development, Harmonizing Our Bodies, Emotions, and Thoughts* and *Technical Manual of Deep Wholistic Bodywork.* Both are available from the International Center for Release and Integration.

Additional information and an international directory of postural integration practitioners is also available from the center.

❦ | PRANIC HEALING | ❧

Pranic Healing is one of the oldest and most widespread systems of natural healing. This technique utilizes a form of energy sometimes called prana, magnetism, or vitality to treat various ailments.

Prana is a Sanskrit word meaning "to breathe forth." It is the universal vital life energy force that is found in the sun, the air, and the earth that keeps the body alive and healthy. It is also known as *chi* in Acupuncture and *ruah* or "breath of life" in the Old Testament.

Pranic Healing works with the "bioplasmic" or etheric body. Also known as the "aura," it is the energy field that surrounds and penetrates the physical body.

The philosophy of Pranic Healing is that by healing the etheric body, the physical body will also be healed in the process. It acts as a catalyst to initiate the body's innate ability to heal itself.

In a Pranic Healing session, the practitioner scans or "feels" the individual's etheric body to diagnose disease energies and then remove them. No physical contact is made between the practitioner and subject, who remains fully clothed.

The practitioner or healer utilizes her own chakras to assimilate prana. She then converts it into healing energy and sends it to the receiver's body. When vital life energy is transferred from the practitioner or healer to the receiver's etheric body, it serves to vitalize his physical body, especially the endocrine glandular system.

Pranic Healing increases the body's natural healing rate by stimulating the cells and tissue back to normal activity. It can be used to vitalize the immune system, relieve headaches, menstrual pains, muscle and back pain, and relieve ailments related to other body systems.

Although it can be used alone, it is only an adjunct to orthodox medical care—not a replacement for it. Pranic Healing can also be used as a self-healing technique. It is used by physicians, nurses, bodyworkers, chiropractors, hypnotherapists, and other health care workers as a supplement to their main modality.

Pranic Psychotherapy uses Pranic Healing techniques to help alleviate psychological and emotional problems. Traumatic and negative experiences held in various parts of the etheric body as negative energy can be removed and dissipated with the help of Pranic Psychotherapy.

Problems such as anxiety, grief, phobias, compulsive behaviors, alcoholism, and others can be treated with Pranic Healing. Pranic Psychotherapy is not meant to replace professional psychiatric care but rather to enhance and complement it. It is used by psychiatrists and psychological therapists.

For additional information concerning training in Pranic Healing and Pranic Psychotherapy, contact the American Institute of Asian Studies. The institute also has available the book *Pranic Healing* by Master Choa Kok Sui, the world's foremost authority on Pranic Healing.

PRIMAL THERAPY

Primal Therapy, a type of psychotherapy, is sometimes mistakenly known as Primal Scream Therapy. It is a slow, precise, systematic, and predictable method of experiencing pain from repressed feelings, and then releasing these repressed feelings.

Primal Therapy was developed by Dr. Arthur Janov, who wrote *The Primal Scream* in 1970; the therapy has remained unchanged since that time. In the decades since, it has been carefully examined at research facilities throughout the world. Studies have shown that heart rate and other vital signs improved in patients who received Primal Therapy.

Primal Therapy is based on the concept that all people experience traumatic events in life, beginning at the time of birth and continuing through to the present. Sometimes the pain from these events is more than we can absorb or integrate at the time it occurs. When this happens, it is necessary to repress a good part of the trauma and store it for future reference.

Dr. Janov feels that repression is the number one killer in the world today. This accumulated reservoir of pain from lack of love, unfulfilled or poorly met needs, and a host of other reasons can produce many serious medical problems. Repression can manifest itself disguised as many different ailments, including cancer, heart disease, diabetes, anxiety, high blood pressure, ulcers, depression, sexual difficulties, sleep disorders, and a host of others.

The way Dr. Janov found to reverse the process of repressed feelings is to have the patient go back and relive the original overwhelming experience. Each scene, feeling, or need relating to the experience is recounted bit by bit over a period of time until it is resolved and out of the patient's system.

In a session, a patient is led back into her unconscious to relive the most recently occurring events first, and then works back to the time of birth. The traumatic events are removed one layer at a time over a period of months to years. Crying is an essential part of the therapy.

Primal Therapy is able to reduce or eliminate a variety of physical and psychic ailments in a relatively short period of time with lasting results. The process enables individuals to become more feeling human beings whose bodies are no longer strangers to their minds.

Treatment usually begins with a patient receiving individual therapy almost every day for three weeks to open her defense system. Primal therapists believe individuals set up a defense system to guard and protect their deeply repressed feelings. A defense system is developed for each traumatic event that an individual experiences and cannot deal with.

Primal Therapy opens the defense system in two ways. First, the defense system is identified and then dispersed. Second, the therapist helps direct the patient to the feeling, which releases the defense system.

After three weeks of individual therapy, patients enter a group. It usually comprises thirty to forty people and meets once a week for six to twelve months. After six months of group therapy, another week of individual therapy is scheduled to monitor progress. The patient then returns to the group. At the end of twelve months, additional individual therapy is scheduled if necessary.

Because an avalanche of painful traumatic experiences can be quickly released and may overwhelm a patient, therapists must have the proper training and experience to be able to deal with these situations. Dr. Janov warns of the dangers of therapists practicing Primal Therapy without sufficient training. Therapists trained by him are required to go through Primal Therapy themselves in addition to receiving two to three years of education.

For a complete and detailed description of Primal Therapy, Dr. Janov's book, *The New Primal Scream: Primal Therapy Twenty Years On*, is available in bookstores and libraries.

❧ | PRITIKIN DIET | ❧

The Pritikin Diet, also called the Pritikin Lifetime Eating Plan, is the nutritional half of the Pritikin Program, which also includes aerobic exercise.

The Pritikin Diet is not vegetarian, but it is low in fats, cholesterol, protein, and highly refined carbohydrates such as sugar and bleached white flour. It stresses foods high in unrefined, fiber-rich carbohydrates like vegetables, fruits, and grains.

Basically, these are "foods as they are grown" or minimally processed and eaten raw or cooked. Meat and fish intake is restricted to under one-quarter pound per day. These principles are not new. For centuries the hardiest, longest-living people in the world have thrived on these foods, a diet similar to many eaten in Third World countries. People in these countries have a minimum of diseases associated with modern Western culture such as heart attack, stroke, arthritis, gout, and diabetes.

Ideally the Pritikin Lifetime Eating Plan should be started at age two and followed for a lifetime. It is a maintenance diet designed to keep good cardiovascular health and body weight.

For those who need to control or even reverse heart disease, high blood pressure, or diabetes there is a variation of the Lifetime Eating Plan. Called a "therapeutic modification" to the Lifetime Eating Plan, it is used at the Pritikin Longevity Center. This variation is more restrictive than the maintenance diet. It limits high protein intake to three and one-half ounces per week and lowers the total daily caloric intake.

As an additional benefit the Pritikin Diet has been shown to make people look and feel younger, with greater energy, vitality, and increased sensory acuity. It mitigates many of the devastating effects of the aging process.

During World War II Nathan Pritikin reviewed classified documents which showed that death from heart disease and diabetes in Europe had dropped significantly during the wartime period. This information piqued his interest because he had been taught that stress caused heart disease. Pritikin reasoned that few situations could be more stressful than war.

In the mid-1950s, after an examination by a cardiologist, Pritikin discovered at the age of forty-two he had substantial coronary heart disease. After extensive research on heart disease, Pritikin was convinced he needed to reduce his cholesterol level below 160. Seeking help at the nutrition department of a major West Coast university, Pritikin was told that cholesterol could not be controlled and that to try to do so would be dangerous. He decided to make diet changes on his own and at his own risk.

By 1958 Pritikin had become a vegetarian and reduced his cholesterol level to 162, but he showed no improvement in heart function. By 1960 his cholesterol was down to 120 and his electrocardiogram was normal.

Pritikin then decided he would try to increase his coronary circulation by expanding his walking program. Later he began jogging and by 1965 he was able to run continuously for an hour.

In 1976 the Pritikin Longevity Center in Santa Barbara, California, was opened. There it was shown that as many as twenty major ailments responded to nutritional therapy.

Today the Pritikin Longevity Center is located near the ocean in Santa Monica, California. It offers closely supervised thirteen- and twenty-six-day programs utilizing diet and exercise for people with "mild" to "serious" heart disease, high blood pressure, and diabetes.

For additional information on the Pritikin Diet and Pritikin Program, two books, *Pritikin Program for Diet and Exercise* by Nathan Pritikin and *The New Pritikin Program* by Robert Pritikin, are available in bookstores and libraries.

For information on the Pritikin residential programs and the Pritikin Longevity Center, contact the center.

❧ | PRITIKIN EXERCISE | ❧

Pritikin Exercise is an exercise program geared toward helping the heart and circulatory system function better. It is one-half of the Pritikin Program and used in conjunction with the Pritikin Diet (Pritikin Lifetime Eating Plan; see above).

Any aerobic exercise will accomplish this but walking is preferred because of its convenience and its involvement of the arms and legs.

Exercise that puts a constant stress on the legs is beneficial because the leg muscles act as a "second heart" by helping to pump blood back to the heart.

At the Pritikin Longevity Center in Santa Monica, participants in the program always begin their exercise with a gentle stretching routine. They then have a choice of walking, aerobic dancing, aerobic weight training, or Yoga. Aerobic exercises coupled with the Pritikin Diet (Pritikin Lifetime Eating Plan) greatly improve an individual's quality of life. This includes looking better, feeling better, and performing better.

❧ | PROPRIOCEPTIVE NEUROMUSCULAR FACILITATION (PNF STRETCHING) | ❧

Proprioceptive Neuromuscular Facilitation, or PNF Stretching, is a unique stretching technique. It is a type of muscular reeducation therapy that utilizes a method of "tricking" the proprioceptors in the body to accomplish specific goals.

Proprioceptors are neurological receptive mechanisms (sensory receptors) located throughout the body. Although found primarily in the soft tissue, they are also located in and around the joints.

The purpose of proprioceptors, which function at the subconscious level, is to monitor every body movement. This information is conveyed through the nervous system to the brain, which is then able to tell us exactly where our body is situated in space.

Proprioceptors in soft tissues are continuously relaying information concerning the status of that soft tissue to the brain. The information includes how short or long a muscle is, its state of contraction, and how much tension is on the muscle tissue. Proprioceptors in joints tell at what angle the joint is, and how much pressure is on it.

All of this information provides a frame of reference from which we can engage in motion. In essence, proprioceptors tell the brain everything it needs to know so that we can coordinate the action of the movements we want to make.

Without information from proprioceptors we would feel as if we were lost in the space we were currently occupying, and it would be impossible to do any of our normal daily tasks.

The human body has a tremendous potential to be flexible and agile. It is able to move into complicated positions which most individuals never use.

A gymnast or circus contortionist is an example of a person that explores the full range of movements available.

Proprioceptive Neuromuscular Facilitation is a Physical Therapy–oriented technique that was developed in the 1940s and 1950s. It was used to treat individuals with neurological impairment.

PNF Stretching is used to "trick" a proprioceptor in order to gain increased flexibility and improvement in physical performance. For example, a therapist puts a client into a stretch that is comfortable for him, then holds the client in that position as the client tries to push out of it. The muscle is tensed during the stretch. When the tensing is released, the muscle is able to stretch a little bit further. This procedure is repeated three to four times. Each time the muscle stretches a little further, with less resistance.

Through some mechanism, the proprioceptors have been trained to accept the new possibility (the further stretching of the muscle). There is a limit to what can be accomplished in one day. Although an individual can gain a significant amount of increased flexibility, the improvement is not always permanent.

PNF Stretching has other applications in Physical Therapy. It can be used as a tool to unlock an injured joint (joints sometimes lock from injury) that is not relearning its ability to bend, and it also has applications in rehabilitation therapy.

This versatile technique is also used outside the Physical Therapy venue. Currently it is receiving extensive use in Sports Massage and sports training.

PNF Stretching can be used by an athlete before an event for increased performance or after a race to keep the body from binding itself up. It makes the body a little lighter and a little easier to move, and can give an athlete a winning edge.

❧ | RADIANCE TECHNIQUE | ❦

The Radiance Technique is a vibrational science of universal energy that allows an individual to access and transmit healing energy through his hands. This form of Reiki (see elsewhere in this book) can be used to benefit yourself or others.

This ancient Tibetan system is not unique but one of several similar energy sciences that have come from the East. The Radiance Technique is related to other forms of energy science such as Transcendental Meditation, Yoga, the science of the mandala, and others.

Although the actual methods, processes, and procedures of these ancient sciences are all different, they share one common purpose—that of empowering an individual to directly access and guide an energy principle known as transcendental, universal cosmic energy.

The inner knowledge of these energy sciences has been passed on for centuries in many different forms, including music, chanting, intonation of mantras such as the universal mantra "om," and complex systems of colors and symbols.

As an energy science, the Radiance Technique is based on a special language of symbols which generate universal, light vibrations. The complete system consists of a series of seven degrees or levels in which students are provided the necessary symbols to learn "attunement." This attunement process opens the student to receive energy. Each higher degree or level of attunement allows the student to receive greater energy.

Through the "laying-on of hands" an individual can use this transcendental universal energy on himself, others, pets, and plants. It can be used as a tool for healing, and for personal growth and transformation.

Benefits may include release of tension; enhancement of creativity, vitality, and productivity; release of negative habits; and promoting positive wellness, love, compassion, peace, and serenity.

The Radiance Technique Association International was formerly known as the American-International Reiki Association. The Radiance Technique Association International is headed by Dr. Barbara Ray, who was initiated by Hawayo Takata. The association can provide the names of authorized instructors who teach in your area.

The association also publishes a magazine, *The Radiance Technique Journal*, and has published several books, including *The Official Handbook of the Radiance Technique, The "Reiki" Factor: The Expanded Edition,* and *The Expanded Reference Manual of the Radiance Technique,* all by Dr. Barbara Ray.

❧ | RADIONICS | ❦

Radionics is a method of diagnosing disease through the use of a Radionic instrument which senses vibration in the human body. Some Radionic instruments can also generate vibrations which are used to treat the disease.

The Radionics practitioner can also use the instrument on a sample taken from the individual's body, such as a spot of blood or saliva (called a "witness") which can transmit the individual's "vibrational energies."

Radionics is based on the assumption that an invisible energy field radiates out from all matter, whether animate or inanimate. The more complex the material, the more complex its pattern or wave form. Living organisms such as human beings exhibit extremely complex patterns, parts of which relate to various organs and systems in the body. Each organ or specific disease vibrates at a specific frequency.

In the early 1900s, Dr. Albert Abrams (1863–1924), Dean of Clinical Medicine at Stanford University Medical School, was the first to discover the principles of Radionics. After receiving his medical degree from Heidelberg, Germany, Dr. Abrams became a prominent San Francisco neurologist. A brilliant and imaginative man, he used inherited wealth to fund his own medical research.

While performing examinations, Dr. Abrams discovered quite by chance that tapping sharply on a specific area of a diseased patient's abdomen would produce a "dull" response. He speculated that the diseased tissue produced some type of "radiation" which caused the muscles in the stomach wall to contract and give the dull response.

Abrams developed a theory that diseased tissue had a molecular structure unlike that of normal tissue. He believed it differed in both atomic and electrical composition. If the diseased tissue were different electronically, then it could be detected with an instrument.

Armed with this theory, Abrams developed a simple variable resistance box to measure it. This entirely new system of diagnosis was initially called "the Electronic Reactions of Abrams" but later became known as "Radionics." He proposed that disease could be treated as an electrical aberration which caused an altered vibratory rate in the tissue.

Using the device, he was able to perform "distance diagnoses" using only a spot of the patient's blood. The device was also able to diagnose a disease in its very early stages, before physical symptoms were evident.

Some years later he developed the "Abrams Generator," a treatment device designed to neutralize abnormal radiations and change the vibratory rate in diseased tissue back to normal. Although Abrams did thorough research and had considerable professional status, the medical community in the United States did not accept his work.

During the 1930s Ruth Drown, a chiropractor in Hollywood, California, and T. G. Hieronymus, a radio expert and engineer, undertook serious research into the potential applications of Radionics. Hieronymus developed and then patented in 1949 one of the best-known Radionic instruments produced in the United States. Drown developed Radionic photography, a process in which the "witness" is streamed across photographic film, leaving images of problem areas in the body. Drown's work was not well accepted either. By the early 1950s the Food and Drug Administration banned the sale of her Radionic devices and she was convicted of medical fraud.

Later in England, several researchers developed a variety of Radionic instruments for diagnosis and treatment, and in 1960 the Radionics Association was founded. Curiously, the field of Radionics has had much greater acceptance there than in the United States.

Some researchers believe that the fundamental principle involved in Radionics is mind energy rather than anything to do with electronics.

Modern Radionics instruments have a variety of dials and gauges which the operator can use for either diagnosis or treatment. Although these devices are more sophisticated than the original that Abrams developed, the accuracy of a Radionics diagnosis or success of treatment is still dependent on the sensitivity and skill of the operator. Some would say this "skill" is a form of psychic ability.

Although the procedure is somewhat detailed, complicated, and variable, a simplified description follows. A sample such as a blood spot, drop of saliva, or hair which contains the person's vibrational energy is put in the instrument. The operator strokes a metal plate and each of two main dials give a numerical reading. The reading on dial number 1 indicates the type of disease and the reading on dial number 2 indicates the organ or area of the body where the disease is located. The hyphenated combination of these two numbers is known as the "rate." By knowing the rate, a chart can be used to determine the problem and the machine can be set for treatment. When the operator encounters an ailment for which there is no established rate, she must use her own intuitive powers to determine a diagnosis and treatment.

Radionics is an extremely controversial method of diagnosing and treating ailments. There are many people who say they have been helped by it while an equal number say they have not. The American Medical Association views it as quackery. While still in use today, Radionics remains controversial and is somewhat of an "underground" movement in the United States.

🌿 | REBIRTHING | 🐚

Rebirthing, as defined by Leonard Orr, is a process of "learning to breathe energy as well as air." It is a simple process of breathing and purification that enhances an individual's "aliveness." It can rejuvenate the body and mind while providing the individual with emotional support and spiritual inspiration.

The word *Rebirthing* is used by many people to mean any emotional release or rush of energy in the body that stimulates breathing. A Rebirthing *experience* usually refers to the release of "psychoanalytical" pain and the receiving of healing energy while practicing a specific breathing technique.

The Rebirthing movement was founded by Leonard Orr in the late 1970s after many years of personal experimentation with the process. Previous to developing Rebirthing, he had been an avid student of spiritual and metaphysical thought and worked with the est (Erhard Seminar Training) organization.

Orr was born in the small dairy farming town of Walton, New York. He was an unwanted child, the last to be born, twelve years after his mother decided she did not want any more children than the three girls she already had. His was a breach birth and he nearly died during the very difficult delivery. Although raised in a beautiful rural setting, Orr did not enjoy it because of these early traumas.

In 1962 Orr's first Rebirthing experience occurred spontaneously while bathing. One morning he stayed in the bathtub for two hours before regaining enough strength to get out. Between 1962 and 1975 he had numerous Rebirthing experiences. During that period he discovered the main component of the process, with the major advance occurring between 1974 and 1975.

During a spiritual psychology seminar in 1974 he described to the audience the birth memories he had experienced and instructed them on how to precipitate these memories while in their own bathtubs.

The people who tried this experiment had powerful results but expressed the wish that there had been someone there to talk with about the experience. This is how Orr developed the idea of Rebirthing in a redwood hot tub.

Completely submerged in the warm water of a hot tub, an individual with nose clips in place and breathing through a snorkel tube would regress to birth and prenatal states of consciousness. This was called wet Rebirthing.

During the Rebirth an individual would relive physiologically, psychologically, and spiritually the moment of his first breath, and release all of the trauma connected with it. Once an individual is free of his birth trauma, he can begin to uncover, identify, and then work on the unresolved issues in his consciousness. During subsequent Rebirth sessions deep emotional discharges are common.

By 1975 Orr had given hundreds of wet Rebirths and noticed people having a "healing of the breath" experience. They all breathed with a specific rhythm in which the inhalation and exhalation of each subsequent breath were merged into one breath. More descriptively called "conscious connected breathing" or "energy breathing," it is a simple connected breathing rhythm in which the inhalation and exhalation of one breath are merged with the inhalation and exhalation of the next breath in a continuous and uninterrupted circle, through the mouth. It differs from the normal breathing rhythm, in which there is a pause between one breath and the next, and breathing takes place through the nose rather than the mouth.

Orr experimented with this connected breathing out of water and found it was better to give people a series of connected breathing sessions before putting them into the water. Thus dry Rebirthing was born.

Today, because of convenience and other factors, the most popular and widely practiced method of Rebirthing is dry Rebirthing. In this process an individual usually lies flat on the floor, cushioned by a pad of some type, and breathes in a sustained in-and-out manner.

A Rebirth takes approximately one to two hours. During this time the professional Rebirther coaches and monitors the individual's breathing rhythm. The rhythm is relaxed and must be intuitive because the purpose of breathing is to breathe in life energy as well as air. Breathing life energy cannot be done with a mechanical breathing technique. Success at conscious breathing requires that it be soft and gentle.

Rebirthers believe the process of conscious connected breathing integrates body, mind, and spirit, and helps an individual maintain a perpetual state of health, happiness, and abundant energy. Full and free breathing, combined with the creative power of thought, can produce major transformational improvements in the physical body through oxygenation and reju-venation of the cells. Rebirthing is the principal medium for putting divine life energy back into the human body and mind.

Rebirthing is usually done in a series of ten to twenty sessions with a professional Rebirther. The ultimate goal is to teach the individual how to Rebirth himself in order to enjoy Rebirthing's benefits of relaxation, clarity, and well-being for his entire life.

Because a person tends to live his life in a way similar to how he breathes, by freeing the breath he can produce a corresponding release of the natural life force within himself.

Since its beginning in a Northern California hot tub, Rebirthing has evolved greatly, and today it is practiced throughout the United States and in many parts of the world. Over 10 million people have been Rebirthed and there are over one hundred thousand professional Rebirthers. The first Rebirther training center was opened in Walton, New York in 1975.

Currently there are two organizations that train Rebirthers. They are Loving Relationships Training International and Clarity Productions.

Loving Relationships Training International offer Rebirthing seminars around the world, as well as books on related subjects. For additional infor-mation contact LRT International.

✑ | REFLEXOLOGY | ✎

Reflexology, sometimes called Zone Therapy, is a form of bodywork which utilizes the principle that there are reflex points, also called "areas" or "zones," on the soles of the feet (or palms of the hands) that represent or correspond to every major organ, gland, and area of the body.

The basic idea of Reflexology is not new. A pictograph over 2,300 years old shows Egyptians massaging their feet. We know from ancient texts and illustrations that the Chinese, Japanese, and Indians worked on their feet to promote good health.

In the early 1900s the American physician William H. Fitzgerald, M.D., coined the term "Zone Therapy," referring to his theory that certain areas of the body directly correspond to other areas. Fitzgerald's colleague, Edwin Bowers, M.D., further popularized Zone Therapy by demonstrating that a volunteer felt no pain after being stuck in the face with a needle, if he first applied pressure to a point on the hand that corresponded to the area of the face where the needle was inserted.

In the 1930s physiotherapist Eunice Ingham, while in the employ of a physician, used Zone Therapy on patients. Through her work she concluded that the feet were the most responsive areas for working the zones because of their sensitivity. She created a map of the entire body as represented on the feet.

At that time the function of Zone Therapy, as developed by Drs. Fitzgerald and Bowers, was limited to the reduction of pain. Ingham then discovered that by alternating pressure on the various points she was able to achieve much greater therapeutic effects than with Zone Therapy. This work developed into what she called the Ingham Reflex Method of Compression Massage. Later it became known as Reflexology. In 1938 Ingham published her first book on Reflexology.

Currently called the Original Ingham Method of Reflexology, it is the combined work of the late Eunice Ingham-Stopfel and her nephew, Dwight C. Byers, the world's current leading authority on Foot Reflexology.

Reflexology views the soles of the feet as miniature representations (mirrors) of the whole body. In addition to the soles, there are reflex points on the tops and sides of the feet, and points up the sides of the legs as well. All of these locations have been graphically charted.

Reflexology is not foot massage. No equipment or instruments are used in Reflexology, only the hands. It consists of a specific type of steady, even pressure with the fingers, thumbs, and palms to a reflex point on the foot.

Although Reflexology does not treat specific diseases, Reflexologists believe that the proper stimulation of reflex points can affect a particular organ, gland, or area of the body to improve or alleviate many health problems. It also contributes to the health and harmony of the total person in a natural way.

Similar in principle to Oriental Acupressure methods, Reflexology works with subtle energy flows to revitalize the body and activate the natural internal mechanisms to help the body heal itself.

Reflexology is used primarily to reduce stress and promote deep relaxation, which cause all systems of the body to function more efficiently. Other benefits include improved circulation of blood and lymphatic fluid, which brings more oxygen to tissue and removes metabolic waste products, and a normalizing of the whole body system to a state of homeostasis or equilibrium.

For over fifty years, thousands of practitioners have been taught the Original Ingham Method. Currently, two-day seminars are presented throughout the United States. Although the Original Ingham Method is the oldest and best-known form of Reflexology, there are other schools that offer instruction in Reflexology and Zone Therapy.

Some practitioners specialize in Reflexology although most do other types of bodywork as well. Practitioners of the Original Ingham Method can be located through the International Institute of Reflexology. Other information on Reflexology is available from the American Reflexology Certification Board and Information Service, and the Foot Reflexology Awareness Association.

Numerous books can be found on the subject, including *Better Health Through Reflexology* by Dwight C. Byers, *Feet First: A Guide to Reflexology* by Laura Norman, and *Reflexology: Art, Science and History* by Christine Issel.

✌ | REICHIAN THERAPY | ✍

Reichian Therapy, sometimes called Reichian Release Therapy, is a method of clinical bodywork that can also include psychoanalysis. It uses a variety of original techniques to dissolve the "muscular armor" which holds sexual-emotional energy in the body and interferes with the energy's natural free flow.

Another important purpose of Reichian Therapy is to develop an individual's ability to build up and release full energy at the time of orgasm. This aptitude to reach what is called "full orgastic potency" (full sexual functioning) is central to Reichian Therapy. Reich believed, as did Freud, that the cause of neurosis is repressed sexual energy.

In our society open expression of sex and sexual matters is neither encouraged nor condoned. For an individual to resist these natural, primal sexual urges requires a "holding back" or "contraction" that affects the entire organism. This leads to pain and frustration, which require even more contraction to suppress. As these contractions become more deeply imbedded, the individual becomes rigid, somber, and less animate, and loses much of his childhood openness and "aliveness." He develops chronic muscle tension and becomes "armored."

Armoring and the negative feelings of guilt, shame, etc., prevent the complete convulsive discharge of orgasm. When energy remains from an incomplete orgasm, the surplus remains held inside the body. It is this "pool" of restrained sexual energy that causes a variety of neuroses because it has no other outlet.

Habitual armoring also causes chronic muscular contractions leading to spasms, pain, and other physical dysfunctions. Muscles in this state of tension cannot be relaxed voluntarily. Suppressed emotions and memories, resting dormant in the muscles like a "capsule of energy," are now responsible for contributing to additional armoring—and the cycle continues until broken.

Austrian psychoanalyst Dr. Wilhelm Reich (1879–1957) is considered "the father of most body-oriented therapies" currently in use. He graduated from the University of Vienna and spent the following six years with Sigmund Freud at the Vienna Psychoanalytic Polyclinic as his clinical assistant.

By the late 1920s Reich had separated from Freud and the psychoanalytic movement over differences in theories. He was at odds with Freud's ideas concerning man's need to control sexual drive for the good of society. Reich then began expounding controversial theories and doing pioneer work in relating neurosis to its physiological basis.

In contrast to Freud's treatment of physical and emotional problems by verbal means, Reich developed a therapeutic viewpoint and developed ingenious techniques for treatment based on the anatomy.

According to Reich, sexual drive was the source of "life energy" in the human body. He called this "orgone energy." He wanted to treat physical problems—especially chronic conditions—by restoring the free flow of this energy in the patient.

A brilliant writer, thinker, and researcher, Reich was a man far ahead of his time, which unfortunately caused him many problems throughout his life. He was repeatedly forced to move from city to city in Europe because the sexual contents of his lectures and the laboratory experiments he performed on vital energy met with public disfavor.

Acceptance of an assistant professorship at the New School for Social Research brought him to the United States, and in 1939 Reich established the Orgone Institute in New York City. He began working with orgone, or life energy, which he believed could treat health problems, especially chronic conditions.

Reich spent more than ten years experimenting and creating different apparatuses to utilize orgone energy. He developed a "box," large enough to hold a person, which would accumulate and concentrate this "energy." He believed a person in the box could be cured of various medical conditions by restoring the natural flow of orgone in the body.

He also developed a blanket consisting of several layers of organic and inorganic materials containing orgone, claiming it would prevent and cure colds, rheumatism, and other ailments.

Reich was very unpopular with the American Medical Association, which actively tried to curb his activities. In 1954 he was arrested by the Food and Drug Administration for selling orgone devices. The government obtained an injunction, based on the nonexistence of orgone, which specified that he was to refrain from further work. Refusing to heed the injunction, he was prosecuted under the Pure Food and Drug Act in 1956 and sentenced to two years in a federal penitentiary. In 1957 he died while incarcerated in a Pennsylvania prison.

Reich's earlier work, before the sensationalism of orgone, involved therapeutic techniques which he called "vegetotherapy," which means a primitive, involuntary level of biological functioning. The idea behind vegetotherapy techniques was to remove chronic muscular tension and liberate an individual's life energy, especially his sexual energy.

The following techniques are typical of those used in Reichian Therapy to melt away the muscular-emotional armoring. Although there is a sequence to the therapy and the techniques are practiced in a certain progression, it is always adjusted to meet the needs of each client.

Deep breathing is used for increased oxygenation of the body; it can also produce spontaneous emotional releases.

Deep massage to areas of the body holding muscular armoring (spasms), in concert with deep breathing, can also produce spontaneous eruption of repressed emotion. Through screams or facial expressions the client can outwardly manifest the pain being experienced.

Working with the gag reflex involves such reactions as coughing, yawning, or other convulsive reflexes, which work well in breaking up deep internal armoring.

Facial expressions, or "unmasking," include the movement of parts of the face such as rolling of the eyes or opening of the mouth and making faces while in eye contact with the therapist.

Pushing down on the chest of the client while he is screaming or exhaling helps remove the block to complete expiration involved in breathing armoring.

Maintaining stress positions or postures utilizes various body configurations such as leaning backward with the knees bent and the back arched; this can produce a release when held for a period of time.

Making "bioenergetic" movements such as kicking, stamping, pounding, shaking the head or limbs, and other movements along with breathing, facial expressions, and generated sounds.

The work of Reich was continued after his death. Bioenergetics, developed by Alexander Lowen, is the most popular and well known branch of Reichian Therapy practiced today. Another body-oriented psychotherapy called the Hakomi Method, developed by Ron Kurtz, also has its roots in Reich's original work. Body-oriented psychotherapies treat the body and mind as one, not to be separated.

At the present time, unfortunately, there is no restriction on the use of the name "Reichian Therapy," and anyone can use it. There are no specific credentials to identify a well-trained practitioner from one who is not as well trained.

Wilhelm Reich wrote more than thirty books, including the *Orgone Energy Accumulator* and *Selected Writings: An Introduction to Orgonomy*.

❧ | REIKI | ❧

Reiki is a powerful system of healing that utilizes specific techniques for restoring and balancing the natural life force energy within the body. It is a holistic, natural, hands-on energy healing system that touches individuals on all levels: body, mind, and spirit.

Reiki (pronounced ray-key) is a Japanese word representing universal life energy, the energy which is all around us. It is derived from *rei*, meaning "transcendental spirit" or "universal" and *ki*, meaning "vital life force energy."

Although various accounts relate slightly different versions of its history, it is thought that Reiki began in Tibet several thousand years ago. In ancient times seers in the Orient studied energies and developed a system of sounds and symbols for universal healing energies. Various healing systems, which crossed many different cultures, emerged from this single root system. Unfortunately, the original source itself was forgotten.

Dr. Mikao Usui, a Japanese Christian educator who was part of a Christian seminary in Kyoto, Japan, is acknowledged for rediscovering the root system in the mid- to late 1800s.

Responding to a challenge from his students, after hearing about healing miracles, Usui began an extensive twenty-one-year study of the healing phenomena of history's greatest spiritual leaders to discover how to perform similar miracles. Later he came to the United States to study at the University of Chicago. After receiving his doctoral degree in theology, Usui returned to Japan and resumed his search.

After entering a Zen monastery near Kyoto, Usui spent seven years studying ancient sutras (Buddhist teachings written in Sanskrit). It is there that he discovered ancient sounds and symbols that are linked directly to the human body and nervous system which activate the universal life energy for healing.

Usui then underwent a metaphysical experience and became empowered to use these sounds and symbols to heal. He called this form of healing Reiki and taught it throughout Japan until his death around 1893.

An advanced student of Usui, Dr. Chujiro Hyashi, operated a Reiki clinic in Tokyo. He was the second grand master after Usui. In the 1930s a seriously ill Japanese-American woman, Hawayo Takata, came to Japan for a healing. After Takata was helped by the treatments, she trained in Reiki and returned home to her native Hawaii.

In 1941 Hyashi died and Hawayo Takata became the third grand master. She continued as a Reiki healer but did not start training and initiating students until the 1970s. Before her death in the early 1980s, Takata passed on the tradition to her granddaughter, Phyllis Lei Furumoto, who became grand master.

Currently, Phyllis Lei Furumoto is the head of the Reiki Alliance, located in Cataldo, Idaho. This organization promotes "the Usui System of Natural Healing."

Another form of Reiki, called the Radiance Technique (described elsewhere in this book), is promoted by the Radiance Technique Association International, based in St. Petersburg, Florida. This organization is headed by Dr. Barbara Ray, a former student of Takata's.

Reiki was introduced to the Western world in the mid-1970s. Since then its use has spread dramatically worldwide. It is now used by thousands, both laypeople and practitioners in the healing professions, to help themselves and others.

The Usui System of Natural Healing balances and strengthens the body's energy, promoting its ability to heal itself. Besides the obvious use in serious illness, Reiki promotes the natural healing process in many other areas. Problems like sports injuries, cuts, burns, internal diseases, emotional disorders, and stress-related illnesses are helped through the use of Reiki.

While Reiki is complete within itself, it also maximizes the effect of other forms of therapy such as massage, Chiropractic, physiotherapy, Acupuncture,

Rebirthing, Homeopathy, Meditation, psychotherapy, and other forms of physical and energy body therapies.

Reiki is not a massage technique. A treatment involves the placing of the practitioner's hands on the recipient's body in a passive way. Treatments are carried out in an environment as quiet and comfortable as possible. The recipient remains clothed during the hands-on healing touch. Most people experience a gentle warmth or tingling coming from the practitioner's hands. The position of the hands is changed about every five minutes, and a treatment lasts about one hour.

Reiki cannot be learned from a book. Through a series of attunements, part of the initiation process for new Reiki practitioners, a Reiki master employs the ancient sounds and symbols that attune an individual's nervous system to a higher level of energy. A level is reached in which the student-initiate, neither highly trained nor especially gifted, can then experience more energy flowing through her hands, giving her the power to heal herself and others.

Reiki is taught in three levels or degrees. In Level I or First Degree, the participant receives attunement or initiation to the Reiki energy by the Reiki master. This permanently guides her to greater healing power. She learns how to do full body treatments on herself and others.

In Level II or Second Degree, the participant receives attunements which increase the strength of the practitioner's Reiki energy. This primarily involves learning the sounds and symbols which are used in advanced Reiki bodywork and absentee healing.

In Level III or Third Degree, the participant receives third-level empowerment and the final symbol. It is taught mainly for personal growth. They are also able to give the Level I Reiki attunement.

Reiki practitioners and Reiki classes are available in many cities throughout the world. For additional information on the Usui System of Natural Healing and a list of practitioners and teachers worldwide, contact the Reiki Alliance.

❧ | RICE DIET | ☙

The Rice Diet, also known as the Kempner Rice Diet, is the original high-carbohydrate, low-fat, high-fiber, low-sodium dietary plan used for therapeutic purposes.

It is not a simple do-it-yourself regime, but the most scientific approach to improving and maintaining an individual's health through proper diet, rest, and exercise.

The principles of the Kempner Rice Diet have been modified into other well-known therapeutic diets such as the Pritikin Diet, the Macrobiotic Diet, the McDougall Plan Diet, and the Reversal Diet of Dr. Dean Ornish of the University of California.

The Kempner Rice Diet was originated by Walter Kempner, M.D., who graduated from the University of Heidelberg, Germany, in 1926. The son of a prominent medical researcher, in 1933 he was recruited from the University of Berlin Medical School by Duke University in Durham, North Carolina. Kempner's duties at the medical school were research and teaching. He was the first to advocate dietary treatment of cardiovascular disease, as well as the importance of exercise.

In 1939 Dr. Walter Kempner was treating a thirty-three-year-old female patient with high blood pressure, kidney disease, and associated symptoms. Upon her release from the hospital, Dr. Kempner prescribed the Rice Diet for two weeks. The woman misunderstood Dr. Kempner's German accent and did not return for two months.

After examining the woman, it was determined that amazing results had taken place during the two months she was on the diet. Her blood pressure was drastically reduced, a retinal hemorrhage had healed, and there was a marked decrease in the size of her heart.

Because of the success achieved with this patient, Dr. Kempner began to prescribe prolonged dietary therapy to other patients with kidney disease and hypertensive vascular disease.

Dr. Kempner received national recognition in 1944 after reporting the clinical results of the first 150 patients to the American Heart Association meeting in Chicago. The results were amazing. Patients showed improvement in kidney function, decrease in blood pressure, reduction in heart size, lowered cholesterol level, loss of edema, improvement in electrocardiogram readings, and improvement or disappearance of vascular retinopathy. This proved that certain chronic diseases could be retarded and/or reversed by dietary therapy.

Dr. Kempner reported three years later the disappearance of the signs and symptoms of congestive heart failure. In 1958 he proved that dietary therapy could be used to reduce or eliminate the need for insulin therapy in many diabetics to normalize blood sugar levels.

During the 1950s the Kempner Rice Diet became well known for the treatment of obesity, and Durham, North Carolina, began its rise as the diet center of the world.

In 1991, this same type of diet was recommended by the Physicians Committee for Responsible Medicine in order to reduce the risk of heart disease and cancer.

In May 1992, Dr. Kempner retired as a professor of medicine emeritus at the Duke University Medical Center at the age of eighty-nine. He served as director of the Rice Diet Program for more than fifty years.

The Rice Diet is a residential program. Upon arrival, each patient undergoes a complete diagnostic evaluation. Treatment begins immediately following the examination.

There is no standard duration for treatment. Although a patient's length of stay may be only a few weeks, it is more often several months, and occasionally a year or more. Most patients are told to plan on a minimum of three to four months.

The patient remains in residence and on the basic diet without interruption until her blood pressure, cholesterol, blood sugars, kidney function, heart and lung size, and weight are at their optimal levels. The basic diet consists solely of unsalted rice, fruit, and limited amounts of fruit juices, tea, or decaffeinated black coffee. Sugar is frequently permitted.

Additions to the basic diet begin with other grains and vegetables. Then nonfat dairy products (milk and yogurt) may be added as long as all health factors remain optimal.

While in residence, each patient is given an individual exercise prescription, usually based on walking or swimming.

After a patient has completed the residential program, she returns home with a therapeutic diet.

Today the Kempner Rice Diet remains a viable and effective alternative to the new drugs and technologies available in the treatment of high blood pressure, congestive heart failure, angina pectoris, high cholesterol, diabetes mellitus, kidney failure, and obesity.

For additional information on the Rice Diet Program, contact the Duke University Medical Center, Kempner Clinic (Rice Diet).

✍ | ROLFING | ✍

Rolfing, or Structural Integration as it was called by Ida P. Rolf, is a precise and sophisticated technique for manipulating the body's myofascial system, which is composed of the muscles and the fascia (connective tissue which surrounds and penetrates the muscles and all other structures of the body).

Rolfing was developed by Ida P. Rolf, Ph.D. (1896–1979). Born in New York, she received her bachelor of science degree from Barnard College at Columbia University in 1916 and her doctorate in biochemistry from Columbia University's College of Physicians and Surgeons in 1920. She later worked for the Rockefeller Institute (later called Rockefeller University) as an organic chemist. In the late 1920s, family problems compelled her to leave their employ.

An incident involving a hand injury to her children's piano teacher started Dr. Rolf on an investigation into the relationship between body structure and an individual's well-being. She taught the woman some Yoga exercises in an attempt to return the hand to normal. Rolf soon realized that the Yoga exercises would not provide the effect she was looking for, which led her to search for other methods.

She explored the Alexander Technique and later studied Osteopathy. Holding the view that function is determined by structure, she observed that a structural problem in one part of the body would upset the balance of the entire body. From her studies she also knew that if a body is distorted, it cannot physiologically function properly. To further add to her work, Rolf incorporated exercises she learned from an osteopath in California.

During the 1950s Rolf was teaching what she called Structural Integration in the United States as well as in Canada and Great Britain. Many of the practitioners who learned the method wanted to use only certain techniques from it. She designed it as a systemic approach to balancing the entire body rather than a "fix-it" for specific parts.

Rolf's work came into prominence after she worked on Fritz Perls, founder of Gestalt therapy, while he was at the Esalen Institute in Big Sur, California. Perls's heart condition improved after receiving Structural Integration. He later wrote about the experience with Rolf in his book *In and Out of the Garbage Pail*.

From that time on Ida Rolf spent her summers at Esalen teaching and applying her Structural Integration methods to grateful recipients. Rolf's connection with Esalen led to her inclusion in publicity on the institute and the human potential movement going on there.

The Rolf Institute was started in 1970 to relieve Ida Rolf of unproductive tasks, freeing her to train advanced students and to write and lecture. In

1975 she published a booklet, *What in the World Is Rolfing,* and in 1977 a major work describing her modality in detail, titled *Rolfing: The Integration of the Human Structure.*

Ida P. Rolf was truly an innovator. The originality of Rolfing's principles are the basis for many of the so-called New Age bodywork modalities developed by her students and in widespread practice today. An example is Hellerwork, developed by Joseph Heller, who was trained as a Rolfer and served as the first director of the Rolf Institute.

The body must deal with the effects of gravity just like any structure on earth. For example, a great deal of engineering and construction effort has been spent trying to keep the Leaning Tower of Pisa upright. Because the tower is out of balance, the force of gravity is continually pulling it downward.

The same is true for the human body. When the body is out of balance, gravitational forces become a burden. Energy must be expended to resist the pull of gravity when the skeleton is not upright. The body can become unbalanced from chronic muscular tension and permanent shortening of the fascial structure due to factors such as habitually poor posture, disease, physical trauma, repeated patterns of self-use (such as in a job), surgery, emotional distress, and environmental elements such as shoes, chairs, and desks.

An unbalanced body is "at war" with gravity, and as a result, the body experiences pain, stress, and depleted energy. Outward signs may include a slouched body with the head too far forward, an overly erect body which bows backward, flat feet, high arches, or excessive spinal curvature. These manifestations of strain are caused by tightness and thickening in the muscles and fascia.

Rolfers, practitioners of the Rolf System of Structural Integration, view the body as an integrated series of segments or blocks—the head, thorax (torso), pelvis, and legs. For the body to be in balance and get the most economical energy usage, the gravity centers of these big blocks must be stacked on top of each other so that a line running through their centers would approximate a vertical line.

The Rolfing System of Structural Integration realigns these body segments so that they are in vertical alignment within the field of gravity. Ideally the segments, stacked with their centers of gravity over each other, would approximate a straight line drawn through the ear, shoulder joint, hip, knee, and ankle.

To accomplish this alignment, Rolfers use their fingers, open hands, fists, and elbows to manipulate the major muscle groups and fascia.

The fascial system is a densely woven sheet of connective tissue that lines and covers nearly every muscle, bone, nerve, artery, and vein, as well as the internal organs including the heart, lungs, brain, and spinal cord.

Not just a system of separate coverings, the fascia is actually a single structure that extends from the top of the head to the tip of the toes; it plays an important role in the support of the body. Fascia is composed of two types of fibers: collagenous fibers, which are tough and have little ability to stretch, and elastic fibers, which are stretchable.

In the normal healthy state, fascia is relaxed and has the ability to move without restriction. When the body experiences factors such as habitually poor posture and the others mentioned above, the effect on the fascia is cumulative over time. Eventually, as the fascia loses some of its pliability, it thickens and hardens.

Pressure, mechanical friction, and the heat from the Rolfer's hand causes the hardened, thickened fascia to become elastic and pliable once again. This allows the muscles to lengthen and return to their normal state. As the muscles are lengthened, the body rights itself effortlessly in gravity.

The results of Rolfing vary greatly depending on the individual. In general, the body becomes lighter as the head and chest are raised and the torso is lengthened. As the pelvis aligns horizontally, the stomach and buttocks are pulled in. The legs and feet track forward more, and the soles of the feet meet the ground more squarely.

Although the benefits of Rolfing can include pain relief, greater freedom of joint movement, and conserved energy available for other purposes, it is not considered a cure for any particular disease or physical problem. Pain from emotional trauma, anger, and resentment also disappears as blocked emotional energy is released from the body.

The Rolf technique consists of a series of ten sessions. Each is about one hour in length, and the sessions are usually spaced a week or more apart, which is adequate for most people. If the need for additional work arises after a few months to a year, advanced Rolfing sessions are available to meet the individual's needs.

Rolfing practitioners are trained and certified only by the Rolf Institute of Structural Integration. For additional information and a list of certified Rolfers in your area, contact the Rolf Institute.

✑ | ROLFING MOVEMENT INTEGRATION | ❧

Rolfing Movement Integration is a system of movement education for the development of balance, support of action in the gravitational field, and harmonious movement with gravity.

Based on the concepts developed by Ida P. Rolf, Ph.D., the creator of the Rolfing process, Rolfing Movement can be used alone or in conjunction with Rolfing Structural Integration (Rolfing). When combined with Rolfing, the two processes complement each other.

Rolfing Movement Integration explores an individual's movement patterns such as walking, standing, sitting, and a multitude of other activities while at home, in the workplace, and during recreation. Its goal is a freer, more balanced movement through release of specific holding patterns in different parts of the body. Those parts are then integrated, through movement, with the whole body.

During a series of eight private sessions, an individual learns a series of centering movements that can be used in her daily life to ease pain and stress, and to improve work and recreational activities.

Rolfing Movement teachers are trained and certified only by the Rolf Institute of Structural Integration. For additional information and a list of certified Movement teachers in your area, contact the Rolf Institute. For additional information and a list of certified Rolfers in your area, contact the Rolf Institute.

✑ | ROSEN METHOD | ❧

The Rosen Method is a therapeutic, hands-on form of bodywork that utilizes gentle touch with verbal communication to relieve pain, increase vitality and health, and gain physical and emotional awareness.

It is not for people in acute physical pain, but is very effective for alleviating muscular pain and the manifestations of stress.

The Rosen Method was developed by Marion Rosen, who was born in Nuremberg, Germany, in 1914 to a moderately prosperous family.

Because she was Jewish, Rosen was denied a university education in then-Nazi Germany. As an alternative she became an apprentice to Lucy Heyer, assisting her with massage and breathing sessions. Heyer had been a student of Elsa Gindler, the principal investigator of body/mind integration in Europe during the early 1900s.

Rosen trained and worked as a physical therapist in Sweden while awaiting emigration to the United States. During World War II, she worked as a physical therapist in San Francisco; she later entered the Mayo Clinic in Rochester, Minnesota, for the clinic's advanced Physical Therapy course. Returning to the Bay Area, she opened a private practice in Oakland.

While working as a physical therapist Rosen began to realize that some individuals did not respond to Physical Therapy, while others simply would not spend the time required for the entire series of treatments. In cases where individuals did improve, she noted that they often needed to return for additional treatments to maintain the corrected condition.

Marion Rosen wanted to know what happened when they "healed" and why their condition deteriorated again. She looked for the cause of the problem instead of working on the symptomatic level.

In the early 1970s she had a revelation. From her previous training Rosen realized the importance of relaxation. When she worked on people it relaxed their muscles, and while they were in this state people began to talk. They would tell her deep emotional things they had never told anyone.

Rosen asked herself why people were telling her these things. She wanted to know what the link was between a client's free verbalization and the improvement of his physical condition.

Rosen realized that patients were relinquishing their pain and changing for the positive through this work. These experiences helped her put together the ideas which formed the foundation of the Rosen Method.

The heart of Rosen Method bodywork is to facilitate the connection between the body, mind, and spirit by allowing relaxation with easy and full movement of the breath.

Rather than the patient being worked on by a massage therapist, as in the case of ordinary massage, the Rosen practitioner creates an environment where it becomes possible for the client to know himself in a deep and profound way. He finds the place where body, mind, and spirit meet.

The Rosen Method is not meant to "fix" anything in the body; it merely allows for a transformation which in turn brings about healing. It allows a person to be who he really is.

Memories and experiences are stored in the body as stress. The Rosen Method practitioner touches in a gentle, nonintrusive way which leads to relaxation of chronic muscular tension. This pattern of tension and stress is unique and specific to each individual's life experiences.

As relaxation occurs, information moves from the unconscious to consciousness through internal physical sensations, images, and memories. People find components of themselves they have never really known or have forgotten were there. This awareness provides an insight—that is felt—into oneself and allows contracted muscles to return to a relaxed state. Thus anxiety is reduced and a greater ease of physical movement occurs.

By learning to follow a client's breath as an indicator of change or release, a Rosen Method practitioner notices and responds with touch and/or words to what is occurring in the client's body. These changes relate to the client's inner experiences.

During a session of Rosen Method bodywork, the practitioner usually begins work on the diaphragm and surrounding muscles. When the diaphragm is chronically tense it restricts the body's breathing capacity and its ability to get oxygen to muscles and organs.

The Rosen Method is a process of gently showing people to themselves. It is not a substitute for psychotherapy, but is known as an effective addition to it. Neither is it recommended for people suffering from severe emotional disturbances.

Students of the Rosen Method are taken through the same process as a client would be. They are worked on by both instructors and classmates. It is through the work itself that their knowledge and awareness increases. The Rosen Method also helps to precipitate the release of limitations and barriers they have imposed on themselves.

For additional information and the name of a practitioner in your area contact the Rosen Method Practitioner Referral Service.

❧ | RUBENFELD SYNERGY METHOD | ❦

The Rubenfeld Synergy Method is a dynamic system for the integration of body, mind, emotions, and spirit. Through gentle touch each of these four levels can be accessed, simultaneously releasing pain and fears which are held in the body/mind.

It utilizes principles from several well-known therapies, including the Alexander Technique, the Feldenkrais Method, Gestalt therapy, and Ericksonian hypnosis.

The Rubenfeld Synergy Method was developed by Ilana Rubenfeld. She was born in Palestine in the 1930s to Russian immigrant parents; her family moved to New York City when she was five years old.

In the 1950s Rubenfeld entered the Juilliard School of Music. She studied with Pablo Casals and played the piano, viola, and oboe. She also became an orchestral and choral conductor.

Juilliard training was rigorous. Rubenfeld would practice four to five hours a day rehearsing the student orchestra and choir with baton in hand. Along with many other students, she developed back spasms. Going from doctor to doctor, she received only temporary relief to complete a performance; then the pain would return.

She realized that although Juilliard provided excellent musical education, no instruction on how to use the body was given. The correct way to stand, move, or conserve energy was not explained. To accomplish this, a friend recommended that Rubenfeld investigate the Alexander Technique, a method of learning to use the body more efficiently.

A series of Alexander lessons improved her condition. Then one day, in the middle of a lesson, while being gently touched Rubenfeld began to cry, sobbing from very deeply within. Several more lessons evoked the same response. At that point the Alexander instructor recommended she see a therapist.

Rubenfeld realized that although the Alexander lessons made her body feel better, she could not control her emotions. She went to a therapist who was very helpful. Unfortunately, by the time she got to him the emotions released in the Alexander lesson were a distant memory.

Rubenfeld was now receiving help from one person who touched her but would not talk about the emotions released, and another person who would talk about the released emotions but would not touch her. Between the therapist and the Alexander instructor she had created her own body/mind therapist. She wondered why a therapist could not work with both the verbal and nonverbal expressions of their clients.

Like F. M. Alexander and Moshe Feldenkrais, who had cured themselves of health problems, Ilana Rubenfeld set out to heal herself. She studied the Alexander Technique and became a teacher of it. In 1965 she worked with Fritz and Laura Perls to learn Gestalt therapy. In the summer of 1971 she trained with Moshe Feldenkrais at the Esalen Institute in the two-tier method of Functional Integration and Awareness Through Movement. Later Rubenfeld added Ericksonian Hypnotherapy to her body of knowledge.

Buckminster Fuller suggested the word *synergy* to her. He felt that her work with the Alexander Technique, Gestalt therapy, and the Feldenkrais Method had gone beyond integration and perhaps even synthesis into a true synergy.

Having used her approach for several years with clients and in various workshops, she offered the first Rubenfeld Synergy Method training program in 1977.

Painful memories, regardless of how old, are still alive in the body. The Rubenfeld Synergy Method approach of using multiple modalities is a key to lasting change. It helps an individual integrate previously unassimilated traumatic experiences which are still active in subtly destructive ways.

The Rubenfeld "synergist" (practitioner of the Rubenfeld Synergy Method) acts as a facilitator or guide to help an individual heal himself.

At the heart of every session is a four-stage metaprocess. Stages are awareness, experimentation, integration, and reentry. They occur separately and simultaneously on all four interrelated levels of body, mind, emotion, and spirit. The body movements and verbal interventions of the synergist are simultaneous, and the integration process occurs continuously.

The synergist, or practitioner, uses what is described as a touch that "listens" and "talks." Practitioners often begin a session by touching the head very gently, enabling them to sense where a client is physically and emotionally. The synergist's hands can also transmit information back to the client by teaching him to distinguish between what he considers to be relaxed and what is a genuinely relaxed part of the body. This knowledge helps the client release tension.

The desire for change starts from within the client and moves outward toward the synergist, who acts primarily as a catalyst in the change process. The synergist's touch moves inward to meet with the client. During a session it may appear that the synergist is doing something to the client, but it is actually the client who initiates and allows the change.

Change cannot occur without the client's own awareness. Clients may explore alternate choices and develop possibilities for psychological change after unconsciously held habitual patterns are brought out. Every touch can bring about awareness at all levels.

It is Ilana Rubenfeld's philosophy that mastery does not come from taking several introductory courses in a smattering of methods and then mixing them together. Mastery comes from a commitment to in-depth learning and training.

To become a Rubenfeld synergist requires a minimum of three years of study, and trainees often take up to six additional years.

Currently there are several hundred Rubenfeld synergists practicing in the United States. For additional information and the name of a Rubenfeld synergist in your area contact the Rubenfeld Center.

❧ | SCHUESSLER CELL SALTS | ☙

Schuessler Cell Salts, also known as Schuessler's Biochemic Cell Salts and Tissue-Salts or Twelve Schuessler Remedies, are among the most popular and best-known homeopathic remedies on the market today. They have been successfully used by physicians and laymen throughout the world to help prevent illness as well as alleviate it. Their simple application and safety make them especially useful to the layman for self-treatment of a wide variety of disorders that would be regarded as responsive to home treatment.

Dr. Wilhelm Heinrich Schuessler, born in Oldenburg, Germany, in the nineteenth century, was a practicing homeopathic physician and founder of the Schuessler Biochemic System of Medicine. Inspired by the important work of the time in the field of organic and inorganic cell chemistry and cellular physiology, he postulated that when one or more of these mineral salts was missing from the body some abnormal condition would result.

He then began his own research. Using symptoms exhibited by patients, Dr. Schuessler was able to determine which salts would improve certain conditions. Dr. Schuessler believed that most diseases could be cured by restoring the cellular equilibrium with minute homeopathic doses of essential mineral salts normally found in the body.

The Schuessler Biochemic System of Medicine is based on the physiological fact that body tissue and organs are dependent on certain essential inorganic salts, in the proper proportion (based on chemical analysis of ashes from the blood and various other body tissues), for health and vitality.

The twelve different Scheussler Cell Salts are: Ferrum phos. (iron phosphate); Kali sulph. (potassium sulfate); Kali phos. (potassium phosphate); Kali mur. (potassium chloride); Magnesium phos. (magnesium phosphate); Natrum sulph. (sodium sulfate); Nature phos. (sodium phosphate); Nature mur. (sodium chloride); Silica (silicic oxide or sand); Calc. sulph. (calcium sulfate); Calc. phos. (calcium phosphate); and Calc. fluor. (calcium fluoride).

Schuessler Cell Salts, which are taken in infinitesimally small quantities, work at the cellular level. They restore the cell's ability to utilize that particular mineral salt more effectively and are not meant to replenish deficiencies of that salt in the body.

Each mineral salt, or remedy, has specific applications. For example, Ferrum phos. (iron phosphate) is required by the body to make red blood cells, which carry oxygen. A deficiency of this salt causes an anemic condition and gives rise to fever and inflammation. Use of the salt relieves the condition.

To understand the wide scope of usefulness of these remedies, a book such as *The Biochemic Handbook* or one of the many others available is recommended reading. For additional information on Schuessler Cell Salts also contact the Luyties Pharmacal Company.

❧ | SHAMANISM | ☙

Shamanism is an ancient healing tradition. A deeply spiritual practice, it is used for healing or achieving well-being and helping others. Used by tribal cultures all over the world, Shamanism is based on the belief that all healing includes the spiritual dimension.

The basic uniformity displayed in shamanic methods throughout the world suggests that different cultures, through trial and error, arrived at the same end result.

The history of Shamanism goes back forty thousand years or more to North Asian, Ural-Altaic, and Paleo-Asian peoples, making it the oldest of all healing therapies.

The term *shaman* is derived from the Tungusu-Manchurian word *saman*, which means "to know." Stone Age hunter-gatherers of the Tungus tribe in Siberia called their healer-priest or medicine man "shaman."

Shamanism or similar practices can be found in the cultures of Native Americans (North and South), and in the cultures of central Asia, Africa, the Pacific Islands, Australia, and southeast India.

Survival in ancient hunting, gathering, and/or fishing tribes was an everyday struggle. Although their role may have varied from tribe to tribe, shamans were respected leaders involved with many different functions in tribal life. Most likely they acted as a "religious" leader, healer, artist, seer, interpreter of dreams, and more.

Shamans designed rituals that included song, chanting, dance, story-telling, and art. These rituals were used to help the hunter-gatherers find game and edible food, assist the tribe members in their mysterious journey from birth to death, and heal the sick.

They were the first healers to discover and use medicinal herbs. By observing what animals ate and by using others on a trial-and-error basis, they found plants with healing properties. In this way they discovered plants with mind-altering properties which were sometimes used in ritual ceremonies.

As the hunting, gathering, and/or fishing tribes developed into sedentary cultures and became dependent on agriculture over the millennia, the role of the shaman changed. Shamans gave up their religious duties to priests and became shaman-healers.

Shamanism is a form of trance healing. The shaman can be a man or woman who enters an altered state of consciousness, at will, to contact and utilize an ordinarily hidden reality. He communicates with the spirit realm while in a trance state. During a ritual or ceremony he seeks guidance and answers to help heal the sick.

This altered state is achieved either through meditation, chanting, drumming, or the use of natural hallucinogenic substances. Shamans of the Huichol Indian tribe in Mexico use peyote derived from cactus, and Siberian shamans use the amanita mushroom.

The rituals or ceremonies, most of which are conducted at night by firelight, are usually performed in sacred locations such as on a mountaintop or in a cave, with the tribe member to be healed usually part of the ceremony. The shaman may make use of accompaniments such as rattles, symbolic objects, or special clothing. The ceremony may last from several hours to several days.

Shamanic tradition embodies a strong connection between people and nature. It draws tremendous healing power from direct connection with the earth, sky, plants, and animals.

Various forms of shamanic healing are practiced throughout the world today. It is used by many tribes of Native Americans and by the Hawaiian shamans or kahunas, who have practiced healing for centuries. Both make use of medicinal plants, and kahunas work to clear "energy blocks" in the person, a concept well known in Oriental medicine.

Today, modern shamanic healers of many Native American tribes incorporate both shamanic methods and conventional medicine into their healing. They find that some categories of illness are best treated by Shamanism and others respond better to allopathic medicine.

There is a movement to bring ancient shamanic knowledge into the "civilized" world. Information has come from anthropologists Michael Harner and Carlos Castaneda. Harner wrote an excellent book titled *The Way of the*

Shaman (Third Edition). Lynn V. Andrews, author of *The Jaguar Woman*, completed a seven-year apprenticeship with a Cree Indian medicine woman, Agnes Whistling Elk, who wanted to share her knowledge.

Shamanism has recently experienced a resurgence in interest as Native American shamans are beginning to share with outsiders their once secret knowledge about healing the sick. Rolling Thunder, a Cherokee-born shaman, and Sun Bear, a Chippewa medicine man, have done much to spread the word of Native American cultural healing.

Today various lectures, weekend Medicine Wheel gatherings, Sun Dances, Vision Quests, use of sweat lodges, and other activities are available in different parts of the United States. One of the themes taught through these activities is the relationship of people living in balance with the earth and a planetary healing.

With the increased interest in Shamanism, workshops in so-called New Age Shamanism are being taught. Students learn how to use traditional shamanic techniques such as the classic shamanic journey to enter nonordinary reality. In this state they are able to explore the hidden universe to obtain knowledge, answer personal questions, achieve personal goals, and contribute to their own health, the health of others, and the health of the planet.

For additional information on seminars, workshops, pilgrimages, and other programs dealing with Shamanism contact the Foundation for Shamanic Studies and the Dance of the Deer Foundation.

As of this writing there are no organizations that represent shaman healers or any type of certification program. Caution in the form of self-education should be exercised before one utilizes the services of a shaman.

For additional reading, some good books include *Healing States* by Alberto Villoldo and Stanley Krippner, *Shamanism: An Expanded View of Reality*, edited by Shirley Nicholson, and the books by Michael Harner and Lynn V. Andrews mentioned above.

✑ | SHEN THERAPY | ✍

SHEN Therapy is a unique hands-on energy/bodywork system that releases deeply embedded, painful emotions directly from the body. SHEN is the acronym for *Specific Human Energy Nexus*.

Although SHEN is a recent development in the West, some elements of its theories can be found in the distant past. They are contained in the ancient Egyptian concept of "life force," the early Chinese knowledge of emotions and *chi*, and in the Indian ideals of *prana* and *chakras*.

In 1977 Richard R. Pavek made a chance discovery while researching the effects of the human energy field on emotions held in the body. It was conclusively demonstrated that there was a normal direction to these energy flows in the arms, legs, and sides of the torso.

SHEN evolved from these observations and discoveries through research on the bioenergy field, its flow patterns, and its central role in the formation and experience of emotion.

Pavek identified the Auto-Contractile Pain Response (ACPR) as the physiological mechanism by which painful emotions become trapped in the body and disrupt normal bodily functioning. This established a new cause for many disorders previously presumed to be psychosomatic.

At the same time, specific SHEN protocols were developed to nullify various physio-emotional dysfunctions. With energy flow restored, normal physiological and behavioral functioning returned. SHEN Therapy is not derived from any other process.

SHEN Physio-Emotional Release Therapy can be used as a stand-alone treatment, or as an adjunct to other therapy. Psychotherapists, counselors, physical and occupational therapists, deep tissue workers, nurses, and physicians have included SHEN Therapy in their practice.

During a typical SHEN Therapy treatment session the practitioner, without applying pressure, places her hands in paired positions on the fully clothed client while the client is lying on a table. The practitioner ascertains the locations of somatically held emotions and determines an appropriate physio-emotional release plan.

Energy (*chi*) then flows from the practitioner's hands through the emotional centers of the client's body in a precise way to discharge debilitating emotions. This procedure is repeated at several different areas on the client's body in a carefully planned pattern. Once the deeply held emotions are experienced and flow out of the client, the submerged or forgotten feelings of love, joy, and confidence begin to emerge. Sessions usually take about one hour and there is little dialogue between client and practitioner.

SHEN Therapy is an intensive, short-term process that can be effective for a variety of physical and emotional problems.

In the area of physical problems, SHEN Therapy can provide complete or partial relief of chronic digestive disorders, the release of pain associated with old injuries, the reduction of swelling of sprained wrist, knee, and ankle joints, and easing of physio-emotional disorders such as menstrual or PMS distress, eating disorders, migraine headaches, and others.

For emotional problems, SHEN can provide access to emotional awakening, and spiritual and emotional growth. It can also provide relief from emotional depression, anxiety attacks and nightmares, chronic stress, and chronic pain without organic cause.

For additional information on SHEN Therapy, including a number of SHEN techniques, *The Handbook of SHEN* by Richard R. Pavek is available in bookstores or from the International SHEN Therapy Association. The association is also able to provide a list of recommended SHEN practitioners in your area.

❧ | SHIATSU | ❦

Shiatsu is traditional Japanese finger pressure massage therapy. It is similar to Acupressure and is used to improve the flow of vital life energy or *chi* in the body. This system of Oriental bodywork is derived from Amma, a technique of body manipulation which started in India, and Do-In, a system of self-massage with roots which can be traced back to China.

The word *Shiatsu* is derived from the Japanese words *shi*, which means finger, and *atsu*, which means pressure. Shiatsu literally means finger pressure in Japanese.

Origins of this ancient health art goes back to ancient man, whose instinctive urge was to touch or hold a body part that was injured or in pain. We still make the same instinctive type of move today.

Over five thousand years ago Chinese Taoist monks made formal observations of this human instinct of touch for self-healing. It was adapted into a system called Tao-Yinn. Derived from two Chinese words, *Tao* meaning "the way" and *Yinn* meaning "a gentle approach," it was used to sustain overall health and treat specific physical problems. Today it is known as Do-In.

Historically recorded nearly three thousand years ago in central China, the roots of Shiatsu go back to the Yellow Emperor's dynasty. At that time it was called Tien-An, and early recordings of it correspond with the first mention of Acupuncture. Tien-An was later introduced to the Japanese in about the sixth century A.D. and was called Shiatsu. For centuries it remained under the control of Buddhist monks.

It was in the Edo period, beginning in 1830, that Western medical practices (allopathic) were brought to Japan; this influence dominated Japanese medical thinking for over one hundred years. During this time Shiatsu fell into disuse.

In 1930 Dr. Tokujiro Namikoshi revived Shiatsu, and he founded the Nippon Shiatsu Institute in the middle twentieth century. Dr. Namikoshi influenced legislators in Japan to reestablish it as an accepted science with the national licensing board. Currently it is accepted by the Japanese Ministry of Health and Welfare as an authorized health treatment.

Both a do-it-yourself self-help method and a therapy practiced by a professional practitioner, Shiatsu is oriented toward prevention of illness. Its goal is to keep the body in good condition and to prevent the development of sickness rather than to cure it. As a therapy it stimulates the body's inherent natural curative powers and ability to recuperate from illness.

There are 660 neural trigger points or zones (*tsubo*) on the skin used in Shiatsu treatment. Invisible to observation, these points are located on energy pathways or meridians. It is in these areas where the blood vessels, lymph vessels, and ductless glands of the endocrine system tend to concentrate or branch.

Shiatsu practitioners use palpation of the abdomen and other tissues to diagnose a person's condition and determine the specific type of therapy he requires. This procedure is called *hara* diagnosis. A fine sense of touch allows discovery of abnormalities in blood and lymphatic circulation, abnormal internal secretions, skeletal deformities, excessive pressure on nerves, and the condition of the muscles and skin.

The practitioner then uses carefully judged pressure, properly applied to specific points on the body's surface with the fingers, knuckles, hands, elbows, knees, feet, or other body parts. The amount of pressure, method of pressing, and frequency of pressing are all variable. The points are held for only a few seconds. There is little or no massage done per se, although the practitioner may manipulate various parts of the body.

Therapy is pleasant and without a sensation of pain, even for those with stiff muscles. It is a total treatment applied to all parts of the body, with emphasis on those areas manifesting symptoms of pain or discomfort. A treatment can be relaxing or stimulating and is accomplished with the client fully clothed and lying on the floor.

Muscle tension causes energy blocks, and by stimulating certain points, energy blocks are removed. With energy flowing freely once again, the body is able to remove waste products such as lactic acid and carbon monoxide which have accumulated in the tissues. It is this accumulation of waste products that causes muscle stiffness and pain.

Shiatsu treatment may be used to release muscular tension throughout the body, to relieve pain from arthritis, to relieve pain from tension, sinus, and migraine headaches, to reduce discoloration caused by surface bruises, to reduce the severity of deep tissue and bone bruises, and to treat many other problems.

Today, certain bodyworkers specialize in Shiatsu. Local massage schools that teach Shiatsu are a good referral source for practitioners.

For additional information on Shiatsu, contact the American Oriental Bodywork Therapy Association. Additionally, the Ohashi Institute offers classes at locations around the United States. Many books on Shiatsu can be found in libraries and bookstores.

✍ | SOMATOEMOTIONAL RELEASE | ✍

SomatoEmotional Release is a therapeutic process, the objective of which is to rid the mind and body of the residual effects of past injuries and negative experiences.

Between 1977 and 1980, at Michigan State University's Department of Biomechanics in East Lansing, researchers Dr. John E. Upledger and Dr. Ziv Karni developed the concept. The name SomatoEmotional Release was suggested by Dr. Elmer Green of the Menninger Foundation after he observed their work using this process.

The concept that developed from the work of Upledger and Karni was that physical forces absorbed by a victim's body at the time of an accident or injury may be dealt with by the victim's body in one of two ways.

The injured body may immediately begin to dissipate these forces, and the natural healing process will follow; or the physical forces imposed upon the victim's body may be retained rather than dissipated.

If these forces are retained by the victim's body, it must adapt to this deposit of abnormal physical force. The adaptive response is to surround this abnormal force so that a pocket of energy is formed. It is called an "energy cyst" by Dr. Upledger.

The energy cyst becomes a dysfunctional area unable to perform its usual work, which thereby inhibits normal body function. A normally healthy person can work around the area of dysfunction by utilizing extra adaptive energy. As years pass, the adaptive patterns become less effective, and symptoms and dysfunctions appear that become increasingly more difficult to ignore and suppress.

Studies by Upledger and Karni have shown that if a person is harboring powerful negative feelings such as anger, resentment, or fear at the time of injury, the forces imposed on the body by the inquiry will be retained as energy cysts. Correspondingly, once these negative feelings are discovered and released, the body's dysfunctions and its accompanying symptoms are free to leave the body.

During the therapeutic process of SomatoEmotional Release the practitioner acts as a facilitator to encourage the positive aspects of the mind/body and discourage the negative aspects. These positive aspects help to release the energy cyst from the body by facilitating the body's memory of the injury, thus ending suppression.

To accomplish facilitation, the practitioner, who requires extreme sensitivity, touches the person and tunes into what the "positive body" would like to do, then assists in this process. The usual result is that the body will assume the position it was in when the external injury forces were imposed on it. As this occurs the energy cyst is expelled. Heat radiates from the area where the energy cyst was, and the tissues relax.

During the therapeutic session the release of the energy cyst frequently results in a reexperiencing of the pain, fear, anguish, resentment, etc., that were attendant upon the original incident. For more information contact the Upledger Institute.

❧ | SPORTS MASSAGE | ❧

Sports Massage is a specialty within the field of Massage Therapy which focuses on the muscles pertinent to a particular athletic activity. Although geared toward athletic performance for the professional, amateur, and recreational athlete, it is also used by dancers, fitness enthusiasts, and others. Sports Massage plays an important role in the treatment of sports-related injuries.

Sports Massage is an eclectic therapy utilizing classic Swedish Massage and specialized techniques including Cross-Fiber Friction Massage, Deep Compression Massage, Hydrotherapy, Cryotherapy, and Trigger Point Therapy.

- *Cross-Fiber Friction Massage* is a technique in which the massage therapist applies friction to the muscle by rubbing across or perpendicularly to the muscle fibers.
- *Deep Compression Massage*, or Compression Massage, is a specialized bodywork technique that utilizes a "pumping" action on the muscle.
- *Hydrotherapy* is the use of water, hot or cold, fresh or mineral, for therapeutic or healing purposes.
- *Cryotherapy*, also known as Ice Therapy, is the application of cold to various parts of the body for therapeutic purposes. It can range from immersion in ice water to the application of ice cubes, crushed ice (in containers), or frozen commercial gel packs directly to the problem site.
- *Trigger Point Therapy* is the use of various techniques to sedate, desensitize, or eliminate "trigger points." A trigger point is defined as a hypersensitive area in the myofascia (muscle and connective tissue) which is very painful to the touch.

A complete description of each of these methods can be found elsewhere in this book under its individual subject heading.

In Russia and European countries, massage has long been an integral part of athletic training, with some top sports figures receiving Massage Therapy on nearly a daily basis.

Dr. Myk Hungerford, former national director of education for the American Massage Therapy Association, founder and director of the Sports Massage Training Institute in Costa Mesa, California, and president of the International Sports Massage Federation, has been committed to the professional training and clinical practice of Sports Massage throughout her life.

Dr. Hungerford, who was trained as a physiotherapist and practiced Massage Therapy for nearly thirty years, worked diligently to bring Sports Massage into the Olympic arena. This finally occurred in 1984 at the Los Angeles Games; many consider this to be the beginning of Sports Massage in the United States. Currently, the American Massage Therapy Association has a national Sports Massage team which provides Massage Therapy at events such as the Olympic Games, the Iron-man Triathlon, the Boston Marathon, and others.

Sports Massage has numerous applications. During training it is used to improve performance through increased flexibility and coordination, to remove fascial limitations, to help prevent the occurrence of injuries, and for rehabilitation to overcome injuries. Before an athletic event, Sports Massage, combined with stretching, loosens and prepares the muscles for intense usage. After an event, Sports Massage helps to mitigate pain and stiffness by increasing blood circulation, which brings nutrition to the cells and removes lactic acid from the soft tissue. Sports Massage tends to be more vigorous and shorter in duration than a regular full-body massage.

Currently, there are numerous massage schools throughout the United States that teach Sports Massage; they are a good source of practitioners in your area. Additionally, there are massage therapists in private practice that specialize in or offer Sports Massage.

For additional information on Sports Massage contact the American Massage Therapy Association. They have a certification program in Sports Massage, and can provide the name of a certified practitioner in your area. Additionally, the Sports Massage Training Institute offers classes and a certification program in Sports Massage therapy.

For additional reading on Sports Massage, Dr. Hungerford's book, *Beyond Sports Massage: Injury Prevention and Care Through Sports Massage*, considered the definitive work on Sports Massage, is available from the International Sports Massage Federation and Training Institute.

❧ | ST. JOHN'S NEUROMUSCULAR THERAPY | ❧

St. John's Neuromuscular Therapy, also known as St. John's Neuromuscular Pain Relief and as Neuromuscular Therapy, St. John Method, is a system of bodywork to treat soft tissue pain and dysfunction. It is a unique approach to neuromuscular therapy that is Physical Therapy–oriented and uses many rehabilitation-oriented techniques.

Evolving like many other therapies, St. John's Neuromuscular Therapy was developed by Paul St. John as a result of trying to alleviate pain from his own body. In 1970, he returned to his home in Geneva, New York, after serving in Vietnam.

In 1974 he was severely injured in a devastating automobile accident. In constant pain, he was unable to continue his job as a trash collector.

Over the next four years constant pain changed his life. Aside from the damage caused by the automobile accident, he began to reexperience pain from previous injuries. In high school he had broken his back, and while in Vietnam he was in a helicopter that was shot down. Now, every morning he would wake up with a severe headache and other pain.

During this time he spent over fifty thousand dollars on orthopedists, neurologists, and chiropractors. Muscle-relaxing drugs did not help. Although his low back pain was severe, his neck and shoulders were much worse. As a natural reaction to get some relief, he began to squeeze the tissue in that area.

Although unaware of the principle of trigger points at that time, he discovered that touching a point on his neck would cause pain in other parts of his head. Medical practitioners he went to seemed to discount St. John's "discoveries." Finally one neurologist sent him to a psychiatrist, who concluded his pain was the result of a conflict with his mother, an explanation St. John would not accept.

St. John now realized that he must take action on his own behalf if he were to become healed. By 1976, he began to read literature related to soft tissue at the University of South Florida's Medical School Library. At this time his friend Richard Hamilton, while in Chiropractic training, took a workshop from Dr. Raymond Nimmo. Dr. Nimmo had developed what he called "receptor tonus technique," later known as the Nimmo technique.

Although not terribly interested in the technique, Hamilton decided to try it on his dog when her hind legs became paralyzed after being hit by a car. To his amazement, the dog began to walk again after the treatment. Knowing how much pain his friend Paul St. John was in, he wanted to try this technique on him.

After being treated by Hamilton, St. John woke the next morning without a headache, the first time in several years. St. John then went to Palmer College to take Dr. Nimmo's course. After completion, he realized there was still more to learn, so he returned to the literature.

He began further research into the functioning of the pain mechanism and developed neuromuscular techniques to treat pain. St. John taught these techniques to his friends so they would be able to treat him.

Over a period of about a year, Paul St. John's body began to heal and grow pain-free. After spending thousands of hours in medical libraries and doing extensive clinical research, Paul St. John developed his own approach to neuromuscular therapy. In 1978 he began teaching seminars nationally to train health care professionals in the "St. John Method."

There are five principles of neuromuscular therapy: biomechanics, ischemia (localized tissue anemia due to obstruction of arterial blood), trigger points, nerve entrapment/nerve compression, and postural distortion. All of these neurological concepts can interrupt the nervous system's normal functioning and eventually cause physiological dysfunction and pain.

The goal of St. John's Neuromuscular Therapy is to bring about homeostasis between the nervous system and the musculoskeletal system, thereby relieving pain and dysfunction. Techniques can be used to treat soft tissue pain in virtually all parts of the body, including the neck, shoulders, upper torso, spinal column, extremities, hands, and feet.

Benefits of St. John's Neuromuscular Therapy include relief from low back pain, neck and shoulder pain, pain from whiplash, chronic headaches, migraines, TMJ syndrome (a painful condition in the jaw), pain resulting from poor posture, and many others.

Today, Neuromuscular Therapy, St. John Method, is a very popular and very effective therapy. Paul St. John has put together some of the most effective therapeutic methods in the field and offers an excellent training program. It is taught throughout the United States in a series of four seminars. For additional information contact the St. John's Neuromuscular Pain Relief Institute.

❧ | STRAIN-COUNTERSTRAIN THERAPY | ❧

Strain-Counterstrain Therapy is an osteopathic method of soft tissue manipulation to relieve pain. It was developed by an osteopath named Lawrence Jones.

Strain-Counterstrain Therapy is a neuromuscular technique that involves identification of a trigger point, a hypersensitive area in the muscle and connective tissue that is painful to touch. Stimulation of a trigger point "refers" a sensation of pain to some other part of the body. This elaborate neuromuscular mechanism is the result of nerve connections that developed embryologically between the skin, muscles, and organs.

In Strain-Counterstrain Therapy, the practitioner passively moves the patient's body into a position that relieves the referred pain and holds that position for ninety seconds. When the body is moved back into the original position and the trigger point is pressed, the referred pain is gone.

Although the patient is sometimes required to bend or twist like a contortionist to secure a position of comfort, for the most part patients report enjoyment of the procedure.

Like other specialized bodywork techniques, Strain-Counterstrain Therapy is an extremely effective method of relieving neuromuscular pain when used by a skilled practitioner. For additional information contact the American Osteopathic Association or the American Academy of Osteopathy.

❧ | STRUCTURAL INTEGRATION | ❦

Structural Integration is a technique for manipulating and realigning the body's myofascial system. The myofascial system is composed of the muscles and fascia.

Fascia is the connective tissue which gives shape to the body and holds it together. The fascial system is a densely woven sheet of connective tissue that surrounds, penetrates, lines, or covers nearly every muscle, bone, nerve, artery, and vein as well as all the internal organs, including the heart, lungs, brain, and spinal cord.

The fascia is not just a system of separate coverings, but rather a single structure that extends from the top of the head to the tip of the toes; it plays an important role in the support of the body. Fascia is composed of two types of fibers: collagenous fibers, which are tough and have little ability to stretch, and elastic fibers, which are stretchable.

In the normal healthy state, fascia is relaxed and has the ability to move without restriction. When the body experiences habitually poor posture, disease, physical trauma, repeated patterns of self-use (such as in a job), surgery, emotional distress, and other factors, the effect on the fascia is cumulative over time. Eventually, as the fascia loses some of its pliability, it thickens and hardens. This leads to stiffness, restricted motion, pain, and an overall loss of freedom in the body.

Fortunately, connective tissue has a physical structure that is like gelatin. It becomes amorphous (having no definite shape) when energy is applied to it. While in the amorphous state, it can be re-formed into any position or shape desired. Then, as the energy is removed, the fascia solidifies and retains the new shape.

The original concept of Structural Integration was conceived by Ida Rolf, Ph.D., who developed the concept into her own form of bodywork, called Rolfing. The work of Rolf also gave rise to several other forms of structural bodywork that utilize her original principles of Structural Integration. These include Hellerwork, Aston-Patterning, Postural Integration, and several others.

The objective of Structural Integration is to soften and then realign the fascia, thereby releasing the pressure (tension) from muscles, blood vessels, lymphatic channels, and nerves.

Once the limitations caused by the hardened fascia are removed, the body is more free and coordinated. Movement becomes smoother and lighter, and requires less force, yet the body has more energy and greater strength and power.

An overall increase in energy allows the entire body to function more efficiently, and enhances life through greater comfort, ability, and self-confidence. In addition, there are internal benefits to every system of the body, which tends to improve general health, often freeing energy to heal chronic pain and health problems.

Structural Integration utilizes the application of physical pressure, mechanical friction, and heat from the practitioner's hands to cause the hardened, thickened fascia to become elastic and pliable once again. This allows the muscles to lengthen and return to their normal state. As the muscles are lengthened, the body becomes balanced and moves effortlessly in the gravitational field.

When Structural Integration was first developed, a series of ten one-hour sessions was the standard treatment. However, movement limitations usually develop over the course of a lifetime and exist for twenty, thirty, forty, or more years before being treated. In addition to severe adhesions in the fascia, most individuals have strong habits of movement which are difficult to change. Currently, some practitioners consider fifteen one-hour sessions to be the standard.

In the early days of Structural Integration the procedure was to push with great force to make the changes occur, which was often an extremely painful process. The problem with this procedure was that the physical tissue was stretched and released so rapidly that the client was unable to assimilate the change. Although improved for a while, he eventually fell back into his original way of moving and tensing, and the pain returned.

Today, the goal of Structural Integration is permanent improvement. Although a point is reached where deep, forceful work is no longer needed, the body never loses its need for bodywork (therapeutic touch). Only lighter forms of bodywork are then needed to maintain healthy body function.

Anecdotal evidence has shown Structural Integration to be effective in treating such problems as arthritis, scoliosis, lumbago and sciatica, allergies, digestive weakness, temporomandibular joint (TMJ) syndrome, whiplash, tennis elbow, flat feet, knee problems, and many others.

Structural Integration is taught at many massage schools throughout the country and is part of the curriculum for holistic health practitioners. The names of local practitioners can be obtained from these massage schools.

❧ | SUBLIMINAL THERAPY | ❧

Subliminal Therapy is a self-help tool that uses subliminal perception, both audio and visual, for therapeutic and beneficial purposes including health-related matters and behavior modification.

Perception is a natural way that people receive impressions from the environment. Subliminal refers to information that is perceived below the level of conscious awareness.

Although we consciously ignore them, sounds of every description constantly bombard us. Traffic noise, singing birds, closing doors, or someone coughing is perceived below conscious awareness by a very receptive and sensitive subconscious mind.

Interest in subliminal communication developed around the turn of the century, shortly after Sigmund Freud introduced his revolutionary idea that every person has a hidden, unconscious mind.

In 1917 Dr. O. Poetzel, one of Freud's contemporaries, was the first scientist to demonstrate the relationship between subliminal stimuli and posthypnotic effect. He discovered that subliminal perceptions evoke dreams and actions days or weeks after the original perception.

In 1957 a well-publicized experiment took place at a movie theater in Fort Lee, New Jersey. While the movie was being shown subliminal messages ("Hungry? Eat Popcorn. Thirsty? Drink Coca-Cola") were flashed on the screen for a fraction of a second between frames of the film *Picnic*. As a result, popcorn and cola sales skyrocketed during the six-week period these subliminal messages were shown.

In later years it was learned that subliminal messages could be masked in music and other audio programs. Subsequently, subliminal messages were used very effectively by department stores in the United States and Canada to reduce shoplifting and employee theft.

A supermarket chain found that pilferage dropped drastically and cashier shortages were reduced to an amazing low when subliminal messages about honesty were broadcast in the store.

Countless scientific studies conducted during decades of research clearly indicate that subliminal perception does occur and information that is perceived subliminally does affect the unconscious or subconscious mind.

Research indicates that subliminal perception takes place when the unconscious or subconscious portion of the mind is exposed to messages below the level of conscious awareness.

Psychologists have found that behavioral improvements result from the use of subliminal messages. Subliminal Therapy effectively helps people in a wide variety of personal transformations, especially in ridding themselves of alcohol, drug, and tobacco addictions.

A typical subliminal program utilizes a script of strong positive messages that are "masked" by a musical selection or by sounds from nature such as ocean surf, a thunderstorm, singing birds and rustling trees, and others.

Through the use of sophisticated electronic technology, the subliminal voice-track messages are integrated into the musical selection but not heard on the conscious level. The music or other sounds effectively hide the voice messages. The reason that subliminal audio- and videotapes are proving to be so effective is that the positive messages go directly to the subconscious mind.

Today subliminal programs are a popular self-help method of dealing with a wide variety of behavioral and health-related problems. They provide an effective, low-cost way to pain relief, relaxation and stress management, strengthening of the immune system, enjoyment of exercise, speeding recovery by enhancing the body's own natural ability to heal itself, relief of insomnia, and weight reduction.

A book that covers the field of subliminal tapes and evaluates available products is *Subliminal: The New Channel to Personal Power* by Lee M. Schulman, Ph.D., and Joyce Schulman, Ph.D., with Gerald P. Rafferty. It can be found in bookstores.

There are numerous brands of subliminal tapes available through mail order and at retail stores. A list is provided in the resource section.

❧ | SWEDISH MASSAGE | ❧

Swedish Massage, also known as Swedish Circulatory Massage, is a fairly vigorous style of bodywork that is designed to energize, invigorate, or "wake up" the body through increased blood circulation. It is geared toward relaxation and pleasure and does not directly address specific physical problems.

Per Hendrik Ling (1776–1839), born near Reashult, Sweden, was known as the "Father of European Physical Culture." In 1813 he founded the first gymnasium in Stockholm, and built the first swimming pool in Europe.

During the last half of the sixteenth century, French physician Ambroise

Pare and other French physicians and surgeons began to explore the benefits of body manipulation techniques for treatment. While a student at the University of Stockholm, Ling studied the writings of Pare and others. This combined information formed the basis for Ling's development of Swedish Massage.

Ling wanted to create a system of body manipulation that would reproduce the movements and associated benefits of Swedish gymnastics and other types of exercise. Swedish gymnastics is an exercise regimen that stimulates circulation, increases muscle tone, and creates balance in the musculoskeletal system. It contains forty-seven positions and eight hundred movements for stimulating and relaxing the body.

Ling's system was not well received by the Swedish government or the established medical profession. In 1812 he applied for a license to teach and practice massage. Although he was turned down at first, popular acceptance of the technique and his own perseverance finally led to the acquisition of a license in 1814. Eventually, numerous Ling institutes were established in Sweden and throughout the world.

Swedish Massage is characterized by several different types of strokes and manipulations.

Effleurage is light stroking, either superficial or deep. Centripetal strokes move toward the heart to increase circulation. Rotating or spiraling strokes stimulate circulation in the skin.

Petrissage is kneading. The muscle is lifted, pulled away from the bone, and then squeezed (kneaded). It stimulates circulation in deeper blood vessels and lymphatics, and exercises the muscle.

Tapotement, or percussion strokes, is performed as hacking, tapping, cupping, or clapping over the muscle. These strokes produce both sedating and stimulating effects to muscles and nerves.

Friction strokes use pressure applied down into the tissue. This movement raises temperature in the area and is useful in breaking down adhesions.

Vibration is a stroke during which shaking or pulsating motions at different speeds and amplitudes are created in the massaged tissue. Depending on the force and strength of the vibration, the effects can be felt on the surface or deep within the muscle tissue.

Generally, the entire body surface or "full body" (that which is legally allowed) is rubbed in a mostly superficial manner. Oil or lotion is used as a lubricant to make the bodyworker's hands glide easily over the skin. Swedish Massage is the least specialized form of Massage Therapy practiced.

It is probably the most familiar form of massage known to or recognized by a majority of people. It is the type of massage an individual would receive at a spa or health club unless he requested some specialized technique.

Swedish Massage is the foundation of the Western approach to massage. It is especially popular with athletes and forms the foundation of Sports Massage. Swedish Massage is usually used in combination with other massage techniques, which increases its effectiveness and benefits.

Benefits from Swedish Massage include relief from sore and stiff muscles, reduction of stress, reduction of swelling, and a better general overall feeling in the body.

Today, there are massage practitioners available in most cities. The numerous massage schools around the country are a good source for referrals.

Two organizations, the American Massage Therapy Association and the Associated Bodywork and Massage Professionals, are able to provide therapist referrals. Currently, laws concerning training and licensing of massage therapists vary from state to state.

❧ | TAI CHI CHUAN | ☙

Tai Chi Chuan was originally designed as a system of self-defense. As it is currently practiced in China, it is a system of physical exercises or gymnastics that is based on principles of rhythmic movement, equilibrium of body weight, and effortless breathing.

It is characterized by a technique of moving slowly and continuously, without strain, through a varied sequence of contrasting movements. Each movement develops from what it was previously joined to and evolves into the oncoming movement. In simplest terms Tai Chi Chuan is exercise controlled by the mind.

In the sixth century A.D. an Indian Buddhist, Dharuma, founded the Zen school of Buddhism in China. He originated the Shao-lin school of boxing in Shao-lin temples. At this time boxing was thought of in terms of physical strength and courage.

Most historians have concluded that Tai Chi Chuan originated near the end of the Sung dynasty (A.D. 960–1270) with the famous Taoist boxer

Chang San-feng. A man of great strength, he applied the philosophy of the Yellow Emperor (twenty-seventh century B.C.) and Lao-Tzu to boxing.

Chang San-feng developed the rhythmic exercises of Tai Chi Chuan as an accompaniment to boxing to increase pliability in the body rather than to develop muscular power. This was a digression from the original idea of boxing, which was based on physical strength for hard hitting.

Tradition tells that Chang San-feng, while in the semitrance state of mystical meditation, envisioned how every part of the human body works simultaneously in cooperation with every other. He realized how a guiding vital principle within the body works to affect metabolism and facilitate the circulation of blood.

Through repeated personal experiences he understood that one should follow or obey nature in every movement rather than use artificial exercise as a means of invigorating the body. This led him to advance a system beneficial not only to his followers but to the average person as well.

Over the centuries Chang San-feng's original system has been greatly expanded into its more elaborate present-day form. Although the complete system comprises 128 different movements, a modern Tai Chi Chuan authority and author named Cheng Man-Ch'ing has simplified the system.

His earliest teachings had reduced the number to 13 movements. His revised system now has 37 movements. These 37 essential movements preserve all of the fundamental elements and original sequence of the 128-movement system.

The objective of Tai Chi Chuan is to achieve health and tranquillity while developing the mind and body, through movement. It teaches an individual how to control her nervous system in order to put the entire body to rest, which is an effective way to stay healthy.

Tai Chi Chuan is an exercise that initially demands no physical strength and is suitable for men and women of all ages in almost any state of health. A key element is performance of the exercises in a relaxed state by first loosening the muscles and releasing stored tension.

The essence of Tai Chi Chuan lies in maintaining perfect body balance at all times. To accomplish this, most movements are done from a semicrouch position to preserve maximum stability.

Although not intended for presentation to an audience, Tai Chi Chuan appears to be a dance form. It is a synthesis of form and function complete unto itself and is not derived from any other art-dance form.

There are five essential qualities to Tai Chi Chuan; *slowness* helps to develop awareness; *lightness* aids in flowing movement; *balance* places the body in an unstrained position; *calmness* is created by an even-flowing continuity; *clarity* is cleansing the mind of intruding thoughts.

Two essential elements of Tai Chi Chuan are softness and circular motion. Movements appear "soft" due to the continuous flow from one to another without any strain during execution. The circular motions are composed of geometric patterns such as circles, arcs, spirals, and curves in various sizes and in many directions. Circular motion creates evenness, evokes calmness, and creates energy.

The benefits of practicing Tai Chi Chuan are both physical and mental. It enables the mind to function with greater awareness, clarity, and concentration; it increases blood circulation to nourish the muscles; and it stimulates the nervous system and glandular activity, and helps joint movement. All of this is accomplished without an increase in heart activity or change in breathing rhythm. Because of its emphasis on balance, Tai Chi Chuan provides the added benefit of good posture.

As a healing tool, Tai Chi Chuan has been an effective remedy for high blood pressure, anemia, joint disorders, and gastric disturbances.

On any given day in China, millions of Chinese emerge at daybreak onto streets, public squares, parks, and rooftops to practice Tai Chi Chuan.

An excellent book for the beginner is *Tai Chi Chuan: A Simplified Method of Calisthenics for Health and Self Defense*, by Cheng Man-Ch'ing. The popularity of Tai Chi Chuan is on the rise and many types of schools offer classes in it.

ॐ | THAI MASSAGE | ॐ

Thai Massage, also called Thailand Massage or Thailand Medical Massage, is a therapeutic type of bodywork. The main focus of Thai Massage is to unblock energy that is trapped in the body.

It is based theoretically on the energy lines or meridians that run throughout the body. Of the seventy-two thousand energy points or vessels that are said to exist to distribute the vital life energy force known as *chi* or *prana*, Thai Massage focuses on the ten major lines, called *sens*.

The ten *sen* lines are more closely related to the Indian system than to the Chinese or Japanese systems of meridians. Important Acupressure points are found along the *sen* lines.

Massage has a long history of therapeutic healing in Thailand. Thai Massage was created over two thousand years ago and is still practiced today.

The roots of Thai Massage are traced back to India although the original source of knowledge that led to Thai Massage was traditional Chinese medicine, in which were developed the Acupuncture and Acupressure theories. The oldest known text on this subject, the *Huang-ti Nei-Ching (The Yellow Emperor's Classic of Internal Medicine)*, dates back to 2600 B.C.

In the second century B.C. the Indian king Ashoka sent Buddhist missionaries to Thailand. They built great temples where the practice of massage flourished. Many of the postures and movements used in Thai massage communicate the adaptation of yogic techniques from Hinduism.

The knowledge of massage and traditional massage in Thailand has been handed down orally or by the practical demonstration of touch from one generation to the next within the family. It is usually passed from parent to child and teacher to student.

In 1776 the royal capital of Ayuthaya was destroyed by the Burmese, and with it nearly all of the ancient medical texts. The remaining information was literally carved in stone and set into the walls of the Wat Poh temple in Bangkok. These towering temple walls depict various Yoga and massage postures. Part of the Wat Poh temple today serves as a medical clinic to treat Thai and foreigners alike. It also functions as a school to teach traditional medicine and massage.

When the flow of vital life energy is impeded, certain points along the meridians accumulate blockage. These blockages can be caused by physical injury, emotional stress, improper diet, and lack of exercise, and ultimately result in pain and disease when left untreated.

To clear blocked meridian points the practitioner uses pressure exerted with fingers, thumbs, hands, forearms, elbows, and feet. Stretching all the muscles of the body and integrating Yoga-like stretches using a rocking motion are integral parts of the treatment. Once the stagnated energy is flowing freely, tensed muscles relax and dysfunctional organs heal themselves.

A unique feature of Thai Massage is that it is given on the floor. This is to accommodate the Yoga-like stretches. Also, the person remains clothed during the massage.

Thai Massage is increasing in popularity in the United States, and more massage schools are teaching it. For additional information contact the American Oriental Bodywork Therapy Association.

ॐ | THERAPEUTIC TOUCH | ॐ

Therapeutic Touch is a derivative of the ancient technique of "laying on of hands." Although religious faith is not required by either the healer or the person receiving the touch, the healer does use his hands with the intent to heal.

The underlying premise of Therapeutic Touch is that healing is promoted when the energy (vital life force) enveloping the body is in balance. The disease process is thought to be manifested when this energy is in a state of imbalance.

By passing his hands lightly over the person's body, the healer can feel any energy imbalances. These usually show up as one of several sensations: heat, cold, tingling, pulsation, electric shock, or tightness.

Proponents of Therapeutic Touch believe that anyone can be taught to sensitize himself and feel the unnamed and unmeasured energy that they claim envelops every person. And, with the proper intention, the healer can direct his healing energy to the person he is working with or he can fine-tune and balance that person's own energy.

Cave paintings in the Pyrenees Mountains dating back fifteen thousand years show man helping man through the use of the hands. Carvings from ancient Egypt, India, and Tibet, and from medieval Roman Catholic churches serve to illustrate that the laying-on of hands has been valued for many centuries.

In early England and France the laying on of hands was known as the "King's Touch," as the touch of the king was considered good for curing certain ailments.

Therapeutic Touch was developed by Dolores Krieger, a professor of nursing at New York University, and Dora Kunz, a clairvoyant and gifted healer in her own right. Krieger grew up in Brooklyn, New York, and while in her early twenties enrolled in nursing school. Personal interests led her to study the theories of the major religions and later explore Eastern esoterica.

In the early 1950s Krieger joined a meditation group led by Dora Kunz, who became her friend, mentor, and eventual collaborator in developing Therapeutic Touch. In the late 1960s and early 1970s Kunz was studying the laying on of hands as practiced by world-renowned healer Colonel Oscar Estebany.

Kunz invited Krieger to meet Colonel Estebany, a seventy-one-year-old former Hungarian cavalry officer. Krieger carefully observed Estebany session after session as he would sit quietly next to each patient brought to him by Kunz, and gently allow his hands to move to the spot he felt needed healing.

Krieger was amazed as she watched Estebany alleviate and seemingly cure a wide variety of illnesses, and she realized the only discernible action between healer and healee was the touch, the laying on of hands.

Dolores Krieger attempted to imitate what Estebany was doing. She would have Dora Kunz interpret for her, as Estebany spoke little English, and give her feedback on her attempts. Through this method Krieger and Kunz developed what is now known as Therapeutic Touch.

Studies Krieger carried out on patients receiving Therapeutic Touch showed that their hemoglobin value (ability of red blood cells to carry oxygen) was significantly raised afterward. Krieger taught several nurses her technique and tested patients they treated. The results were the same: raised hemoglobin value.

Now convinced of the efficacy of Therapeutic Touch, she began to give workshops on the technique to thousands of health care workers; in 1976 she was allowed to teach a master's level course at New York University (where she was a tenured professor) in Therapeutic Touch.

In Therapeutic Touch the healee can be sitting or lying down while receiving the treatment and can either be in a conscious or unconscious state while the healing takes place.

The healer, a nurse or other health care practitioner, becomes centered in a meditative state before touching the receiver. With compassion and motivation the healer focuses her consciousness with a strong intent to help or heal the individual. This is an important part of the process.

The practitioner then accesses the individual's energy field and transmits energy to her as appropriate. This requires that the healer's hands be sensitive to temperature change, pressure, and other sensations to indicate the location of energy blocks. This is a skill that is developed with experience.

After the areas of energy imbalance have been determined, the practitioner begins to move or redistribute the energy around the body, relieving parts that are congested and enhancing those that are lacking energy.

Therapeutic Touch is noticeably useful for two purposes: It elicits a rather profound relaxation in the patient, and it is very good at relieving pain.

Ultimately it is the patient who heals herself. The healer's role is only to accelerate the patient's own healing process by giving her a boost of energy until her recuperative system can take over. It can also be used as a self-healing technique.

In addition to the excellent book *Therapeutic Touch: How to Use Your Hands to Heal* by Dolores Krieger, Ph.D., R.N., there is another, titled *Therapeutic Touch: A Practical Guide*, by Janet Macrae. For additional information contact the Nurse Healers–Professional Association or the American Holistic Nurses Association.

✺ | TOUCH FOR HEALTH | ✺

Touch for Health, an easily applied and practical system of natural self-health care, is a synthesis of methods and techniques which includes Acupuncture principles, Acupressure, muscle testing, massage, and dietary guidelines.

Although health care professionals, many of them chiropractors, use Touch for Health as an adjunct to their regular practice, it is primarily intended for the layperson to learn and use on others.

Touch for Health promotes the idea that many methods of treatment and therapy cannot be done by an individual to himself, but require a second person. It is through the involvement of the second person and the use of touch that a greater degree of communication and trust is developed between people as they begin to help each other. This is true for both family members and friends.

Also, it shares a philosophy with Chiropractic regarding the idea that health comes from within, and focuses on promoting and maintaining good health rather than treating illness.

In the 1960s, Chiropractic physician Dr. George Goodheart developed a system called Applied Kinesiology which is based on a highly systematic charting of muscle reflexes and their effect on corresponding organs. It uses a series of tests to ascertain muscles' relative strength and weakness.

Based on this information, a course of treatment to strengthen the muscle or related organ using Acupressure, massage, prescribed herbs, and nutritional guidelines is then recommended.

Touch for Health was developed by Dr. John F. Thie, a chiropractor in Pasadena, California, in the 1970s as a simplified version of Applied Kinesiology that the average person could learn and apply to his daily life.

Muscle testing is the fundamental element to the Touch for Health system. It determines which muscles are strong or weak, indicating the areas of the body that need work. Each separate muscle group that is tested correlates to a muscle function, body function, or their related organs.

A muscle that tests weak indicates that a physical problem or organ malfunction exists. This indication can often expose a physical problem before the individual is aware of its existence. More commonly, the procedure is used to confirm that symptoms such as pain are actually the manifestation of a physical problem.

When it is determined which muscles are weak, a program of muscle strengthening is begun. To accomplish this, a variety of methods is used, including massage of points on Acupuncture meridians, pressure on Acupressure holding points, finger pressure on neurovascular holding points on the head, deep massage of the neurolymphatic massage points, and separation of the skull bones to facilitate the movement of cerebrospinal fluid.

After various methods have been used to strengthen a muscle, it is rested. This serves a twofold purpose: First, it tests the effectiveness of the strengthening treatment; and second, activating the muscle once it has strength helps realign the body to a more normal internally balanced position.

When all muscles are strong and functioning properly the body is in homeostasis; it does not need to compensate for weak muscles to maintain structural balance. Energy then flows through the body, without blockage, giving rise to improved vitality and enhancing the body's natural ability to maintain good health.

Today Touch for Health classes are taught by trained and certified Touch for Health instructors in colleges, schools, health centers, recreation centers, and homes throughout the United States and Canada, and around the world.

For additional information contact the Touch for Health Association. The association can provide the names of teachers and practitioners in your area, and has available a book that describes the process in detail, *Touch for Health* by John F. Thie, D.C. Other books, charts, and teaching aids that deal with Touch for Health are also available.

❧ | TRAGER APPROACH | ❧

The Trager Approach, also known as Tragerwork, is an innovative system of movement reeducation that combines bodywork and movement sequences. It combines Trager Psychophysical Integration with Mentastics Movement Education. Although Tragerwork is therapeutic, it is a learning experience rather than a medical treatment.

Milton Trager, M.D., created and developed the Trager Approach over a period of more than fifty years. At the age of eighteen, Trager was a professional boxer in Miami, Florida. He began to realize that his hands were especially talented after a boxing trainer commented on how good his rubdowns were. He then turned his talented hands on friends, neighbors, and his father, who suffered from sciatica. Later Trager quit boxing to save the wear and tear on his hands.

After becoming a dancer and acrobat, Trager decided to attempt a new type of movement one day while practicing jumping with his brother on the beach. He would try jumping "softer" rather than higher. This opened a new area of interest for him, one in which the emphasis was on performance of movements in an effortless manner.

Trager's interest in physical health gained momentum, and in 1941 he graduated from the Los Angeles College of Drugless Physicians with a Ph.D. in physical medicine. He then began to work with victims of polio.

In 1949, by then in his early forties and wanting to become a physician, Trager applied to medical school but was summarily rejected by schools in the United States. He was eventually accepted by a medical school in Mexico.

While attending medical school, Trager demonstrated the techniques he had used earlier on polio patients. Impressed by his work, the school opened a rehabilitation clinic and let Trager operate it while he attended classes.

After receiving his degree, Trager went to Hawaii and opened a medical practice which gave him the opportunity to practice and refine his techniques. This continued for nearly twenty years before his work was "discovered."

Recognition finally came to Dr. Milton Trager in 1975 after a demonstration at the Esalen Institute in Big Sur, California, where Ida P. Rolf had introduced her Structural Integration work some years earlier.

The objective of Trager Psychophysical Integration (Trager bodywork) is to alleviate neuromuscular holding patterns which serve to block, inhibit, or distort the body's natural free-flowing motion. These patterns are often the result of physical or emotional traumas such as accidents, injury, surgery, emotional upset, poor posture, muscular tension from the stress of daily living, illness, and poor movement habits sometimes associated with occupation.

Within the Psychophysical Integration segment of Tragerwork, the client lies on a table while the practitioner, in a relaxed meditative state, uses light, nonintrusive movements to help release deep-seated physical and mental patterns stored in the body.

An important aspect of Tragerwork is the mind-link communication between client and practitioner. While working in a relaxed, meditative state, the practitioner is able to connect with the client on a deep level. Dr. Trager calls this state of consciousness "Hook-up."

During the sixty- to ninety-minute session of Pyschophysical Integration, the client, usually wearing swimwear, stays passive. During the session his torso and limbs are moved in a gentle rhythmic way, such as rocking or shaking, without unnecessary force. This produces an experience in the client of being able to move each part of the body freely, effortlessly, and gracefully on his own. No oils are used during a session.

"Mentastics" is a word coined by Dr. Trager for mental gymnastics. It is a system of simple, effortless, dancelike movement sequences developed by Dr. Trager.

These exercises are usually given to clients as "homework" after a session, so they can recreate for themselves the sensory feelings they received on the table while being manipulated by the practitioner.

Mentastics helps the client recall the pleasurable state or feeling he experienced during the session while positive change was taking place in his tissue. Each time this pleasurable feeling is recalled it reinforces the positive change that took place and becomes more permanent.

Based on the client's experiences, the effect of a Trager session penetrates below the level of conscious awareness and continues to produce results long after the session is completed.

The benefits of a Trager session can include deep relaxation, increased physical mobility, mental clarity, enhanced energy, improved posture, and the reduction or elimination of chronic pain, stiffness, and muscular tension.

The Trager Institute gives introductory training seminars throughout the United States and in Europe. Additional information and a list of certified Tragerwork practitioners in your area is available from the institute.

Although relatively little has been published on Tragerwork, one book by Dr. Milton Trager, *Trager Mentastics: Movement as a Way to Agelessness*, is currently available.

❧ | TRANSCENDENTAL MEDITATION | ❧

Transcendental Meditation, or TM, is a natural technique for reducing stress and expanding conscious awareness. It is neither a religion, a philosophy, nor a way of life.

The use of Meditation for healing is not new, and its value to alleviate suffering and promote healing has been known and practiced for thousands of years.

An East Indian teacher named Maharishi Mahesh Yogi was the first to introduce the technique of Transcendental Meditation to the world. Born in 1918, he was the son of a forest ranger in what was then British India. He graduated from Allahabad University in 1942 with a degree in physics. His family belonged to the Kayasthe caste, which destined him to become a clerk, shopkeeper, merchant, or scribe.

But in the 1940s he met Swami Brahmananda Saraswati, the Jagad-guru Bhagwan Shankaracharya or Guru Dev (divine teacher), a major religious leader in India at that time. Wanting to become the Guru Dev's disciple, he received his parents' permission to follow this calling and was accepted by the Guru Dev. Quickly becoming the master's favorite disciple, he was given the name, Mahout. He stayed with Guru Dev for over thirteen years.

Before his death in 1953, the Guru Dev asked Mahout to continue his work on developing a simple form of meditation which could be learned and used by everyone. After agreeing to continue the Guru Dev's work, Mahout went into a two-year seclusion in Utter Kasha in the Himalayan Mountains and emerged with the system he called Transcendental Meditation.

In 1958 in Madras, India, a memorial celebration of Guru Dev's eighty-ninth birthday was held. At this event Maharishi Mahesh Yogi, after delivering a eulogy, announced to the crowd of followers his intention to teach the benefits of TM to the world.

In 1959 he established the International Meditation Society in London and began to formally teach TM. It gained popular notoriety after the Beatles rock group heard the somewhat unknown Indian guru speak in London, and soon after became disciples. During April of that same year the Maharishi came to San Francisco and TM was introduced into the United States.

The next year saw extensive media coverage. Major magazines and

Sunday newspaper supplements ran articles on the TM movement and its founder, Maharishi Mahesh Yogi.

In 1961 he began teacher training courses in India. There was only one TM teacher in the United States until 1966, when approximately thirty Americans became teachers. In 1967 the Maharishi toured the United States and lectured at Harvard, Yale, Berkeley, and UCLA. Students became interested in the practice and requested classes in TM. By the end of the 1960s, several hundred thousand people were practicing TM.

In the early 1970s, TM was firmly established in the United States and was taught in more than fifty countries around the world. Scientific research at the Stanford Research Institute and the Harvard University Medical School showed that individuals practicing TM experienced profound physiological changes while meditating.

In the United States today, Transcendental Meditation is probably the most well known and widely practiced form of meditation.

TM is not a theory or an idea, but a unique and specific practice. This simple, natural, and effortless technique is experiential in nature. TM allows activity in the mind to quiet down while an individual sits comfortably with her eyes closed. It allows the mind to reach subtler levels of thinking until the thinking process is transcended and the mind comes into contact with the source of thought.

Therapeutic benefits can be derived from TM when it is practiced for fifteen to twenty minutes each morning and evening. These sessions allow the body to rest deeply and the mind to expand its awareness. The benefits of TM are numerous and can be divided into three categories: mental, physical, and those derived from the integration of body and mind.

Mental benefits for those in school include increased learning ability and the ability to solve problems accurately with more speed and improved academic performance. Benefits in the workplace include increased productivity, increased job satisfaction, improved relations with supervisors and co-workers, and many others.

Physical benefits include greater stability of the autonomic nervous system, faster reaction time, lower heart rate and blood pressure, increased auditory discrimination, reduction of stress, decreased anxiety, relief from insomnia, and many others.

Through the integration of body and mind an individual may become more creative; his comprehension is broadened, his ability to focus attention is improved, his self-actualization is improved, and more.

Although there are numerous books on the subject of Transcendental Meditation which explain and provide an overview of how it works, the techniques cannot be learned from a book. To begin practicing TM requires personal instruction from a trained TM teacher.

Today, Transcendental Meditation classes can be found in almost any city in the United States. The easiest way to find a TM class is to consult the telephone directory. Additional information can be obtained from the Maharishi Vedic University.

❧ | TRIGGER POINT THERAPY | ❦

Trigger Point Therapy is the use of various techniques to sedate, desensitize, or eliminate "trigger points." A trigger point is defined as a hypersensitive area in the myofascia (muscle and connective tissue) which is very painful to the touch. Stimulation of this point also "refers" a sensation of pain to some other part of the body.

By sedating pain in the trigger point, the myofascia is allowed to relax and let the area normalize, which in turn stops pain in the referred area.

Trigger Point Therapy is used by medical doctors, physical therapists, massage therapists, trigger point myotherapists, and alternative healers. Bonnie Prudden developed it for use by the layman under the name Myotherapy (see elsewhere in this book).

Dr. Janet Travel was called the "Trigger Queen" by noted British rheumatologist Dr. W. S. C. Copeman, in reference to her mapping of uncharted patterns of "referred pain" in the body from "trigger areas."

Although this was the major part of her life's work, she is probably best known for being John F. Kennedy's physician while he was a senator and during his presidency.

Dr. Travel was born into a medical family in New York City in 1901. Her father, Willard Travel, M.D., was a pioneer in physical medicine. Especially skilled in treating musculoskeletal and neurological pain, he still practiced medicine at the age of eighty-five. Her sister, Virginia Travel Weeks, became a pediatrician.

In 1922 Dr. Janet Travel graduated from Wellesley College and entered Cornell University Medical College. In 1926 Dr. Travel received her M.D. and won the Polk Memorial Prize for highest scholastic standing in her class.

It was due to a chance set of circumstances which began in 1939 that Dr. Travel became interested in the phenomenon of trigger areas. She read a scientific article, published in 1936, which was of great interest to her and would greatly influence the future of her work. In it the authors described what they called a "trigger-zone" in the shoulder blade area of two patients. Pressure applied to this area produced pain that radiated into the patient's shoulder, neck, and down the arm. They also reported there was no effective treatment for this condition.

Dr. Travel had developed a very painful right shoulder and arm of her own from overuse of muscles in writing longhand and performing precise laboratory procedures. One day while trying a self-massage on the muscles in her shoulder, she reproduced the pain previously experienced in her arm. Dr. Travel then realized that this referred pain she had felt in her own body was not her imagination. It was this incident that started her work in "trigger points."

In her medical practice Dr. Travel became aware of patients who would feel severe muscular pain in an area or "reference zone," often a considerable distance from the site in the muscle where the actual pain originated. She then realized that knowing specific referred pain patterns would assist in accurately locating the trigger areas.

While working at a tuberculosis hospital on Staten Island, she noted that some of the patients with life-threatening pulmonary disease complained more about the pain in their neck and shoulders. Through a palpation examination, she discovered the patients' trigger areas.

After reading articles on the use of intramuscular injections of procaine (Novocain) into trigger areas to alleviate pain in the referred areas, Dr. Travel sought approval to try the technique on selected patients with painful shoulder syndrome. The procedure tested gave prompt and lasting relief of pain and the shoulder joint was returned to its normal range of motion.

In 1941 Dr. Travel began to study referred skeletal muscle pain. Joining her was Dr. Seymour H. Rinzler; their collaboration would last for twenty years. During that time they published numerous papers on this work in prestigious journals.

Wondering how a short-term anesthetic like procaine could cause a permanent effect, she set about to understand the process. Through experimentation and observations, Dr. Travel determined that stimulation of the fascia (connective tissue) as well as of muscle in the trigger area would cause referred pain. Terminology was then modified to "myofascial" pain to reflect this.

Different procedures were tested to eliminate the trigger areas. These included injection of procaine, injection of saline solution, and multiple punctures with a dry needle. For several reasons, the procaine injections seemed to be most effective.

Dr. Travel then set about to map these trigger points and referral patterns by injecting them with saline. In other words, what she did specifically was to identify those areas where you press *here* (e.g., a hip) and a referred pain is experienced *there* (e.g., a leg).

A medical treatment plan was developed for physicians desiring to use this technique. Injection of a local anesthetic such as procaine or a counterirritant such as lydocaine would desensitize the trigger point and permit it to relax. This would break the self-sustaining cycle of muscle spasm in the trigger area, allowing the referral area to stop hurting.

Although this medical treatment was successful, it was later discovered that finger pressure could affect these points very much the way Acupressure works. A light or heavy touch sedates the trigger point pain and eliminates pain in the area of referral.

Once the trigger point is eliminated, massage techniques can be used on the area to move stagnated lymph and restore blood circulation, which prevents the trigger point from coming back.

Trigger Point Therapy works especially well with acute musculoskeletal problems such as bursitis or tendonitis. Physical problems that are considered untreatable or difficult to treat are often not due to organic deterioration, but rather are caused by trigger points.

Sometimes bursitis, as has been discovered, is referred from somewhere other than the shoulder. When the trigger point is eliminated, the bursitis can be alleviated and the area will respond to Massage Therapy.

It is thought that some trigger points involved with tendonitis refer their pain to the internal organs. Some internal organ pain can be alleviated by eliminating trigger points in the abdominal wall or on the back. A common sore throat can sometimes be alleviated by a trigger point in the neck.

❧ | TUI NA MASSAGE THERAPY | ❧

Tui Na Massage Therapy is an ancient Chinese system of healing and Acupressure massage. It uses a variety of hand techniques to effect changes in the physical and energetic systems of the body. *Tui* means "to push" and *na* means "to grasp."

The origin of Tui Na Massage goes back to ancient China. Written records from the Shang dynasty describe massage methods for treating infants. About 2500 B.C., the *Huang-ti Nei-Ching (The Yellow Emperor's Classic of Internal Medicine)* mentions the use of Tui Na along with Acupuncture, herbs, moxabustion, and Qi Gong exercises as major methods of treatment.

During the Tang dynasty, A.D. 618–907, Tui Na Massage Therapy was included in the curriculum of the Imperial Medical College.

Some people in the field of bodywork believe that Tui Na, which was brought to Europe by Marco Polo, eventually became Swedish Massage. The two disciplines have many similarities and share some of the same techniques, such as stroking, kneading, and working on specific points.

In 1976, at the Taoist Institute in Los Angeles, Taoist master Share K. Lew became the first teacher of Tui Na Massage in the United States.

Today, Tui Na Massage Therapy is more widely known in the United States and is included in the curriculum of many massage schools and Oriental medical colleges.

In the People's Republic of China, Tui Na Massage is taught in traditional medical colleges. It is widely used to treat soft tissue damage, joint and tendon diseases, and internal disorders, and enjoys the same status as Acupuncture or Herbal Medicine.

Traditional Chinese medical theory believes that all disease is a result of an imbalance between the yin and yang energies *(chi)* within the body (see page 7). These energies circulate freely throughout the body in main channels called "meridians" and in smaller channels called "collaterals." Each channel relates to a specific body organ, and along the channels are located focal points called "acupoints" which affect the energy moving through them. An acupoint also influences the organ related to it and the tissue surrounding it.

When the flow of energy is interrupted (obstructed) at any of these points, the yin/yang balance is disturbed and certain characteristic symptoms result; stagnation is the most common condition. When energy and blood are stagnant, pain, inflammation, and physiological dysfunction in a specific area of the body result.

The objective of Tui Na Massage Therapy is to restore the free flow of energy and blood in the affected area by removing the obstruction that is causing the stagnation. Depending on whether there is an excess or deficiency of energy in the area, techniques are employed to either sedate (reduce) or tonify (build up) the existing energy.

The primary features used in Tui Na Massage techniques include grasping, pressing, penetrating, and rubbing. Each Tui Na technique uses these features in a certain way. A therapist makes use of his fingers, different surfaces of his thumb, knuckles, palm, and elbow to stimulate the acupoints, activate the meridians and collaterals, and perform various manipulations on the soft tissue and the joints.

To properly apply Tui Na Massage Therapy, the therapist must develop the strength and sensitivity in his hands. Also, the practice of Chi Kung exercises is used to increase the flow of energy to his hands.

Although their effect on energy is of principal concern, Tui Na Massage techniques are also effective on the physical body, including the nervous, circulatory, respiratory, digestive, lymphatic, and musculoskeletal systems.

Tui Na Massage Therapy is used to treat a myriad of conditions including asthma, allergy, hay fever, painful menstruation, arthritis, rheumatism, sore throat, infant crying, back pain, and others.

For additional information on Tui Na Massage Therapy including classes, contact the Taoist Institute of Los Angeles or the Taoist Sanctuary of San Diego. An illustrated book that describes the Tui Na technique in detail, *Tui Na: Chinese Healing and Acupressure Massage* by Share K. Lew and Bill Helm, is available from either organization.

URINE THERAPY

Urine Therapy is the use of one's own water (urine) for therapeutic purposes. It is an entirely drugless system of healing that encourages overall health and is not a specific treatment for any particular disease.

The history of Urine Therapy goes back to the ancient Greeks, some of whom used urine exclusively to treat wounds. *Salmon's English Physician*, a book published in 1695, denotes the use of urine to heal wounds and treat numerous other conditions. For centuries European Gypsies have known about the curative properties of urine. They have used cow's urine to cure Bright's disease (several acute and chronic diseases of the kidneys which produce albumin in the urine). It has been claimed that the yogis and lamas of Tibet reach extended ages by drinking their own urine.

A book from the early 1800s, *One Thousand Notable Things*, describes the use of urine to cure scurvy, relieve skin itching, cleanse wounds, and for many other treatments. An eighteenth-century French dentist praised urine as a valuable mouthwash. In England during the 1860s and 1870s, the drinking of one's own urine was a common cure for jaundice. In more modern times, Alaskan Eskimos have used urine as an antiseptic to treat wounds.

The main proponent of Urine Therapy in modern times is Britisher John W. Armstrong, author of *The Water of Life: A Treatise on Urine Therapy*. He was rejected as unfit for military service during World War I due to consumption. Advised to seek the advice of a physician, Armstrong was diagnosed as being more catarrhal than consumptive. Put on a regimen of sunshine, fresh air, and nutritious food, he gained nearly thirty pounds in the ensuing year.

Still unsatisfied with his condition, Armstrong consulted another physician, who diagnosed him as actually consumptive in both lungs. The prescribed diet high in starches and sugars gave him diabetes. This new condition called for yet another regimen more drastic than the previous ones.

Armstrong was allowed a light snack three days a week and only water for the remaining four days. After sixteen weeks his physical condition improved and his cough and catarrhal condition withdrew. In spite of his improvement, his diet also produced many physical and emotional side effects which he considered worse than the disease. Losing faith in doctors, Armstrong set about to effect his own cure.

Feeling week and ill, Armstrong recalled the Bible proverb, "Drink waters out of thine own cistern." This led him to recall the case of a young girl who was successfully treated for diptheria by drinking her own urine and the cases of others who were treated for jaundice by the same means.

Holding to his biblical interpretation of this proverb and other passages, Armstrong decided to pursue his belief, and fasted on his urine and tap water for forty-five days. After breaking the fast, he ate cautiously and continued to drink his urine. This treatment proved to be his deliverance. He gained weight, his energy increased, and his skin was rejuvenated.

In 1918, convinced that this knowledge should be shared with others, Armstrong began to advise others and supervise their fasts. Those suffering from a variety of aliments, including medically diagnosed cases of cancer, Bright's disease, gangrene, and others, were treated with Urine Therapy.

Contrary to the medical opinion that urine contained dead tissue and could not be assimilated by the body as such, Armstrong believed that urine perhaps contained "flesh, blood, and vital tissues in a living solution."

In his book, *The Water of Life: A Treatise on Urine Therapy*, Armstrong details numerous case histories of people suffering with gangrene, various types of cancer, diabetes, consumption, disease of the heart valves, Bright's disease, bladder problems, malaria, fevers, wounds, burns, bronchial asthma, and many other afflictions who were cured with urine-fast therapy. During the fast, urine taken orally helps to rebuild and recondition vital organs, including the intestines. Urine Therapy for virtually every aliment is the same; therefore, no diagnosis is required.

Besides drinking it, urine is used to bathe the skin. The entire body is rubbed with urine several times a day with emphasis on the face, neck, and feet. This is followed by washing the skin with warm tap water. Urine-soaked compresses placed on various parts of the body are also used for treatments. These two procedures are used because urine is absorbed by the skin.

Armstrong believed that a healthy, well-balanced diet was essential in maintaining health and fighting disease. Because man is omnivorous, Armstrong did not recommend a strictly vegetarian diet. He felt that it would not agree with people unless they were raised from birth on such a diet.

He recommended a diet comprised of meat, fish, poultry, eggs, steamed vegetables, salads, fresh seasonal fruits, brown rice, and whole-wheat bread. Butter and honey for sweetening could be used in moderation. All processed and highly refined foods such as white sugar and white bread were to be avoided.

For additional information consult *The Water of Life: A Treatise on Urine Therapy* by John W. Armstrong.

❧ | VISCERAL MANIPULATION | ☙

Visceral Manipulation is a hands-on therapy that utilizes manipulative techniques to encourage normal movement, muscle tone, and inherent tissue motion of the viscera (organs located in the abdominal cavity) and their connective tissues.

It is a well-known fact that tension, caused by stress, can accumulate in skeletal muscles. The idea behind Visceral Manipulation is that in addition to skeletal muscles, the so-called involuntary muscles associated with the visceral organs respond to stress as well.

When these involuntary muscles accumulate tension, deformation of the organ can result. Additionally, the many membranes (connective tissue) that suspend the organs and keep them in place are affected as well. These membranes are responsible for maintaining the visceral cavity in an organized fashion.

If organs become distorted from tension and are pulled off-center (out of normal position) for a long period of time due to chronic tension, the connective membranes can "dry up" and stick together. This prevents the organs from returning to their normal, functional position on their own.

The visceral organs are dependent on their ability to move freely in the visceral cavity to work correctly and efficiently. When they are pulled out of their effective positions, they cease to function properly.

For example, digested food is squeezed through the intestine in a highly coordinated way. If this coordination is disrupted in any way, stagnated pockets of decomposing food can result in the intestine. As the decomposing food lingers in the intestine, it rots, releasing toxins in the body. Thus, restoration of function to the intestine or other organs is very important.

The technique used in Visceral Manipulation is much like the basic CranioSacral Therapy technique, an extension of the cranial unwinding effect. In Visceral Manipulation, practitioners deal with what they believe to be a balanced "pulse" (inherent CranioSacral rhythm) in each organ. The practitioner will try to induce the "out-of-position" organ to come back to "center" (the normal, balanced position).

Workshops in Visceral Manipulation techniques are given by the Upledger Institute. For further information contact the institute.

❧ | VITAMIN THERAPY | ❧

Vitamin Therapy is the use of specific vitamins, minerals, or combinations of the two for a wide variety of therapeutic purposes. Vitamins and minerals can be used for both the prevention and cure of disease and other physical and mental problems.

For therapeutic use, vitamins and minerals are usually taken in quantities greater than the recommended daily allowance (RDA) established by the U.S. government. Taking large quantities of vitamins is sometimes called megavitamin therapy (See Orthomolecular Therapy elsewhere in this book).

Vitamins are a class of organic substances which are essential to human nutrition. Thirteen are currently recognized as such. Although they do not provide energy to the body, vitamins are necessary in minute quantities for the metabolic process to take place.

Throughout history natural foods which contain vitamins and minerals have been used as a therapy to prevent and cure diseases. Hippocrates noted that the symptoms of bleeding gums and hemorrhage, common to scurvy, were found in armies that ate only dried rations for long periods of time.

During the fifteenth and sixteenth centuries Spanish and Portuguese sailors were also ravaged by scurvy due to a lack of fresh foods. In 1747 James Lind, a surgeon in the British navy, treated scurvy patients with different foods and drinks. He found that patients given two oranges and one lemon each day had the most rapid recovery from the disease's symptoms. Although vitamin C was yet to be discovered at that time, it is now known that the vitamin C in citrus fruit prevents scurvy. And this is how the British came to be called "Limeys."

The disease beriberi appeared in the rice-eating areas of the world, such as India, Japan, South China, the Philippine Islands, and the Dutch East Indies, during the nineteenth century, after the introduction of polished rice. This severe and fatal malady is characterized by weakness, gastric irritation, extreme emaciation, and painful nerve degeneration, eventually leading to death.

It was later concluded that something in the rice polishing (the brown coating that covers the rice grain) prevented beriberi. This substance was thiamin, or vitamin B_1.

The malady called rickets is caused by a lack of vitamin D. Rickets was a scourge from medieval times until well into the twentieth century. It produced twisted limbs, curved spines, and swollen joints in its victims.

Pellagra, a disease characterized by scaly skin, diarrhea, and dementia (symptoms similar to schizophrenia) is caused by a lack of vitamin B_3, niacin.

Although some physicians in the past believed that taking vitamins only created expensive urine, that view is changing. As more and more research produces encouraging results, scientists are beginning to believe that traditional medical views have been too restricted. Currently the medical establishment is growing more aware of vitamins' potential therapeutic benefits.

Nobel Prize–winning chemist Linus Pauling stirred the vitamin controversy beginning in the 1970s when he championed the use of vitamin C for a variety of ailments. This increased public awareness of vitamins and their potential therapeutic uses. With the proliferation of health food stores and books on the subject, vitamins became a self-help therapy as the results of more positive research became available.

The use of vitamins and minerals is also a prominent part of the Life Extension movement (see elsewhere in this book) which began in the late 1970s and gained notoriety through the work of Durk Pearson and Sandy Shaw. Life Extension makes extensive use of vitamins and minerals.

Today, there is an ever increasing awareness of vitamins by the general public, as is shown by the cover story of the April 6, 1992, issue of *Time* magazine: "The Real Power of Vitamins." Vitamins, minerals, and nutrient supplements are almost a "subculture" within the health food industry.

New research has shown that vitamins and minerals may help fight cancer, heart disease, and the ravages of aging. Other research and studies have shown that low levels of certain vitamins or minerals in the body are correlated to a specific disease or precondition for a disease.

A recent University of Alabama Medical School study shows that women with low levels of the vitamin folic acid in their blood, after being exposed to the virus that causes cervical cancer, are five times more likely to develop a precancerous lesion. Schizophrenic patients have been successfully treated with a combination of vitamins B_3, C, and B_6.

Studies have shown that the mineral zinc has been successful in reversing night blindness in men. Also, men suffering from enlarged prostate glands experienced an easing of symptoms after taking zinc.

Vitamins and minerals are effective in preventing physical problems. For example, an individual who lives in severe air pollution can mitigate its harmful effects by taking extra vitamin A. And an individual who is subjected to heavy stress on a daily basis needs to replace the pantothenate, a B vitamin, that is rapidly depleted from her body.

In her book *The Way Up from Down*, Priscilla Slagle, M.D., describes how vitamins and minerals can influence moods. Amino acid nutrients along with vitamin supplements can provide a nutritional approach that has decidedly positive effects on depression, low moods, and overall general health.

Research continues into the possible benefits of vitamins and minerals on health and longevity.

Although there are numerous books available, it is recommended that an individual consult a physician, one who understands the therapeutic use of vitamins, before starting any vitamin supplement program. Also, contact the Linus Pauling Institute of Science and Medicine.

❧ | WHEATGRASS DIET | ❧

The Wheatgrass Diet, as it is sometimes called, is not a specialized dietary regimen, but the use of wheatgrass juice as a food, medicine, and an overall tonic for various ailments.

Blades of wheatgrass are actually the tops of young wheat plants which grow to a length of six to nine inches after seven days. The deep green juice squeezed from wheatgrass contains an abundance of natural vitamins, minerals, enzymes, chlorophyll, and vital life energy.

Wheatgrass juice was first used for human health purposes in the 1950s by Ann Wigmore, founder of the Hippocrates Health Institute in Boston. Plagued by personal health problems, Wigmore recalled as a child in Europe how her grandmother had used grasses to heal wounded soldiers during World War I.

Wigmore experimented with different grasses and began feeding them to animals. For a variety of reasons, wheatgrass proved to be the most satisfactory. After seeing how wheatgrass increased her pets' well-being, she sought the opinion of Dr. G. H. Earp-Thomas, an expert in plants and soils who was familiar with grasses and chlorophyll. After a lengthy research into the literature as well as a thorough laboratory analysis, Dr. Earp-Thomas determined that wheatgrass contained many vital nutrients which would be beneficial to human health.

Also, while searching the literature, Dr. Earp-Thomas read scientific papers written by Dr. C. Schnable, whose research supported the use of wheatgrass and other grasses for human and animal nutrition. Schnable determined that it would take 350 pounds of the choicest fresh vegetables to equal the nutritional value of only 15 pounds of wheatgrass.

Armed with this promising information, Wigmore set about to test wheatgrass on herself. She attempted to cure an intestinal problem developed from eating a typical American diet for over twenty years. She began by chewing on and drinking the juice from young wheatgrass plants. Within weeks her physical condition improved, and eventually Wigmore was completely cured. As an added benefit, she began to feel more energetic.

Wigmore believes that a great deal of the disease and degeneration suffered by many people is due to a lack of vital nutrients in the overcooked, highly processed foods most people eat. The use of wheatgrass juice combined with other raw foods can help to counteract these deficiencies and fight illness by stimulating the body's immune system. She is a proponent of "live foods" such as fresh vegetables, fruits, sprouts, nuts, and seeds because they retain the nutrients and enzymes that are either reduced or destroyed by cooking and/or processing.

Wigmore prefers fresh-squeezed wheatgrass juice to the dehydrated or tablet forms. In fact, she recommends drinking or using wheatgrass juice immediately after it is cut and juiced. Fresh-squeezed wheatgrass juice is available at many health food stores, juice bars, and health clubs. Wheatgrass plants, ready for juicing, can be obtained from commercial growers in most major cities in the United States, or an individual can grow the plants easily and inexpensively at home.

The key ingredient in wheatgrass juice is chlorophyll. Some years ago, research on red blood cells by Dr. Hans Fischer and his associates led to a Nobel Prize. In their work they noticed that hemoglobin, the oxygen-carrying component of human red blood cells, and plant chlorophyll were almost identical at the molecular level.

One research project by Dr. A. Zin in the 1930s showed that animals with normal hemoglobin counts, after receiving injections of chlorophyll, had increased numbers of red blood cells. Another study done in England showed that anemic animals given raw chlorophyll regenerated hemoglobin more than 50 percent faster than those not receiving it.

Today, many naturalists believe that wheatgrass and other green sprout juices generate red blood cells. This raises the hemoglobin count, which allows the blood to carry more oxygen to every cell in the body. With more oxygen available, the body is able to function better.

Drinking wheatgrass juice has numerous positive benefits. Laboratory tests have shown that enzymes in wheatgrass juice are an effective blood cleanser. Also, because of the high enzymatic content, wheatgrass juice is a powerful detoxifying agent that helps the body eliminate internal waste such as hardened mucus and decaying fecal matter from the colon. It can also stimulate and regenerate the liver, a main organ of detoxification.

Because wheatgrass juice is a powerful detoxifying agent, it is recommended that an individual start with a one-ounce portion and work up to portions of four ounces or more per serving, as the body becomes conditioned and more purified. It can be diluted with vegetable juice or water.

Wheatgrass juice can also provide long-lasting energy throughout the day compared to beverages high in sugar or stimulants, such as caffeine, which only provide an immediate benefit but quickly fade as the day progresses.

In addition to drinking it, wheatgrass juice has numerous other applications. Used topically, it can help heal cuts, wounds, scrapes, and insect bites, or be used as a skin cleanser and astringent. In bathwater, it stimulates circulation. Wheatgrass juice can be inserted directly into the rectum with a small bulb syringe. Called an "implant," one to two ounces of wheatgrass juice are used as a purge, or retained and absorbed into the body in conjunction with a wheatgrass fast.

In her informative book *The Wheatgrass Book: How to Grow and Use Wheatgrass to Maximize Your Health and Vitality*, Ann Wigmore describes the many uses of wheatgrass juice and how to grow and juice wheatgrass plants. Another good book by Wigmore is *The Hippocrates Diet and Health Plan*. Both are available at many libraries, booksellers, and health food stores. For more information, contact the Ann Wigmore Foundation.

WHOLE FOODS DIET

The Whole Foods Diet is a nutritional plan that utilizes whole, pure, and natural foods to fight disease, maintain good health, and keep the body in proper chemical balance. It is based on the idea that foods contain certain chemicals which, when quantities are either deficient or in excess in the body, can cause physical problems.

The philosophy of the Whole Foods Diet was developed by Dr. Bernard Jensen, a world-renowned nutritionist and author of more than twenty-five books. At the age of eighteen, after graduating high school, Jensen entered the West Coast Chiropractic College. The demands of study combined with outside work to support himself and a less than desirable diet led to his physical collapse shortly after completing his Chiropractic education.

Jensen was diagnosed with an incurable lung disease, often fatal back in the late 1920s before the advent of antibiotics. Fortunately, at that time, he was introduced to a Seventh-Day Adventist physician.

Jensen was told his physical problem stemmed from nutritional deficiencies and the doctor enlightened him as to the importance of a proper diet. In place of the junk food that had become his usual fare, Jensen was placed on a diet of healthful foods combined with breathing exercises. This regimen put Jensen back on the road to health by increasing his energy and filling out his body. Nutrition and exercise cured his lung disease.

Although trained as a chiropractor, Jensen's personal experience with the recuperative powers of a proper diet impelled him to make nutrition a part of his healing methods. Jensen's dietary philosophy, developed over the years, is based on the original work of Hippocrates and V. G. Rocine, as well as on Jensen's own studies.

Hippocrates (460–377 B.C.) laid the foundation for modern medical and nutritional science. Previous to his work, healing relied heavily on superstition and magic.

From his quote "Let food be thy medicine," it seems obvious that Hippocrates knew the healing potential of nutrition. He realized proper nutrition was an integral part of health care and necessary for medical therapy to be effective. In his writings, Hippocrates stressed that a balanced diet and a sensible lifestyle were the way to prevent disease.

Victor G. Rocine was a Norwegian homeopath who had emigrated to the United States. He began to study the work, by a number of European biochemists, on quantitatively measuring the chemical constituents in man's common foods.

Rocine readily assimilated this information and proposed that most human disease, maladies, and mental problems were due to either a deficiency or an excess of certain chemical elements in the body. By expanding on Hippocrates' idea that food could be used as a medicine, Rocine believed that foods could be classified as to their function. Since certain foods affect the body in a particular way, they could be used to help treat a disease.

In the 1930s Jensen attended a lecture given by Victor Rocine, and was so impressed by what he had to say that Jensen became Rocine's student. For the next ten years, in Oakland, California, Chicago, Illinois, and Portland, Oregon, Jensen studied food and nutrition with him. This developed into a long-lasting personal friendship and professional relationship.

Dr. Jensen took what he had learned from the works of Hippocrates, his training with Rocine, and his own nutritional research, then refined it so he could share it with the world.

One of the premises behind food's ability to heal is based on the fact that food is composed of organic compounds, just as human beings are. Chemical elements found in food are obtained from the soil and used for specific purposes in the body. Food alone is able to rebuild tissue damage caused by disease or trauma. This makes nutritional therapy an indispensable tool for accomplishing repairs to the body. No known drug or medical therapy can accomplish this feat.

When an individual consumes fresh, whole, unprocessed plant food grown without pesticides, wild game, or organically fed livestock, he is receiving the purest natural source of these chemical elements without consuming harmful impurities carried through the ecological food chain.

Green plants are at the bottom of the ecological food chain, and the "lower" on the food chain we eat, the better. Recent research has shown that the more whole, fresh, pure, and natural foods we eat the better our chances of maintaining good health and avoiding disease.

Dr. Jensen recommends a diet that is composed of 60 percent vegetables, 20 percent fruits, 10 percent starch, and 10 percent protein. Of these foods consumed, 60 percent should be eaten raw and 40 percent cooked. This creates an 80 percent alkaline to 20 percent acid ratio in the body, which is ideal for nutrition and guards against disease. This corresponds to the ratio in human blood, which contains 80 percent alkaline nutrients and 20 percent acid nutrients. The reason for the high percentage of raw foods is that cooking or processing destroys nutrients and enzymes.

To achieve and maintain optimal health, not only is it necessary to eat the proper foods which provide the necessary nutrients in proper quantities, but it is equally important to avoid harmful ones such as smoked, salted, or fried foods, excessive amounts of sugar, most kinds of vinegar, rancid foods, and others.

The benefits of proper nutrition are twofold. Not only will it help cure disease, but it will also provide an individual with increased energy and vitality combined with an overall higher state of wellness. By eating healthy foods and avoiding those that are harmful, all of the glands, organs, and other body tissues function with increased efficiency.

In his excellent book, *Foods That Heal: A Guide to Understanding and Using the Healing Powers of Natural Foods*, available in bookstores and libraries, Dr. Jensen explains in detail how different health disorders can be treated and healed with specific foods.

Dr. Jensen also conducts a residential program of educational seminars called "Radiant Health" at the Feathered Pipe Ranch near Helena, Montana. An extensive number of books, audio- and videocassette tapes, and nutritional supplements are also available. For additional information contact Bernard Jensen International.

❧ | YOGA | ❧

Yoga is a method or system of physical, mental, and spiritual development. It is the practical application of the ancient Indian Vedic teachings.

The techniques of this art and science of living seek to bring into balance all the separate aspects of an individual. Yoga teaches that a healthy person is a harmoniously integrated unit comprising body, mind, and spirit.

The word *Yoga* means to combine, coordinate, harmonize, integrate, and utilize. It is derived from the Sanskrit root *yuj*, which means "union" or "to join." Yoga has many synonyms in Sanskrit and other languages. Often called "the way, "the path," or "the work," it originally referred to the joining of man's physical, mental, and spiritual elements.

There are different styles and paths of Yoga known by such names as Kriya Yoga, Bhakti Yoga, Karma Yoga, Mantra Yoga, Kundalini Yoga, Hatha Yoga, Raja Yoga, and others. The techniques used for achieving better health are based on Hatha Yoga, which is known as the Yoga of the physical body and physical well-being. The word *hatha* means "force."

It is thought that Yoga originated in India some five thousand to six thousand years ago, although some suggest that it may be older than that. It is unknown who originated Yoga, but around 200 B.C., legend states, a mystery man named Patanjali went into the mountains to meditate, and after he emerged wrote of the system now called Yoga.

Although Patanjali is called the Father of Yoga, little is really known about him. Since ancient times, the doctrines of Yoga had been handed down from master to student. Patanjali was the first to collect this knowledge from other yogis. He aligned the information with his own experience and restated it as definite principles and precise techniques in a work titled *Aphorism on Yoga*.

Hatha Yoga is devoted to the thorough care of the human body and all of its functions. Its primary aim is to remove the sources of ill health before they can cause dysfunction. It is believed that insufficient oxygenation, poor diet and nutrition, inadequate exercise, and poor elimination of waste products are the causes of disease.

In Yoga, the goal of good health is accomplished through a combination of techniques including exercises called *asanas* or postures, controlled breathing, relaxation, meditation, and diet and nutrition.

The Yoga postures or asanas are designed to stretch and activate every muscle in the body. Additionally, performing deep breathing techniques while in these postures tends to balance the functions of the entire body, including involuntary functions such as circulation, respiration, digestion, metabolism, and elimination, as well as the glands, organs, and nervous system.

Breathing techniques are of paramount importance to Yoga. Without them Yoga is just another type of physical fitness. These special breathing techniques allow a Yoga practitioner to control not only the body but the mind as well. Controlled breathing can provide relief from tension and negative emotions like anger, impatience, and nervousness. This leads to relaxation, improved concentration, and increased oxygenation of the blood.

Although Yoga is not meant to cure specific diseases or ailments directly, it has been found effective in treating many physical problems. Yoga achieves good health by removing the impurities that obstruct the body's normal functioning, thereby helping the body cure itself.

The practice of Yoga normally is not started before the age of six or after the age of sixty-five, although some individuals starting after the age of sixty-five have found it to be effective. Once the Yoga postures are learned, they can be used throughout an individual's lifetime.

There are numerous how-to books available in bookstores, health food stores, and libraries that teach the various Yoga postures. Since Yoga has been practiced for such a long time, there are many teachers and classes available in many areas. For additional information contact the American Yoga Association or the International Association of Yoga Therapists.

❧ | ZERO BALANCING | ☙

Zero Balancing is a specific and powerful way to align body energy with body structure. Western science has shown that energy and matter are fundamentally coupled. Zero Balancing (ZB) is born out of this perception with roots in Eastern as well as Western concepts of energy, body function, and body structure. Zero Balancing is a unique approach in that it aims primarily at the energetic and structural function of the skeletal system, which often results in the holistic integration of the client.

Zero Balancing was developed by Dr. Fritz Frederick Smith, an osteopathic M.D. born into the manipulative healing arts tradition. His father, at the age of ninety-three, was recognized as the oldest practicing chiropractor in America. Fritz Smith received his doctor of osteopathy degree in 1955 and his doctor of medicine degree in 1961. Later, while engaged in a personal and clinical pursuit of a deeper understanding of illness and health, Dr. Smith became a certified Rolfer, licensed acupuncturist, and a Fellow in the Chinese College of Acupuncture.

In 1975 Zero Balancing coalesced as a system while Dr. Smith was completing his "project of excellence" during his bachelor and master of Acupuncture studies with J. R. Worsley at the Chinese College of Acupuncture in England.

Through the use of touch, Zero Balancing works to create clearer energy fields in the body and expand states of consciousness. It also balances the interface between energy movement and physical functioning with special attention to the body's deepest layer—the skeletal system.

The interface of energy and structure is beneath our level of awareness. When imbalances occur at this level, the body tends to compensate around them rather than resolve them directly. Experience has shown that these imbalances have a direct effect on the physical, mental, emotional, and spiritual health of an individual, but can be altered through the touch of Zero Balancing.

Using her hands, the Zero Balancing practitioner applies gentle vectors of force to the client's body in a pressing, stretching, or bending manner to create "fulcrums," defined by the *American Heritage Dictionary* as "a position, element, or agency through, around, or by means of which vital powers are exercised." The practitioner heightens and follows the client's response to the fulcrums using finely cultivated skills of observing the working energy signs such as eyelid movements, facial expressions, changing breath patterns, and levels of vitality. A Zero Balancing session generally takes thirty minutes and is typically done through clothing.

The impact of studying and learning Zero Balancing will depend on a person's experience. For the clinician with little or no training in hands-on bodywork, Zero Balancing presents an integrated approach to dealing with the body. For the acupuncturist, it offers ways of opening structural blocks which may impede Acupuncture therapy. For the physical therapist, massage therapist, or any person doing body-oriented work, it opens new possibilities of balancing energy through hands-on touch. For the psychologically oriented therapist, it shows how to directly engage and work with personal history, early conditioning, and expanded states of consciousness through touch.

At this writing, Zero Balancing is taught nationally and internationally in seminars designed for licensed health care professionals by twenty-one certified Zero Balancing teachers. The core Zero Balancing program is taught in two thirty-hour segments (ZB I and ZB II), usually separated by four to six months. The intent of ZB I is to give the student a fundamental working knowledge of Zero Balancing, while ZB II is for the student to embody the work and make it an expression of his or her creativity. Students may enter a specific training program which generally takes one and a half to two years and leads to the in-house recognition as a certified zero balancer.

Many of the principles and perspectives within Zero Balancing are described in Dr. Smith's widely available book, *Inner Bridges, a Guide to Energy Movement and Body Structure*, which is a classic in the body energy field. For additional information on Zero Balancing or to order Dr. Smith's book, contact the Zero Balancing Association.

⌗ ⌗ ⌗

Appendix: Illnesses and Therapies

This section has been designed as a guide to matching one hundred diseases/ailments/maladies/illnesses/afflictions with the most applicable alternative therapies described in this book. For each disease, etc., we listed five therapies below it. These five therapies are listed in alphabetical order, so as not to give any one therapy more importance than the others.

Creating this guide was not an easy endeavor, since, for any one disease, etc., there are numerous therapies that could be considered appropriate. We relied on twenty years of experience in the field of Alternative Medicine, and all of the research material compiled for writing this book, to choose five therapies we consider most suitable. But we want to stress that they may not be the *only* effective treatments for that particular disease, etc. Indeed, they are general listings and you may find that any number of therapies are quite effective depending on your body type, predilections, personality, and many other individual variables.

You will note that Acupuncture, Homeopathy, Ayurveda, and Naturopathic Medicine do not appear as one of the therapies/treatments in any of the listings. They are not included because each of these therapies is a complete system of medical treatment and should always be considered when contemplating the use of alternative treatments.

Finally, no matter what therapy you find interesting, it is extremely important to consult a licensed practitioner before embarking on any alternative treatment program.

AIDS (ACQUIRED IMMUNE DEFICIENCY SYNDROME)

Exercise Therapy
Gerson Therapy
Imagery and Visualization
Oxidation Therapy
Wheatgrass Diet

ALLERGIES

Aromatherapy
Environmental Medicine
Herbal Medicine
Mucusless Diet
Vitamin Therapy

ALZHEIMER'S DISEASE

Chelation Therapy
Environmental Medicine
Imagery and Visualization
Life Extension
Vitamin Therapy

ANGINA

Chelation Therapy
Oxidative Therapy
Pritikin Diet
Touch for Health
Vitamin Therapy

ANOREXIA NERVOSA

Autogenic Training

Biofeedback Training
Hypnotherapy
SHEN Therapy
Vitamin Therapy

ARTHRITIS

Dong Diet
Herbal Medicine
Jin Shin Jyutsu
No-Nightshade Diet
Vitamin Therapy

ASTHMA

Manual Lymphatic Drainage
Mucusless Diet
Reflexology
Schuessler Cell Salts
Vitamin Therapy

ATHLETE'S FOOT

DMSO Therapy
Environmental Medicine
Herbal Medicine
Hydrotherapy
Natural Hygiene

AUTISM

Colon Therapy
Color and Sound Therapy
CranioSacral Therapy
Vitamin Therapy
Whole Foods Diet

🐾 BACK PAIN

Egoscue Method
Shiatsu
St. John's Neuromuscular Therapy
Trigger Point Therapy
Yoga

🐾 BAD BREATH

Colon Therapy
Environmental Medicine
Herbal Medicine
Natural Hygiene
Wheatgrass Diet

🐾 BACTERIAL INFECTION

Gerson Therapy
Herbal Medicine
Natural Hygiene
Ozone Therapy
Vitamin Therapy

🐾 BED-WETTING

Amino Acid Therapy
Biofeedback Training
Environmental Medicine
Reflexology
Vitamin Therapy

🐾 BENIGN PROSTATIC HYPERTROPHY

Chi Kung
Herbal Medicine

Imagery and Visualization
Reflexology
Vitamin Therapy

🐾 BODY ODOR

Colon Therapy
Manual Lymphatic Drainage
Natural Hygiene
Schuessler Cell Salts
Vitamin Therapy

🐾 BOILS

Fasting
Manual Lymphatic Drainage
Natural Hygiene
Wheatgrass Diet
Whole Foods Diet

🐾 BRUISE

Amino Acid Therapy
Chi Kung
Chi Nei Tsang
Schuessler Cell Salts
Vitamin Therapy

🐾 BRONCHITIS

Aromatherapy
Herbal Medicine
Manual Lymphatic Drainage
Mucusless Diet
Vitamin Therapy

✎ BUNIONS

Herbal Medicine
Hydrotherapy
Osteopathy
Reflexology
Structural Integration

✎ BURSITIS

Physical Therapy
St. John's Neuromuscular Therapy
Structural Integration
Therapeutic Touch
Trigger Point Therapy

✎ CANCER

Anticancer Diet
Imagery and Visualization
Livingston Treatment
Macrobiotics
Wheatgrass Diet

✎ CANDIDIASIS

Herbal Medicine
Mucusless Diet
Natural Hygiene
Oxidation Therapy
Vitamin Therapy

✎ CATARACTS

Amino Acid Therapy
Herbal Medicine
Life Extension

Vitamin Therapy
Whole Foods Diet

✎ CARPAL TUNNEL SYNDROME

Aston-Patterning
Chiropractic
Myofascial Release Therapy
St. John's Neuromuscular Therapy
Vitamin Therapy

✎ CANKER SORES

Cayce (Edgar) Therapies
Herbal Medicine
Natural Hygiene
Vitamin Therapy
Wheatgrass Diet

✎ CAVITIES (DENTAL)

Ozone Therapy
Natural Hygiene
Vitamin Therapy
Wheatgrass Diet
Whole Foods Diet

✎ CELLULITE

Deep Tissue Sculpting
Exercise Therapy
Macrobiotics
Manual Lymphatic Drainage
Swedish Massage

❧ CEREBRAL PALSY

Biofeedback Training
CranioSacral Therapy
Environmental Medicine
Feldenkrais Method
Reflexology

❧ CHEMICAL POISONING

Chelation Therapy
Colon Therapy
Environmental Medicine
Fasting
Herbal Medicine

❧ CIRRHOSIS

Fasting
Imagery and Visualization
Live Cell Therapy
Orthomolecular Therapy
Oxidative Therapy

❧ CHICKEN POX

Herbal Medicine
Hydrotherapy
Imagery and Visualization
Natural Hygiene
Vitamin Therapy

❧ CHRONIC FATIGUE SYNDROME

Colon Therapy
Herbal Medicine

Manual Lymphatic Drainage
Schuessler Cell Salts
Vitamin Therapy

❧ CHRONIC PAIN

Hellerwork
Imagery and Visualization
Touch for Health
Trager Approach
Trigger Point Therapy

❧ COLDS AND FLU

Fasting
Fit for Life Program
Herbal Medicine
Mucusless Diet
Vitamin Therapy

❧ COLIC

Herbal Medicine
Infant Massage
Jin Shin Jyutsu
Mucusless Diet
Therapeutic Touch

❧ COLON DISORDERS

Colon Therapy
Environmental Medicine
Herbal Medicine
Visceral Manipulation
Wheatgrass Diet

CYSTITIS

Fasting
Herbal Medicine
Orthomolecular Therapy
Oxidative Therapy
Schuessler Cell Salts

DEPRESSION

Bach Flower Remedies
Exercise Therapy
Herbal Medicine
Meditation
Orthomolecular Therapy

DIABETES MELLITUS

Autogenic Training
Gerson Therapy
Herbal Medicine
Orthomolecular Therapy
Whole Foods Diet

DIZZINESS AND VERTIGO

Acupressure Massage
Environmental Medicine
Herbal Medicine
Vitamin Therapy
Whole Foods Diet

DRUG ADDICTION

Aromatherapy
Drama Therapy
Hypnotherapy

SHEN Therapy
Transcendental Meditation

EAR INFECTION

Environmental Medicine
Herbal Medicine
Mucusless Diet
Orthomolecular Therapy
Oxidative Therapy

EATING DISORDERS

Drama Therapy
Meditation
Past Lives Therapy
Rebirthing
SHEN Therapy

EMOTIONAL DISORDERS

Amino Acid Therapy
Bach Flower Remedies
Dream Therapy
Hakomi Method of Body Mind
    Therapy
Orthomolecular Therapy

EMPHYSEMA

Aromatherapy
Live Cell Therapy
Orthomolecular Therapy
Pranic Healing
Wheatgrass Diet

EPILEPSY

Amino Acid Therapy
CranioSacral Therapy
Live Cell Therapy
Orthomolecular Therapy
Pranic Healing

FIBROCYSTIC BREAST DISEASE

Herbal Medicine
Macrobiotics
Manual Lymphatic Drainage
Swedish Massage
Vitamin Therapy

FIBROMYALGIA

Biofeedback Training
Deep Tissue Massage
Herbal Medicine
Orthomolecular Therapy
Structural Integration

FLATULENCE

Colon Therapy
Herbal Medicine
Natural Hygiene
Schuessler Cell Salts
Wheatgrass Diet

FUNGUS

DMSO Therapy
Environmental Medicine
Herbal Medicine

Natural Hygiene
Oxidative Therapy

GALLBLADDER DISORDERS

Colon Therapy
Fasting
Herbal Medicine
Live Cell Therapy
Visceral Manipulation

GASTROINTESTINAL DISORDERS

Acupressure Massage
Fit for Life Program
Herbal Medicine
Macrobiotics
Transcendental Meditation

GOUT

DMSO Therapy
Jin Shin Jyutsu
Orthomolecular Therapy
Oxidative Therapy
Wheatgrass Diet

GYNECOLOGICAL DISORDERS

Exercise Therapy
Herbal Medicine
Vitamin Therapy
Whole Foods Diet
Yoga

☙ HEADACHE

Biofeedback Training
CranioSacral Therapy
Feldenkrais Method
Hypnotherapy
Trigger Point Therapy

☙ HEART DISEASE

Chelation Therapy
Chi Kung
Jazzercise
Mucusless Diet
Pritikin Diet/Exercise

☙ HEAVY METAL TOXICITY

Chelation Therapy
Colon Therapy
Environmental Medicine
Manual Lymphatic Drainage
Wheatgrass Diet

☙ HEMORRHOIDS

Colon Therapy
Fit for Life Program
Herbal Medicine
Hydrotherapy
Whole Foods Diet

☙ HEPATITIS

Gerson Therapy
Herbal Medicine
Live Cell Therapy

Oxidative Therapy
Vitamin Therapy

☙ HERPES

Amino Acid Therapy
Herbal Medicine
Natural Hygiene
Oxidative Therapy
Vitamin Therapy

☙ HIGH BLOOD PRESSURE

Chi Kung
Exercise Therapy
Meditation
Pritikin Diet
Vitamin Therapy

☙ HIATAL HERNIA

Acupressure Massage
Polarity Therapy
Pranic Healing
Touch for Health
Visceral Manipulation

☙ HIVES

Environmental Medicine
Fit for Life Program
Natural Hygiene
Orthomolecular Medicine
Schuessler Cell Salts

☙ HYPERACTIVITY

Biofeedback Training
Fit for Life Program
Herbal Medicine
Transcendental Meditation
Vitamin Therapy

☙ IMPOTENCE

Biofeedback Training
Exercise Therapy
Herbal Medicine
Hypnotherapy
Subliminal Therapy

☙ INSOMNIA

Herbal Medicine
Hypnotherapy
Subliminal Therapy
Transcendental Meditation
Vitamin Therapy

☙ IRRITABLE BOWEL SYNDROME

Colon Therapy
Fit for Life Program
Herbal Medicine
Meditation
Oxidative Therapy

☙ KIDNEY STONES

Fasting
Herbal Medicine
Macrobiotics

Natural Hygiene
Schuessler Cell Salts

☙ LONGEVITY

Colon Therapy
Exercise Therapy/Jazzercise
Life Extension
Vitamin Therapy
Whole Foods Diet

☙ LOW-BACK PAIN

Chiropractic
Egoscue Method
Rolfing
St. John's Neuromuscular Therapy
Thai Massage

☙ LUPUS

Environmental Medicine
Gerson Therapy
Herbal Medicine
Livingston Treatment
Natural Hygiene

☙ MACULAR DEGENERATION

Herbal Medicine
Imagery and Visualization
Orthomolecular Therapy
Oxidative Therapy
Whole Foods Diet

❧ MENOPAUSE

Exercise Therapy
Geriatric Massage
Herbal Medicine
Imagery and Visualization
Vitamin Therapy

❧ MENSTRUAL CRAMPS

Exercise Therapy
Herbal Medicine
Meditation
Visceral Manipulation
Vitamin Therapy

❧ MENTAL HEALTH

Bach Flower Remedies
Hakomi Method of Body Mind
Therapy
Hellerwork
Orthomolecular Therapy
SHEN Therapy

❧ MONONUCLEOSIS

Fit for Life Program
Imagery and Visualization
Manual Lymphatic Drainage
Orthomolecular Therapy
Oxidative Therapy

❧ MULTIPLE SCLEROSIS

Herbal Medicine
Livingston Treatment
Movement Therapy

Mucusless Diet
Vitamin Therapy

❧ NECK PAIN

Chiropractic
Lomilomi Massage
LooyenWork
Structural Integration
Trigger Point Therapy

❧ OSTEOPOROSIS

Arthritis Diet
Exercise Therapy
Herbal Medicine
Life Extension
Orthomolecular Therapy

❧ OVARIAN CYST

Acupressure Massage
Chi Nei Tsang
Herbal Medicine
Jin Shin Jyutsu
Visceral Manipulation

❧ PANCREATITIS

Gerson Therapy
Herbal Medicine
Live Cell Therapy
Livingston Treatment
Oxidative Therapy

🐌 PARALYSIS AND STROKE

Chi Kung
Feldenkrais Method
Geriatric Massage
Movement Therapy
Physical Therapy

🐌 POLIO AND POST POLIO SYNDROME

Benjamin System of Muscular Therapy
Callanetics
CranioSacral Therapy
Feldenkrais Method
Imagery and Visualization

🐌 PREMENSTRUAL SYNDROME (PMS)

Acupressure Massage
Exercise Therapy
Herbal Medicine
Transcendental Meditation
Vitamin Therapy

🐌 PROSTATE DISORDERS

Burton Treatment
Gerson Therapy
Herbal Medicine
Oxidative Therapy
Vitamin Therapy

🐌 RAYNAUD'S DISEASE

Autogenic Training
Biofeedback Training
Chi Kung
Gerson Therapy
Hydrotherapy

🐌 REPETITIVE MOTION DISORDER

Alexander Technique
Deep Tissue Massage
Feldenkrais Method
Movement Therapy
St. John's Neuromuscular Therapy

🐌 SCIATICA

Rolfing
Shiatsu
St. John's Neuromuscular Therapy
Trager Approach
Trigger Point Therapy

🐌 SLEEP APNEA

Biofeedback Training
Color Therapy
Exercise Therapy
Hypnotherapy
Meditation

🐌 SKIN DISORDERS

Environmental Medicine
Hydrotherapy
Mucusless Diet

Oxidative Therapy
Schuessler Cell Salts

SPORTS INJURIES

Deep Tissue Massage
PNF Stretching
Sports Massage
Swedish Massage
Yoga

STRESS

Dance Therapy
Reflexology
Swedish Massage
Transcendental Meditation
Yoga

SURGERY (RECOVERING FROM)

Acupressure Massage
Chi Kung
Imagery and Visualization
Physical Therapy
Vitamin Therapy

TENDONITIS

Acupressure Massage
Aston-Patterning
Cross-Fiber Friction Massage
Deep Tissue Massage
Structural Integration

TINNITUS

Acupressure Massage
Herbal Medicine
Mucusless Diet
Orthomolecular Therapy
Reflexology

ULCERS

Chi Kung
Herbal Medicine
Meditation
Rice Diet
Wheatgrass Diet

URINARY TRACT INFECTIONS

Acupressure Massage
Herbal Medicine
Oxidative Therapy
Touch for Health
Wheatgrass Diet

VARICOSE VEINS

Herbal Medicine
Hydrotherapy
Jin Shin Jyutsu
Manual Lymphatic Drainage
Vitamin Therapy

VISION DISORDERS

Bates Method of Vision Training
Color Therapy
Eye-Robics

Herbal Medicine
Vitamin Therapy

☙ WARTS

Cryotherapy
Environmental Medicine
Herbal Medicine
Homeopathy
Natural Hygiene

☙ WEIGHT DISORDER (OBESITY)

Exercise Therapy
Fasting
Jazzercise
Meditation
SHEN Therapy

❈ ❈ ❈

Glossary

acid: a class of chemical substances that lower pH when added to aqueous solutions. They are characterized by a sour taste.

acute: a disease or malady having a short duration; usually severe in nature.

adrenaline: the name of a chemical produced by the adrenal glands, also called *epinephrine*. A potent stimulator of the sympathetic nervous system, it increases blood pressure, heart rate, and metabolic activities.

aerobic exercise: continuous body movement used to improve the body's ability to deliver and utilize oxygen quickly and efficiently by strengthening the cardiovascular system (heart and lungs).

aerobic: in the presence of oxygen, or requiring oxygen for respiration.

alkali: the residue obtained from the ashes of plant material, usually a sodium or potassium salt.

allergen: a substance capable of producing an immediate allergic reaction.

allergy: a state of hypersensitivity in the body induced by exposure to a particular allergen (antigen).

allopathic: of or pertaining to allopathy.

allopathy: a philosophy of therapeutics in which diseases are treated by producing a condition which is incompatible with or antagonistic to the condition being cured. Opposite of homeopathy.

alpha state: a brain-wave state produced when relaxed, such as when taking a short nap, spending quiet time in nature, or listening to music.

anaerobic: pertaining to or caused by the absence of oxygen.

anatripsis: therapeutic rubbing or friction massage.

anatriptic: of or pertaining to anatripsis.

antibiotic: a chemical substance produced by a microorganism which has the capacity to kill or inhibit the growth of other microorganisms.

antigen: a substance which is capable, under appropriate conditions, of inducing a specific allergic response.

aromatic plant: a plant having a spicy odor.

arteriosclerosis: sclerosis and thickening of the walls of smaller arteries (arterioles).

arthritis: rheumatism in which the inflammatory lesions are confined to the joints; marked by heat, pain, redness, and swelling.

atherosclerosis: a form of arteriosclerosis in which plaque is deposited within the medium and large arteries.

autism: absorption with inner thoughts such as daydreams, fantasies, etc.

autoimmune disease: a disease caused by an immune response directed against its own antigens, such as rheumatoid arthritis.

autointoxication: intoxication by some poison generated within the body.

autonomic nervous system: the portion of the nervous system connected with activity of the cardiac muscle, smooth muscle, and glands.

autonomic: self-controlling, functionally independent.

autosuggestion: the process by which a person induces in himself an uncritical acceptance of ideas, beliefs, or opinions.

Avicenna: (A.D. 979–1037) the greatest of Arab physicians, he systematically compiled all Greco-Arabic medicine. His *Canon*, one of the most famous medical texts ever written, was the standard in Europe throughout the seventeenth century.

balance: a state of homeostasis.

biochemical: the chemical reactions taking place in living organisms.

biologicals: materials of organic origin which are found in the body and used for medicinal purposes.

biomechanic: the application of mechanical laws to living structures.

birth trauma: in some psychiatric theories, the psychic shock produced in an infant by the experience of being born.

body/mind relationship: that which pertains to the physical and emotional connection in the human body.

body/mind/spirit: a term commonly used in alternative therapies to describe the whole or complete person, which encompasses his or her physical, emotional, and spiritual aspects.

bodywork: a term which generally encompasses a wide variety of hands-on manipulative therapies, sometimes used synonymously with massage therapy.

brain waves: measurable electrical impulses given off by brain tissue. Brain-wave states include beta waves, alpha waves, theta waves, and delta waves. The most alert or active state is represented by beta waves; the hierarchy progresses downward to delta waves, which represent deep sleep or the very deepest meditative states.

Bright's disease: a kidney disease marked by mucus or pus and albumin in the urine and pain in the kidneys.

Buddhism: an ancient Eastern religion growing from the teachings of Guatama Buddha.

bursitis: inflammation of the bursa (a sac or saclike cavity filled with fluid, surrounding all ball-and-socket joints), which prevents abnormal friction.

carbon dioxide: a colorless, odorless gas formed in the tissue from the oxidation of carbon during metabolism.

carcinogen: a cancer-producing substance.

carcinogenesis: producing a malignant growth of tissue (carcinoma).

cardiovascular system: the heart and blood vessels which pump blood throughout the body.

cardiovascular: referring to the heart and blood vessels in the body.

catalysis: the causing or accelerating of a chemical reaction by the addition of a substance which is not permanently affected by the reaction itself.

catalyst: a substance which causes catalysis.

cerebrospinal fluid: a fluid that is pumped throughout the brain and spine which nourishes nerve cells with a fresh supply of nutrients to keep them healthy, similar to the way muscles receive nutrients via the blood.

chi: vital life energy which the Chinese believe flows through acupuncture meridians. Also known as *qi* in the *Pinyin* spelling system and as *prana* in Ayurvedic medicine.

chronic: a disease or malady persisting over a long period of time.

clinical: pertaining to or founded on actual observations and treatments of patients as distinguished from theoretical or basic sciences.

collagen: a protein substance found in the collagenous fibers of skin, tendon, bone, cartilage, and all other connective tissue.

congenital: referring to conditions present at birth regardless of cause.

conscious mind: part of the mind that is constantly within awareness.

conventional medicine: also known as Western allopathic medicine.

cranial bones: the bones that constitute the cranial portion of the skull, including the occipital, sphenoid, temporal, parietal, frontal, ethmoid, lacrimal, and nasal bones; in contrast to the facial bones such as the jaw.

cranial dural membrane: or dura mater, is the outermost and toughest of the three membranes covering the brain.

dermatitis: inflammation of the skin caused by a variety of reasons.

detoxification: a process within the body which reduces the toxic properties of a substance through chemical changes rendering it less poisonous or more readily eliminated from the body.

detoxify: to remove the toxic quality of a substance.

diagnosis: the art of distinguishing one disease from another. The determination of the nature of a disease.

diaphragm: the main muscle involved in the breathing process; it is located between the chest and abdominal cavities.

eczema: an inflammatory disease of the skin attended with itching and the exudation of serous matter.

edema: swelling. The presence of large amounts of fluid within body tissue.

electroneuromyography: an electrical test procedure used to study and evaluate the condition of nerves and muscles.

endorphins: any of three opiate-like substances produced in the brain whose function appears to be mediation of pain in the body. Endorphins have been found to be nearly one thousand times stronger than morphine.

enema: the injection of a liquid into the rectum.

enzyme: a protein molecule that catalyzes chemical reactions of other substances without itself being destroyed or altered at the completion of the reaction.

etheric body: also known as the *aura,* it is the energy field that surrounds and penetrates the physical body.

etheric: of or pertaining to the etheric body.

fascia: densely woven connective tissue that lines and covers nearly every muscle, bone, nerve, artery, and vein, as well as all of the internal organs, including the heart, lungs, brain, and spinal cord.

fecal: pertaining to or of the nature of feces.

feces: the excrement discharged from the intestines and consisting of bacteria cells from the intestines, secretions from the liver, and a scant amount of food residue.

Galen: (c. A.D. 129–200) Greek physician, teacher, and author of more than 500 books on philosophy, philology, and medicine. He compiled and systematized Greco-Roman medicine, physiology, and anatomy; 183 medical books survive today.

geriatric: pertaining to the treatment of the aged.

gland: an aggregation of specialized cells which secrete or excrete materials not related to their ordinary metabolic needs.

harmony: a condition pertaining to a state of well-being and peace of mind.

Hippocrates: (460–377 B.C.) Greek physician commonly known as the "Father of Medicine," he was a student and teacher of the medical school at Cos and laid the foundation for modern medical and nutritional science. Previous to his work, healing relied heavily on superstition and magic.

histamine: a chemical compound found in all body tissues, with the highest concentration in the lungs. It plays a major role in allergic reactions.

holistic: that which pertains to the whole body or body/mind/spirit.

homeostasis: a state of balance or equilibrium in which the organs, glands, and all other interdependent body systems are working together in harmony.

immune system: a complete system of cellular and molecular components, the primary functions of which are distinguishing self from not self, and defense against foreign organisms or substances.

inflammation: a localized, protective response caused by injury or tissue destruction which serves to destroy, dilute, or wall off both the injurious agent and the injured tissue. It is normally characterized by pain, heat, redness, swelling, and loss of function.

inorganic: pertaining to substances not organic in origin.

intuitive: inner knowing or feeling pertaining to a specific situation and how to deal with it.

involuntary: performed independently of the will.

ischemia: a deficiency of blood in a part of the body due to functional constriction or actual obstruction of a blood vessel. Localized tissue anemia due to obstruction of the inflow of arterial blood.

kinesiology: the study of motion of the human body. The body of knowledge regarding human motion.

kyphosis: abnormal increased backward convex curvature of the thoracic spine.

lactic acid: the waste produced by glycogenesis (production of sugar) which provides energy in skeletal muscle during heavy exercise.

ligament: a band of fibrous tissue that connects bones or cartilage, serving to support and strengthen joints.

lordosis: the anterior concavity in the curvature of the lumbar and cervical spine as viewed from the side. An abnormally increased curvature sometimes called "swayback" or "hollow back."

lumbago: pain in the lumbar region of the spine.

meridians: in acupuncture theory, the energy channels that run throughout the body.

metabolic waste: waste products produced during normal metabolism.

metabolism: the transformation in which energy is made available for the use of the organism. The sum of all the physical and chemical processes by which living, organized substance is produced and maintained.

migraine: an intense pain specific to one side of the head, often accompanied by nausea, vomiting, constipation, diarrhea, and sensitivity to light.

mind/body relationship: that which pertains to the physical and emotional connection in the human body.

modality: a method of application of, or the employment of, any therapeutic agent, limited usually to physical agents.

mucus: the free slime of the mucous membranes, composed of secretions of the glands along with various other substances.

multiple sclerosis: a neurological disease characterized by speech disturbances, muscular incoordination, weakness, and nystagmus, and caused by sclerotic patches in the brain and spinal cord.

muscular dystrophy: a disease that produces a progressive muscular deterioration and wasting.

muscular tension: prolonged contraction of a muscle usually due to stress or trauma.

musculoskeletal: pertaining to or comprising the skeleton and muscles, such as the musculoskeletal system.

myofibrositis: inflammation of the connective tissue demarcating a fascicle (a small bundle or cluster) of skeletal muscle fibers.

natural healing: that which pertains to healing without drugs or surgery.

neoplasm: any new or abnormal growth, specifically one which is uncontrolled and progressive.

neuritis: inflammation of a nerve, a condition attended by pain and tenderness over the nerves.

neuromuscular: relating to the nervous and muscular systems.

noninvasive: that which does not cause harm to the body.

nurturing: a state of caring.

organic: pertaining to or derived from living plant or animal tissue.

osteoporosis: reduction in the amount of bone mass leading to fractures after minimal trauma.

palpate: examine medically by touch for the purposes of diagnosing.

Paracelsus: (1493–1541) Swiss physician and alchemist known as the "Luther of Medicine." He defied the authority of Galen and Avicenna and condemned all medical teachings not based on experience.

pharmaceutical grade: a substance with the appropriate purity and quality to make it suitable for use as a drug.

physiological; dealing with the functioning of living beings.

postpartum: the period following childbirth.

prana: the universal vital life energy force that is found in the sun, the air, and the earth that keeps the body alive and healthy. It is also known as *chi* or *qi*, and "breath of life" in the Old Testament.

proprioceptor: neurological receptive mechanisms (sensory receptors) located throughout the body. Although found primarily in the soft tissue, they are also located in and around the joints.

psoriasis: a chronic skin disease characterized by scaly patches.

psychiatrist: a medical doctor that specializes in treating mental and emotional disorders.

psychological: pertaining to, dealing with, or affecting the mind and behavior.

psychologist: a practitioner that deals with psychological disorders.

psychosis: a mental disorder characterized by gross impairment in contact with reality.

pulmonary: pertaining to the lungs.

qi: *see* chi or prana.

rheumatism: any of a variety of disorders marked by inflammation or degeneration of the connective tissue structures of the body, especially the joints and related structures, including muscles, bursas, tendons, and fibrous tissue. It is attended by pain, stiffness, or limitation of motion.

rheumatoid arthritis: a chronic systemic disease primarily of the joints, marked by inflammatory changes in the synovial membranes and joints, and by atrophy rarefaction (loss of density and weight, but not size).

sacrum: the triangle of bone just below the lumbar vertebrae, formed usually by five fused sacral vertebrae.

Sanskrit: the religious and literary language or poetry of ancient India.

sciatica: a syndrome characterized by pain radiating from the back into the buttocks and into the lower extremities.

scleroderma: chronic hardening and thickening of the skin, which may be a finding in several different diseases. It can occur in localized form or as a systemic disease.

scoliosis: appreciable lateral deviation in the normal straight vertical line of the spine. Lateral curvature of the spine.

sinusitis: inflammation of the sinus; may be acute or chronic.

soft tissue: normally refers to muscle and connective tissue.

soma: taken from the Greek, *soma* has been used since the eighth century B.C. to mean "living body." A human being may be viewed in two ways: from the outside and from the inside. In conventional medicine or physiology, the person is seen from the outside, a third-person view, as a "body" with a certain size and shape. But when an individual looks at himself or herself from the inside, a first-person view, he or she is aware of internal feelings, movements, and intentions. This is a "soma."

somatic: pertaining to soma.

spasm: a sudden, violent, involuntary contraction of a muscle or group of muscles attended by pain and interference with function.

spiritual: pertaining to spirit or man's connection with his creation.

structural: a mechanical view of the body.

subconscious mind: part of the mind that stores thoughts, events, opinions, dogmas, etc., and is one with the infinite intelligence of the universe.

synthetic: a substance produced by chemical reaction in a laboratory, as opposed to the same substance made in nature, or natural in origin.

Taoism: an ancient religion of China.

temporomandibular joint syndrome: abnormal pathology in the temporomandibular joint characterized by misalignment of the upper and lower jaws, "clicking" of the jaw, jaw pain, and headache.

tendon: a fibrous cord of connective tissue in which the fibers of a muscle end and by which the muscle is attached to a bone or other structure.

tendonitis: or tendinitis, is inflammation of the tendons and tendon-muscle attachments.

TMJ syndrome: *see* temporomandibular joint syndrome.

toxin: a poison, frequently used to refer to a protein produced by some higher plants, certain animals, and pathogenic bacteria which is highly toxic for other living organisms.

trance: hypnotic state of being.

trauma: a wound or injury, whether physical or psychic.

traumatic: pertaining to, occurring as the result of, or causing trauma.

tumor: a new growth of tissue in which the multiplication of cells is uncontrolled and progressive; also called a neoplasm.

unconscious mind: *see* subconscious mind.

vascular: pertaining to blood vessels or indicative of a copious blood supply.

vertebrae: any of the 33 bones of the spinal column comprising 7 cervical, 12 thoracic, 5 lumbar, 5 sacral, and 4 coccygeal.

vital life energy: also known as *chi*, *qi*, or *prana*: it is that which defines life.

voluntary: accomplished in accordance with the will, e.g., moving of the arm.

☒ ☒ ☒

Appellations

The following list of appellations is representative of those found in the field of Alternative Healing, though these are not the only ones being used. It is recommended that caveat emptor, "let the buyer beware," be employed before choosing a health care practitioner. Although practitioners may be "certified," "registered," etc., it is prudent to learn which educational institution, professional organization, licensing bureau, or government agency has granted the title, and what is required of the practitioner to receive and use the title.

A.T.R.—*Art Therapist Registered*
C.A.—*Certified Acupuncturist*
C.A.M.T.—*Certified Acupressure Massage Therapist*
C.C.H.—*Certified Clinical Hypnotherapist*
C.H.—*Certified Herbalist*
C.H.—*Clinical Hypnotherapist*
C.M.A.—*Certified Movement Analyst*
C.M.T.—*Certified Massage Therapist*
D.C.—*Doctor of Chiropractic*
D. Ht.—*Diplomate in Homeotherapeutics*
D.H.A.N.P.—*Democrat of Homeopathic Academy of Naturopathic Physicians*

D.O.—*Doctor of Osteopathy*

D.O.M.—*Doctor of Oriental Medicine*

Dipl.Ac.—*Diplomate in Acupuncture*

H.H.D.—*Doctor of Holistic Health*

H.H.P.—*Holistic Health Practitioner*

L.M.T.—*Licensed Massage Therapist*

L.Ac.—*Licensed Acupuncturist*

Lic.Ac.—*Licensed Acupuncturist*

M.H.—*Master Herbalist*

M.T.—*Massage Therapist*

N.D.—*Naturopathic Doctor or Doctor of Naturopathy*

N.M.D.—*Naturopathic Medical Doctor*

O.M.D.—*Oriental Medical Doctor*

R.Ac.—*Registered Acupuncturist*

R.D.—*Registered Dietitian*

R.D.T.—*Registered Drama Therapist*

R.M.T.—*Registered Massage Therapist*

R.P.T.—*Registered Physical Therapist*

✿ ✿ ✿

Resources

ACUPRESSURE

Acupressure Institute
1533 Shattuck Avenue
Berkeley, CA 94709
(510) 845-1059

**American Oriental Bodywork
Therapy Association (AOBTA)**
Glendale Executive Campus,
Suite 510
1000 White Horse Road
Voorhees, NJ 08053
(609) 782-1616

ACUPUNCTURE

**American Association of
Acupuncture and Oriental Medicine**
4101 Lake Boone Trail #201
Raleigh, NC 27607
(919) 787-5181

**American Foundation of
Traditional Chinese Medicine**
505 Beach Street
San Francisco, CA 94133
(415) 776-0502

**California Acupuncture Association
Referral**
2180 Garnet Avenue, Suite 3G-1
San Diego, CA 92109
(800) 477-4564/(619)270-1005

**National Commission for the
Certification of Acupuncturists**
1424 16th Street NW, Suite 501
Washington, DC 20036
(202) 232-1404

ACUPUNCTURISTS WHO
ARE M.D.'s

**American Academy of Medical
Acupuncture**

5820 Wilshire Boulevard, Suite 500
Los Angeles, CA 90036
(213) 937-5514

ALEXANDER TECHNIQUE

American Center for the Alexander
Technique
129 West 67th Street
New York, NY 10023
(212) 799-0468

North American Society of the
Teachers of Alexander Technique
P.O. Box 517
Urbana, IL 61801
(800) 473-0620

ALTERNATIVE HEALTH
NEWSLETTER

Townsend Letter
911 Tyler Street
Port Townsend, WA 98368-6541
(360) 385-6021

ALTERNATIVE MEDICINE

American Foundation for
Alternative Health Care
25 Landfield Avenue
Monticello, NY 12701
(914) 794-8181

ALTERNATIVE THERAPY
CLINICS (Outside U.S.A.)

American Biologics Hospital
1180 Walnut Avenue
Chula Vista, CA 91911-2622
(800) 227-4458

Gerson Institute
P.O. Box 430
Bonita, CA 91908
(619) 585-7600

Instituto Genesis West-Provida
P.O. Box 3460
Chula Vista, CA 91909-0004
(619) 424-9552

International Medical Center
1501 Arizona Street, Suite 1-E
El Paso, TX 79902
(800) 621-8924

APPLIED KINESIOLOGY

Biokinesiology Institute
5432 Highway 227 - P.O. Box 210
Trail, OR 97541
(503) 878-2080

International College of Applied
Kinesiology, U.S.A.
P.O. Box 905
Lawrence, KS 66044
(913) 542-1801

APPLIED PHYSIOLOGY

International Institute of Applied
Physiology
3014 E. Michigan Street
Tucson, AZ 85714
(602) 889-3075

AROMATHERAPY

Aromatherapy Institute of Research
P.O. Box 2354
Fair Oaks, CA 95628
(916) 965-7546

Flower Essence Society
P.O. Box 459
Nevada City, CA 95959
(916) 265-9163/(800) 548-0075

Pacific Institute of Aromatherapy
602 Fridas Parkway
San Raphael, CA 94903
(415) 479-9121

ART THERAPY

American Art Therapy Association
1202 Allanson Road
Mundelein, IL 60060
(708) 949-6064

ASTON-PATTERNING

Aston-Patterning
P.O. Box 3568
Incline Village, NV 89450
(702) 831-8228

AUTOGENIC TRAINING

International Committee for
Autogenic Training
101 Harley Street
London, W1N 1DF
England

AWARENESS ORIENTED
STRUCTURAL THERAPY

Florida Institute of Natural Health
& Florida Massage School
6421 S.W. 13th Street
Gainesville, FL 32608
(904) 378-7891

AYURVEDA

American School of Ayurvedic
Sciences
2115 112th Avenue NE
Bellevue, WA 98004
(206) 453-8022

Ayurvedic Institute
11311 Menaul NE, Suite A
Albuquerque, NM 87112
(505) 291-9698

Sharp Institute for Mind Body
Medicine
8525 Gibbs Drive, Suite 206
San Diego, CA 92123
(800) 827-4277

Sharp Institute for Mind Body
Medicine
1110 Camino Del Mar
Del Mar, CA 92014
(619) 794-2425

(BACH) FLOWER REMEDIES

Ellon U.S.A., Inc.
644 Merrick Road
Lynbrook, NY 11563
(516) 593-2206

BEE VENOM THERAPY

American Apitherapy Society, Inc.
P.O. Box 54
Hartland, Four-Corners, VT 05049
(800) 823-3460

BENJAMIN SYSTEM OF
MUSCULAR THERAPY

Muscular Therapy Institute
122 Rindge Avenue

Cambridge, MA 02140
(617) 576-1300/(617) 547-5800

BIOENERGETICS

Institute for Bioenergetics and Gestalt
1307 University Avenue
Berkeley, CA 94702
(510) 849-0101

International Institute for Bioenergetic Analysis
144 East 36th Street
New York, NY 10016
(212) 532-7742

BIOFEEDBACK

Association for Applied Psychophysiology and Biofeedback
10200 W. 44th Avenue, Suite 304
Wheat Ridge, CO 80033
(303) 422-8436

Biofeedback Certification Institute of America
10200 W. 44th Avenue, Suite 304
Wheat Ridge, CO 80033
(303) 420-2902

Biofeedback Institute of Los Angeles
3710 S. Robertson Blvd., Suite 216
Culver City, CA 90232
(213) 933-9451

Biofeedback Therapist Training Institute
1826 University Blvd. West
Jacksonville, FL 32217
(904) 737-5821

Biofeedback Training Associates
Dr. Philip Brotman
255 W. 98th Street
New York, NY 10025
(212) 222-5665

Center for Applied Physiology-Menninger Clinic
P.O. Box 829
Topeka, KS 66601
(913) 273-7500 ext. 5373

BODYWORK FOR THE CHILDBEARING YEAR

National Association of Pregnancy Massage Therapists
Ines Benedict, President
P.O. Box 81453
Atlanta, GA 30341
(404) 325-6903

Somatic Learning Associates
Kate Jordan & Carole Osborne-Sheets
8950 Villa La Jolla Drive, Suite 2162
La Jolla, CA 92037
(619) 436-0418/(619) 748-8827

BONNIE PRUDDEN MYOTHERAPY

Bonnie Prudden School for Physical Fitness and Myotherapy
7800 E. Speedway Blvd.
Tucson, AZ 85710
(602) 529-3979

BURTON TREATMENT (Immuno-Augmentative Therapy)

IAT, Ltd. Centre
P.O. Box 590656

Miami, FL 33159-0656
(809) 352-7455

CAYCE (EDGAR) THERAPIES

**Association for Research &
Enlightenment (ARE)**
Edgar Cayce Foundation
67th & Atlantic Avenue
P.O. Box 595
Virginia Beach, VA 23451
(804) 428-3588

ARE Clinic
4018 N. 40th Street
Phoenix, AZ 85018
(602) 955-0551

CAYCE (EDGAR) PRODUCTS

Home Health Products, Inc.
949 Seahawk Circle
Virginia Beach, VA 23452
(800) 284-9123

CHELATION THERAPY

**American Board of Chelation
Therapy**
1401-B N. Wells
Chicago, IL 60610
(312) 787-2228

**American College of Advancement
in Medicine**
P.O. Box 3427
Laguna Hills, CA 92654
(714) 583-7666/(800) 532-3688

CHI KUNG

**American Foundation of
Traditional Chinese Medicine**

505 Beach Street
San Francisco, CA 94133
(415) 776-0502

**Qi Gong Institute/East-West
Academy of the Healing Arts**
450 Sutter Street, Suite 2104
San Francisco, CA 94108
(415) 788-2227

CHIROPRACTIC

American Chiropractic Association
1701 Clarendon Boulevard
Arlington, VA 22209
(703) 276-8800

**Federation of Straight Chiropractic
Organizations**
642 Broad Street
Clifton, NJ 07013
(201) 777-1197

**Foundation for Chiropractic
Research and Education**
1701 Clarendon Boulevard
Arlington, VA 22209
(703) 276-7445

**International Chiropractic
Association**
1110 North Glebe Road, Suite 1000
Arlington, VA 22201
(703) 528-5000

National Directory of Chiropractic
P.O. Box 10056
Olathe, KS 66051
(800) 888-7914

World Chiropractic Alliance
2950 N. Dobson Road, Suite 1

Chandler, AZ 85224
(602) 786-9235/(800) 347-1011

COLON THERAPY

American Association of
Naturopathic Physicians
2366 Eastlake Avenue East, Suite 322
Seattle, WA 98102
(206) 323-7610

California Colon Hygienists'
Society
P.O. Box 588
Graton, CA 95444
(707) 829-0984

International Association for Colon
Therapy
2204 NW Loop 410
San Antonio, TX 78230
(210) 366-2888

National Colon Therapists'
Association
2103 Dorsey Road Avenue
Glen Burnie, MD 21061-3251

COLOR/LIGHT THERAPY

Dinshah Health Society
P.O. Box 707
Malaga, NJ 08328
(609) 692-4686

CRANIOSACRAL THERAPY

Upledger Institute
11211 Prosperity Farms Road
Palm Beach Gardens, FL 33410
(407) 622-4334

CRYSTAL THERAPY

Lifestream Associates
70 Sable Court
Winter Springs, FL 32708
(407) 699-1672

DANCE THERAPY

American Dance Therapy
Association
2000 Century Plaza, Suite 108
Columbia, MD 21044
(410) 997-4040

DEEP TISSUE SCULPTING

Integrative Bodywork Consultants
14961 Budwin Lane
Poway, CA 92064

International Professional School of
Bodywork
1366 Hornblend Street
San Diego, CA 92109
(619) 272-4142

DRAMA THERAPY

National Association for Drama
Therapy
#6 Woods Road
Sherman, CT 06784
(203) 350-1620

DREAM THERAPY

Association for the Study of Dreams
P.O. Box 1600
Vienna, VA 22183
(703) 242-8888

Dream Network Journal
1337 Powerhouse Lane, Suite 22
Moab, UT 84532

Lucidity Association (Lucid
Dreaming)
P.O. Box 170667
San Francisco, CA 94117

EGOSCUE METHOD

T.H.E. Clinic
2775 Via De La Valle
Del Mar, CA 92014
(619) 755-1075

ENVIRONMENTAL
MEDICINE (Clinical Ecology)

American Environmental Health
Foundation
8345 Walnut Hill Lane, Suite 225
Dallas, TX 75231
(214) 361-9515

Environmental Dental Association
10160 Aviary Drive
San Diego, CA 92131
(800) 388-8124

EQUESTRIAN THERAPY

National Center for Therapeutic
Riding
P.O. Box 42501
Washington, DC 20015
(202) 966-8004

North American Riding for the
Handicapped Association
P.O. Box 33150

Denver, CO 80233
(303) 452-1212/(800) 369-7433

EYE-ROBICS (Bates-Corbett
Method of Vision Training)

Vision Training Institute
11303 Meadow View Road
El Cajon, CA 92020
(619) 440-5224

FELDENKRAIS METHOD

Feldenkrais Guild
P.O. Box 489
Albany, OR 97321
(503) 926-0981

GERSON THERAPY and
GERSON DIET

Gerson Institute
P.O. Box 430
Bonita, CA 91908
(619) 585-7600

HAKOMI BODYWORK

Hakomi Institute
P.O. Box 1873
Boulder, CO 80306
(303) 443-6209

HANNA SOMATIC
EDUCATION

Novato Institute for Somatic
Research and Training
(415) 897-0336

HELLERWORK

Hellerwork, Inc.
406 Berry Street

Mt. Shasta, CA 96067
(916) 926-2500/(800) 392-3900

HERBALISM-HERBS

American Botanical Council
P.O. Box 201660
Austin, TX 78720
(512) 331-8868/(800) 373-7105

American Herbalist Guild
P.O. Box 1683
Soquel, CA 95073-1863
(408) 464-2441

American Herb Association
P.O. Box 1673
Nevada City, CA 95959
(916) 265-9552

Herb Research Foundation
1007 Pearl Street, Suite 200
Boulder, CO 80302
(303) 449-2265

Herb Society of America
9019 Kirtland Chardon Road
Mentor, OH 44060
(216) 256-0514

HOLISTIC MEDICINE and HEALTH PRACTITIONERS

American Holistic Medical
Association & American Holistic
Nurse's Association
4101 Lake Boone Trail, Suite 201
Raleigh, NC 27607
(919) 787-5181

International Association of Holistic
Health Practitioners
5010 N. Ridge Club Drive
Las Vegas, NV 89103
(702) 873-4542

HOLOTROPIC BREATHWORK

Grof Transpersonal Training, Inc.
(415) 383-8779

HOMEOPATHY

Homeopathic Educational Services
2124 Kittridge Street
Berkeley, CA 94704
(510) 649-0294/(800) 359-9051

International Foundation for
Homeopathy
2366 Eastlake Avenue East, Suite 322
Seattle, WA 98102
(206) 324-7610

National Center for Homeopathy
801 N. Fairfax Street, Suite 306
Alexandria, VA 22314
(703) 548-7790

HOMEOPATHIC REMEDIES

Arrowroot Standard Direct
83 E. Lancaster Avenue
Paoli, PA 19301
(800) 234-8879

HOSHINO THERAPY

Center For Biotherapeutics/
Hoshino Therapy Clinic
430 So. Dixie Highway
Miami, FL 33146
(305) 666-2243

HOXSEY TREATMENT

Bio-Medical Center
c/o Christina Santo
P.O. Box 433654
San Ysidro, CA 92143
(011) 52 66-84-9011 (Tijuana,
Mexico)

HYPERBARIC OXYGENATION THERAPY

American College of Hyperbaric Medicine
Ocean Medical Center
4001 Ocean Drive, Suite 105
Lauderdale-by-the-Sea, FL 33308
(305) 771-4000

HYPNOTHERAPY

American Academy of Medical Hypnotists
(800) 344-9766

American Association of Professional Hypnotherapists
P.O. Box 29
Boones Mill, VA 24065
(540) 334-3035

American Council of Hypnotist Examiners
700 So. Central Avenue
Glendale, CA 91204
(818) 242-1159

American Psychological Association
Division 30, Psychological Hypnosis
750 First Street, NE
Washington, DC 20002-4242
(800) 374-2721

American Society for Clinical Hypnosis
2200 E. Devon Avenue, Suite 291
Des Plains, IL 60018-4534
(708) 297-3317

International Medical & Dental Hypnotherapy Association
4110 Edgeland, Suite 800
Royal Oaks, MI 48073-2285
(810) 549-5594

National Society of Hypnotherapists
(515) 255-8151

IMAGERY and VISUALIZATION

Academy for Guided Imagery
P.O. Box 2070
Mill Valley, CA 94942
(800) 726-2070

American Imagery Institute
P.O. Box 13453
Milwaukee, WI 53213
(414) 781-4045

American Imagery Association
4016 Third Avenue
San Diego, CA 92103
(619) 298-7502

International Imagery Association
P.O. Box 1046
Bronx, NY 10471
(914) 423-9200

INFANT MASSAGE

International Loving Touch Foundation, Inc.

P.O. Box 16374
10434 S.E. Lincoln Court
Portland, OR 97216
(503) 253-8482

International Association of Infant
Massage Instructors
5660 Clinton Street, Suite #2
Elma, NY 14059
(716) 684-3299

National Association of Pregnancy
Massage Therapists
Ines Benedict, President
P.O. Box 81453
Atlanta, GA 30341
(404) 325-6903

Somatic Learning Associates
Kate Jordan & Carole Osborne-Sheets
8950 Villa La Jolla Drive, Suite 2162
La Jolla, CA 92037
(619) 436-0418/(619) 748-8827

IRIDOLOGY

Bernard Jensen International
24360 Old Wagon Road
Escondido, CA 92027
(619) 749-2727

JIN SHIN DO ACUPRESSURE

Jin Shin Do Foundation for
Bodymind Acupressure
366 California Avenue, Suite 16
Palo Alto, CA 94306
(415) 328-1811

JIN SHIN JYUTSU

Jin Shin Jyutsu, Inc.
8719 E. San Alberto
Scottsdale, AZ 85258
(602) 998-9331

LABAN MOVEMENT ANALYSIS

Laban/Bartenieff Institute of
Movement Studies
11 East 4th Street, 3rd Floor
New York, NY 10003
(212) 477-4299

LIFE EXTENSION

Life Extension Foundation
P.O. Box 229120
Hollywood, FL 33022
(800) 841-5433

LIVE CELL THERAPY

American Biologics
(Books on Cell Therapy)
1180 Walnut Avenue
Chula Vista, CA 91911-2622
(619) 429-8200

Dr. Wolfram Kuhnau
Author: *Live Cell Therapy*
Clinic in Mexico
(011) 52 66-83-5151

LIVINGSTON TREATMENT

Livingston Foundation Medical
Center
3232 Duke Street
San Diego, CA 92110
(619) 224-3515

LOMILOMI MASSAGE

Aunty Margaret School of Hawaiian
Lomilomi
P.O. Box 221
Captain Cook, HI 96704
(808) 323-2416

MACROBIOTICS

George Ohsawa Macrobiotic Foundation
1999 Myers Street
Oroville, CA 95966
(916) 533-7702

Kushi Institute of the Berkshires
P.O. Box 7
Becket, MA 01223
(413) 623-5741

MACROBIOTIC (Natural Foods Cooking Schools)

Natural Gourmet Cooking School
Annemarie Colbin
48 W. 21st Street
New York, NY 10010
(212) 645-5170

Vega Study Center
1511 Robinson Street
Oroville, CA 95965
(916) 533-4777

Kushi Institute of the Berkshires
P.O. Box 7
Becket, MA 01223
(413) 623-5741

MAGNETIC THERAPY

Albert Roy Davis Research Laboratory
P.O. Box 665
Green Cove Springs, FL 32043
(904) 264-8564

Bio-Electro Magnetics Institute
2490 West Moana Lake
Reno, NV 89509
(702) 827-9099

Enviro-Tech Products
17171 S.E. 29th Street
Choctaw, OK 73020
(405) 390-3499

Nikken Products, Inc.
15363 Barranca Pky
Irvine, CA 92718
(714) 789-2000

Pyramid International
414 Manhattan Avenue
Hawthorne, NY 10532
(914) 769-4879

American Magneto-Therapy Association
Ronald Lawrence, M.D., Pres.
17113 Gledhill Street
Northridge, CA 91325
(818) 886-7891

MAHARISHI AYUR-VEDA

Maharishi Ayur-Veda Association of America
P.O. Box 282
Fairfield, IA 52556
(515) 472-8477

MANUAL LYMPHATIC DRAINAGE (Vodder Method)

Dana Wyrick
P.O. Box 99745
San Diego, CA 92169
(619) 273-9764

Medicina Biologica
(Books on Lymphatic Drainage)
2937 N.E. Flanders
Portland, OR 97232
(503) 287-6775

Dr. Vodder School-Walchsee
Alleestr 30
A-6344 Walchsee, Austria
05374-5245

MASSAGE THERAPY/BODYWORK

American Massage Therapy
Association
820 Davis Street, Suite 100
Evanston, IL 60201-4444
(708) 864-0123

Associated Bodywork & Massage
Professionals
P.O. Box 1869
Evergreen, CO 80439-1869
(303) 674-8478/(800) 862-7724
(Referrals)

McDOUGALL PLAN DIET

St. Helena Health
Center/McDougall Plan
P.O. Box 250
Deer Park, CA 94576
(800) 358-9195 outside California

MEDITATION

Center for Spiritual Awareness
P.O. Box 7
Lake Rabun Road
Lakemont, GA 30552-9990

Institute for Noetic Sciences
P.O. Box 909
Sausalito, CA 94966
(415) 331-5650

MUSIC THERAPY

American Association for Music
Therapy
1 Station Plaza
Ossining, NY 10562
(914) 944-9260

National Association for Music
Therapy
8455 Colesville Road, Suite 930
Silver Spring, MD 20910
(301) 589-3300

MYOFASCIAL RELEASE

Myofascial Release Centers
10 So. Leopard Road, Suite One
Paoli, PA 19301
(610) 644-0136/(800) 327-2425

NAPRAPATHY

National College of Naprapathy
3330 N. Milwaukee Avenue
Chicago, IL 60641
(312) 282-2686

NATURAL HYGIENE

Fit for Life
2929 W. Anderson Lane
Austin, TX 78757
(512) 467-6746

International Association of
Professional Natural Hygienists
204 Stambaugh Building
Youngstown, OH 44512
(216) 746-5000

International Association of
Professional Natural Hygienists
Dr. Sabatino at Regency Health
Resort
2000 S. Ocean Drive
Hallandale, FL 33009
(305) 454-2220

Natural Hygiene, Inc.
P.O. Box 2132
Huntington, CT 06484
(203) 929-1557

NATUROPATHY

American Association of
Naturopathic Physicians
2366 Eastlake Avenue East, Suite 322
Seattle, WA 98102
(206) 323-7610

National College of Naturopathic
Medicine
11231 S.E. Market Street
Portland, OR 97216
(503) 255-4860

John Bastyr University
144 N.E. 54th Street
Seattle, WA 98105
(206) 523-9585

NETWORK CHIROPRACTIC

Association for Network
Chiropractic Spinal Analysis
444 N. Main Street
Longmont, CO 80501
(303) 678-8086

NEURO/CELLULAR REPATTERNING

Wellness Institute for Personal
Transformation
8300 Rock Springs Road
Penryn, CA 95663
(800) OK LET GO/(916) 663-3910

NUTRITION

Physician's Committee for
Responsible Medicine
P.O. Box 6322
Washington, DC 20015
(202) 686-2210

ORIENTAL BODYWORK

American Oriental Bodywork
Therapy Association (AOBTA)
Glendale Executive Campus,
Suite 510
1000 White Horse Road
Voorhees, NJ 08053
(609) 782-1616

ORTHO-BIONOMY

Society of Ortho-Bionomy
International, Inc.
P.O. Box 869
Madison, WI 53701
(800) 743-4890

ORTHOMOLECULAR MEDICINE

Academy of Orthomolecular
Medicine
1209 California Road

Eastchester, NY 10709
(914) 337-2552

OSTEOPATHY

American Osteopathic Association
142 E. Ontario Street
Chicago, IL 60611
(312) 280-5800

American Academy of Osteopathy
3500 De Pauw Boulevard,
Suite 1080
Indianapolis, IN 46268
(317) 879-1881

OXIDATIVE THERAPY

International Association for
Oxygen Therapy
P.O. Box 1360
Priest River, ID 83856
(208) 448-2504

ICMA-Physician Referral
P.O. Box 610767
Dallas/Ft. Worth, TX 75261
(817) 481-9772

International Bio-Oxidative
Medicine Foundation
P.O. Box 891954
Oklahoma City, OK 73189
(405) 478-4266

OZONE THERAPY

International Ozone Association
31 Strawberry Hill Avenue
Stamford, CT 06902
(203) 348-3542

PAST LIVES THERAPY

Association for Past-Life Research
and Therapies
P.O. Box 20151
Riverside, CA 92516
(909) 784-1570

PFRIMMER TECHNIQUE

Alexandria School of Scientific
Therapeutics
P.O. Box 287
Alexandria, IN 46001
(317) 724-7745

PHYSICAL THERAPY and PHYSIOTHERAPY

American Physical & Physio
Therapy Association
1111 N. Fairfax Street
Alexandria, VA 22314
(703) 684-2782

POETRY THERAPY

National Association for Poetry
Therapy
P.O. Box 551
Port Washington, NY 11050
(516) 944-9791

POLARITY THERAPY

American Polarity Therapy
Association
2888 Bluff Street,
Suite 149
Boulder, CO 80304
(303) 545-2080

POSTURAL INTEGRATION

International Center for Release
and Integration
450 Hillside Avenue
Mill Valley, CA 94941
(415) 383-4017

PRANIC HEALING

American Institute of Asian Studies
P.O. Box 1605
Chino, CA 91708-1605
(909) 465-0967

PRITIKIN PROGRAM
(RESIDENT)

Pritikin Longevity Center
1910 Ocean Front Walk
Santa Monica, CA 90405
(800) 421-9911

PSYCHOLOGY

Association for Humanistic
Psychology
45 Franklin #315
1772 Vallejo Street
San Francisco, CA 94102
(415) 864-8850

RADIANCE TECHNIQUE

Radiance Technique Association
International, Inc.
P.O. Box 40570
St. Petersburg, FL 33743-0570

REBIRTHING

Loving Relationships Training
International
(800) 468-5578

Clarity Productions
P.O. Box 160
Manhattan Beach, CA 90267
(310) 798-6933

REFLEXOLOGY

American Reflexology Certification
Board & Information Service
P.O. Box 246654
Sacramento, CA 95824
(916) 455-5381

Foot Reflexology Awareness
Association
P.O. Box 7622
Mission Hills, CA 91346
(818) 361-0528

International Institute of
Reflexology
P.O. Box 12642
St. Petersburg, FL 33733-2642
(813) 343-4811

REIKI

Reiki Alliance
P.O. Box 41
Cataldo, ID 83810
(208) 682-3535

Reiki Healing Institute
465 First Street
Encinitas, CA 92024
(619) 944-7013

RICE DIET

Kempner Clinic (Rice Diet)
Duke University Medical Clinic
1821 Green Street
Durham, NC 27705
(919) 286-2243

ROLFING

Rolf Institute of Structural
Integration
P.O. Box 1868
Boulder, CO 80306-1868
(303) 449-5903/(800) 530-8875

ROSEN METHOD THERAPY

Rosen Method Practitioner Referral
Service
(510) 644-4166

RUBENFELD SYNERGY METHOD

Rubenfeld Center
115 Waverly Place
New York, NY 10011
(212) 254-5100

SCHUESSLER'S BIOCHEMIC CELL SALTS

Luyties Pharmacal Company
4200 Laclede Avenue
St. Louis, MO 63108
(314) 652-8080

SHAMANISM

Dance of the Deer Foundation
Center for Shamanic Studies
P.O. Box 699

Soquel, CA 95073
(408) 475-9560

Foundation for Shamanistic Studies
P.O. Box 1939
Mill Valley, CA 94942
(415) 380-8282

SHEN THERAPY

International SHEN Therapy
Association (ISTA)
3213 W. Wheeler Street, Suite 202
Seattle, WA 98199
(206) 298-9468

SHIATSU

American Oriental Bodywork
Therapy Association (AOBTA)
Glendale Executive Campus,
Suite 510
1000 White Horse Road
Voorhees, NJ 08053
(609) 782-1616

Ohashi Institute
12 W. 27th Street, 9th Floor
New York, NY 10001
(212) 684-4190

SOMATOEMOTIONAL RELEASE

Upledger Institute
11211 Prosperity Farms Road
Palm Beach Gardens, FL 33410
(407) 622-4334

SPORTS MASSAGE

American Massage Therapy
Association

820 Davis Street, Suite 100
Evanston, IL 60201-4444
(708) 864-0123

International Sports Massage
Federation and Training Institute
2156 Newport Boulevard
Costa Mesa, CA 92627
(714) 642-0735

ST. JOHN'S NEUROMUSCULAR PAIN RELIEF

St. John's Neuromuscular Pain
Relief Institute
10950 72nd Street, Suite 101
Largo, FL 34647
(813) 541-1900

SUBLIMINAL THERAPY

Gateway Research Institute
P.O. Box 1706
Ojai, CA 93024
(800) 477-8908

Learning Strategies Corporation
900 East Wyzanta Boulevard
Wyzanta, MN 55391
(612) 475-2250

Quantum Quest
P.O. Box 98
Oakview, CA 93022
(800) 772-0090

THERAPEUTIC TOUCH

Nurse Healers–Professional
Association, Inc.
P.O. Box 444

Allison Park, PA 15101
(412) 355-8476

American Holistic Nurses
Association
4101 Lake Boone Trail, Suite 201
Raleigh, NC 27607
(919) 787-5181

Orcas Island Foundation
Box 86, Route 1
East Sound, WA 98245
(360) 376-4526

TOUCH FOR HEALTH

Touch for Health Association
6955 Fernhill Drive, Suite 5-A
Malibu, CA 90265
(310) 457-8342

TRAGER APPROACH

Trager Institute
21 Locust
Mill Valley, CA 94941-2806
(415) 388-2688

TRANSCENDENTAL MEDITATION

Maharishi Vedic University
1401 Ocean Avenue
Asbury Park, NJ 07712
(908) 774-9446

TUI NA CHINESE HEALING AND ACUPRESSURE MASSAGE

Taoist Institute of Los Angeles
(818) 760-4219

Taoist Sanctuary of San Diego
4229 Park Boulevard
San Diego, CA 92103
(619) 692-1155

VISCERAL MANIPULATION

Upledger Institute
11211 Prosperity Farms Road
Palm Beach Gardens, FL 33410
(407) 622-4334

VITAMIN THERAPY

Linus Pauling Insititute of Science
and Medicine
440 Page Mill Road
Palo Alto, CA 94306
(415) 327-4064

WHEATGRASS DIET

Ann Wigmore Foundation
(505) 384-1017

WHOLE FOODS DIET

Bernard Jensen International

24360 Old Wagon Road
Escondido, CA 92027
(619) 749-2727

YOGA

American Yoga Association
Cleveland Ohio Area
(216) 371-0078

American Yoga Association
513 S. Orange Avenue
Sarasota, FL 34236
(813) 953-5859

International Association of Yoga
Therapists
Send a SASE for a referral list
109 Hillside Avenue
Mill Valley, CA 94941

ZERO BALANCING

Zero Balancing Association
P.O. Box 1727
Capitola, CA 95010
(408) 476-0665

⌗ ⌗ ⌗

Bibliography

Author's Note: In preparing this bibliography, every effort was made to provide the reader with as complete an entry as possible. Some entries lack a publication date, but only because such publications were not dated, or a date was not available. Some of the journal citations only include volume and number because they are published at random intervals and did not bear a date. Some information was obtained from pamphlets, brochures, and other small publications produced by an organization representing a particular therapy, which also did not bear a date.

Abramson, David M. "Therapeutic Touch." *New Age Journal*, June 1985.

"Acupuncture without Needles." *Total Health*, April 1992.

Aihara, Cornellia. *Key to Good Health: Macrobiotic Kitchen*. Tokyo: Japan Publications, 1982

Alexandria School of Scientific Therapeutics. *Pfrimmer Deep Muscle Therapy*. Indianapolis, no date.

Altman, Nathaniel. *Everybody's Guide to Chiropractic Health Care*. Los Angeles: Jeremy P. Tarcher, 1990.

American Academy of Environmental Medicine. *What Is Environmental Medicine?* Denver, no date.

American Academy of Medical Acupuncture. *"Doctor, What's This Acupuncture All About?"* Los Angeles, no date.

American Art Therapy Association. *Introduction, History, Organization, and Therapist (Of Art Therapy)*. Mundelein, Ill., 1992.

American Association of Acupuncture and Oriental Medicine. *Facts.* Washington, D.C., no date.

American Association of Ayurvedic Medicine. *Maharishi Ayur-Veda: Review of Scientific Research,* 1990.

American Association of Naturopathic Physicians. *Naturopathic Medicine: What It Is . . . What It Can Do for You.* Seattle, no date.

American Cancer Society. *Eating Smart.* 1987.

American Center for the Alexander Technique. *The Alexander Technique.* New York, 1988.

American College of Advancement in Medicine. *Chelation Therapy.* Laguna Hills, Calif., no date.

American Dance Therapy Association. *What Is Dance/Movement Therapy?* Columbia, Md., no date.

American Health Sciences Institute. *History of Life Science.* Manchaca, Tex., no date.

———. *How Does Life Science Differ from Other Healing Arts?* Manchaca, Tex., no date.

———. *What Does Life Science (or Natural Hygiene) Mean?* Manchaca, Tex., no date.

———. *What Is Natural Hygiene?* Manchaca, Tex., no date.

American Holistic Medical Association. *The Most Asked Questions About Holistic Health and Holistic Medicine.* Raleigh, N.C., no date.

American Institute for Cancer Research. *Dietary Guidelines to Lower Cancer Risk.* 1990.

American Massage Therapy Association. *A Guide to Massage Therapy in America.* Chicago, 1989.

———. *Applications of Therapeutic Massage.* Chicago, 1986.

———. *Massage Therapy.* Chicago, 1986.

———. *Sports Massage.* Chicago, 1986.

———. *Stress.* Chicago, 1986.

American Osteopathic Association. *Osteopathic Medical Education.* Chicago, 1991.

———. *Osteopathic Medicine.* Chicago, 1991.

———. *What Is a D.O.?* Chicago, 1991.

———. *What Is Osteopathic Medicine?* Chicago, no date.

American Physical Therapy Association. *A Future in Physical Therapy: A Hands-On Health Care Profession.* Alexandria, Va., no date.

American Polarity Therapy Association. *Polarity Therapy.* East Arlington, Mass., 1991.

Apsler, Alfred. *From Witch Doctor to Biofeedback: The Story of Healing by Suggestion.* New York: Julian Messner, 1978.

Armstrong, John W. *The Water of Life: A Treastise on Urine Therapy.* 2d ed., Essex, England: Health Science Press, 1971.

Arthritis Foundation. *Arthritis Diet Guidelines and Research.* Atlanta, 1987.

Aston Training Center. *Aston-Patterning.* Incline Village, Nev., 1987.

Bansal, H. L., and R. S. Bansal. *Magnetic Cure for Common Diseases.* no date.

Barnes, John F. "Five Years of Myofascial Release." *Physical Therapy Forum,* September 16, 1987.

Bauman, Edward. "Introduction to Holistic Health." *The Holistic Health Handbook,* 1978.

Bauman, Edward, et al. *The Holistic Health Handbook: A Tool for Attaining Wholeness of Body, Mind, and Spirit.* Berkeley, Calif.: And/Or Press, 1978.

Beck, Mark. "Proprioception: The Seventh Sense." *Massage Therapy Journal,* winter 1992.

"Bee Venom." *Healing and Renewal Newsletter,* vol. 6 (spring 1992).

Benjamin, Ben E. *Are You Tense? The Benjamin System of Muscular Therapy.* New York: Pantheon Books, 1978.

———. "Bee Venom Therapy." *Massage Therapy Journal,* summer 1990.

Binik, Alexander. "The Polarity System." *The Holistic Health Handbook,* 1978.

Bloomfield, Harold H., Michael Peter Cain, and Dennis T. Jaffe. *TM (Transcendental Meditation): Discovering Inner Energy and Overcoming Stress.* New York: Delacorte Press, 1975.

Bond, S. Edgar. "What's in the Hoxsey Treatment?" *Cancer Control Journal,* vol. 3, 1 and 2.

Breaux, Dajawn. "Health and Psychic Awareness." *The Holistic Health Handbook,* 1978.

Brice, Leslie. *What You Should Know About Subliminal Perception and Subliminal Self-Improvement Tapes.* Ojai, Calif.: Gateway Research Institute, 1986.

Bricklin, Mark. *The Practical Encyclopedia of Natural Healing.* Rev. ed. Emmaus, Pa.: Rodale Press, 1983.

Brint, Armand Ian. "Iridology." *The Holistic Health Handbook,* 1978.

Burton, Frank. *Survey of Bodywork Forms Which Are Popular in the East Bay,* 1990.

California Acupuncture Association. *Acupuncture Facts.* San Diego, 1991.

Calvert, Judi, and David Flatley. "Mantak Chia on Chi Nei Tsang: Internal Organ Massage." *Massage Magazine,* January/February 1992.

Calvert, Robert. "Judith Aston: Developer of Aston-Patterning Bodywork." *Massage Magazine,* October/November 1988.

———. "Interview Paul St. John and His Neuromuscular Therapy—Part II." *Massage Magazine,* January/February 1992.

Calvert, Robert, with Noel Abildgaard, comp. and ed. *International Massage and Bodywork Resource Guide.* Davis, Calif.: NOAH Publishing, 1992.

Calvert, Robert, and Judi Calvert. "Interview with Marion Rosen, Founder of the Rosen Method Bodywork and Gloria Hessellund, Rosen Practitioner." *Massage Magazine,* July/August 1991.

Carmona, Victoria. "A Tribute to Thomas Hanna (1928–1990)." *Massage Therapy Journal,* Fall 1990.

Centre for Traditional Acupuncturer. *Is Acupuncture for You?* Columbia, Md., 1989.

Chavis, Geri Giebel. *The Therapeutic Power of Poetry,* no date.

China Sports Magazine. *The Wonders of Qi Gong.* Los Angeles: Wayfarer Publications, 1985.

Chocron, Daya Sarai. *Healing with Crystals and Gemstones.* York Beach, Maine: Samuel Weiser, 1983.

Clark, Linda. *The Ancient Art of Color Therapy.* Old Greenwich, Conn.: Devin-Adair, 1975.

Co, S. *Pranic Healing.* Chino, Calif.: American Institute of Asian Studies, 1991.

———. *Pranic Healing and Pranic Psychotherapy.* Chino, Calif.: American Institute of Asian Studies, 1992.

"Connecting with the Healing Source: An Interview with Patricia Garfield, Ph.D." *Night Visions: A Dream Journal,* vol. 3, no. 1.

Connor, Lew, and Linda McKim. "Reflexology." *The Holistic Health Handbook,* 1978.

"A Course in Dream Healing." *Night Visions: A Dream Journal,* vol. 3, no. 1.

Consumers Guide. *Walking for Health and Fitness.* Lincolnwood, Ill.: Publications International, 1988.

Dachman, Ken, and John Lyons. *You Can Relieve Pain: How Guided Imagery Can Help You Reduce Pain or Eliminate It Altogether.* New York: Harper & Row, 1990.

Davidson-Stinnett, Shirley. *The First Institution of Natural Hygiene since the Late 1800's!* Manchaca, Tex.: American Health Sciences Institute, no date.

Davis, Roy Eugene. *An Easy Guide to Meditation.* Lakemont, Ga.: CSA Press, 1978.

Day, Harvey. *Encyclopedia of Natural Health and Healing.* Santa Barbara, Calif.: Woodbridge Press, 1979.

Delza, Sophia. *T'ai Ch'i Ch'uan.* North Canton, Ohio: Good News Publishing, 1961.

Denniston, Denise, and Peter McWilliams. *The TM (Transcendental Meditation) Book: How to Enjoy the Rest of Your Life.* Allen Park, Mich.: Versemonger Press, 1975.

Devi, Indra. *Yoga for Americans.* Englewood Cliffs, N.J.: Prentice-Hall, 1959.

De Vierville, Paul. "Hydrotherapy: Washes, Wraps, Packs and Herbs." *Massage Therapy Journal,* Winter 1991.

Dorland's Illustrated Medical Dictionary. 27th ed. Philadelphia: W. B. Saunders, 1988.

d'Out, Claire. "Life Changing Chiropractic." *San Diego Resources,* November/December 1992/January 1993.

Diamond, Harvey, and Marilyn Diamond. *Fit for Life.* New York: Warner Books, 1985.

Dobkin, Gene. *Ortho-Bionomy,* no date.

Dong, Colin H., and Jane Banks. *The Arthritic's Cookbook.* New York: Thomas Y. Crowell, 1973.

Doyle, Roger. *The Vegetarian Handbook.* New York: Crown Publishers, 1979.

Dreyfack, Raymond. *The Complete Book of Walking.* Los Angeles: Farnsworth Publishing, 1979.

Duggan, Joseph, and Sandra Duggan. *Edgar Cayce's Massage, Hydrotherapy and Healing Oils.* Virginia Beach, Va.: Home Health Products, 1989.

Duke, Marc. *Acupuncture: The Extraordinary New Book on the Chinese Art of Healing.* New York: Pyramid House, 1972.

Dwyer, James, and David Rattray, senior eds. *Magic and Medicine of Plants.* Pleasantville, N.Y.: Reader's Digest Association, 1986.

Editors of *Prevention* magazine. *Understanding Vitamins and Minerals.* Emmaus, Pa.: Rodale Press, 1984.

Egoscue, Pete. *The Egoscue Method of Health through Motion.* New York: HarperCollins Publishers, 1992.

Ehret, Arnold. *Mucusless Diet Healing System.* Yonkers, N.Y.: Ehret Literature Publishing, 1989.

Eisenberg, Michael. "Traditional Thai Massage (Nuad Bo-rarn)." *Massage Therapy Journal,* Winter 1992.

Ellon Bach USA. *The Bach Flower Remedies.* Lynbrook, N.Y., no date.

Erdmann, Robert, with Meirion Jones. *The Amino Revolution.* New York: Simon & Schuster, Fireside, 1987.

Farr, Charles H., Robert L. White, and Michael Schachter. *Chronological History of EDTA Chelation Therapy,* 1991.

Feldenkrais, Moshe. *Awareness through Movement.* New York: Harper & Row, 1977.

————. *The Feldenkrais Method.* Albany, Ore.: Feldenkrais Guild, no date.

Florida Institute of Natural Health/Florida School of Massage. *Awareness Oriented Structural Therapy: A Psychophysical Approach to Bodywork.* Gainesville, Fla., no date.

Franklin, Neshama. "Bodywork." *Medical Self-Care.* Spring 1984.

Frawley, David. *From the River of Heaven: Hindu and Vedic Knowledge for the Modern Age.* Salt Lake City: Passage Press, 1990.

Free, Valerie H. "Towards A New Era for Total Health: Adapting the Wellness Theme Country by Country." *The Multi-Level Marketer,* 1992.

Fritz, Norman. *The Gerson Therapy: A Brief Summary.* Bonita, Calif.: Gerson Institute, no date.

Fryling, Vera. "Autogenic Training." *The Holistic Health Handbook,* 1978.

Gach, Michael Reed. *Acupressure Health Care: Background, Origins and Current Uses,* 1980.

Gawain, Shakti. "Creative Visualization." *The Holistic Health Handbook,* 1978.

Garfield, Linda Susan. "Ortho-Bionomy: A New System of Healing." *Holistic Health and Medicine.*

Garfield, Patricia. *The Healing Power of Dreams.* New York: Simon & Schuster, 1991.

"Geriatric Massage Training." *Geri News: Day-Break Geriatric Massage Project Newsletter,* Winter 1991/1992.

Gerson Institute. *The Gerson Therapy.* Bonita, Calif., no date.

Gibson, H. B. *Hypnosis: Its Nature and Therapeutic Uses.* New York: Taplinger Publishing, 1977.

Gillespie, Barry. "Dental Considerations of the CranioSacral Mechanism." *Journal of Craniomandibular Practice*, vol. 3, no. 4 (September/December 1985).

Golden, Mary. "Lomilomi: The Loving Touch of Hawaii." *Massage Magazine*, July/August 1992.

Gray, Robert. *The Colon Health Handbook.* 11th ed. Reno, Nev.: Emerald Publishing, 1986.

Greene, William. *est: Four Days to Make Your Life Work.* New York: Pocket Books, 1976.

Griggs, Barbara. *Green Pharmacy: A History of Herbal Medicine.* New York: Viking Press, 1981.

Grow, Gerald. "Improving Eyesight: The Bates Method." *The Holistic Health Handbook*, 1978.

Hakomi Institute. *About Hakomi Therapy.* Boulder, Colo., no date.

Halcyon Health Group. *About Rosen Method Bodywork.* Berkeley, Calif., no date.

Hanna, Thomas. *Somatics: Reawakening the Mind's Control of Movement, Flexibility, and Health.* New York: Addison-Wesley Publishing, 1988.

Harner, Michael. *The Way of the Shaman.* 3rd ed. San Francisco: HarperCollins Publishers, Harper San Francisco, 1990.

Hassin, Vijay. *The Modern Yoga Handbook.* Garden City, N.Y.: Doubleday, Dolphin Books, 1978.

Harris, Robert. "An Introduction to Manual Lymph Drainage: The Vodder Method." *Massage Therapy Journal*, Winter 1992.

Haught, S. J. *The American Experience of Dr. Max Gerson: Censured for Curing Cancer.* Bonita, Calif.: Gerson Institute, 1991.

Health Center for Better Living. *A Useful Guide to Herbal Health Care.* Naples, Fla., no date.

Heimlich, Jane. *What Your Doctor Won't Tell You.* New York: Harper Perennial, 1990.

Heinrich, Steve. "Learning to Let Go: The Role of SomatoEmotional Release in Clinical Treatment." *Physical Therapy Forum*, vol. 8, no. 24.

Heller, Peggy Osna. "The Three Pillars of Biblio/Poetry Therapy." *The Arts in Psychotherapy* 14 (1987: 341–44.

Higgins, Melissa. "Mary Burmeister, Master of Jin Shin Jyutsu." *Yoga Journal*, March/April 1988.

Hilgard, Ernest R., and Josephine R. Hilgard. *Hypnosis in the Relief of Pain.* Los Altos, Calif.: William Kaufmann, 1983.

Hoeffel, Ann, and June Rouse. "Ortho-Bionomy: The Homeopathy of Bodywork." *Conscious Choice*, Summer 1990.

Holt, Paul M. "Cost-Effective Chiropractic." *Health World*, September/October 1991.

Hoshino Therapy Clinic. *Hoshino Therapy.* Miami, no date.

Hunt, Dave, and T. A. McMahon. *America the Sorcerer's New Apprentice: The Rise of New Age Shamanism.* Eugene, Ore.: Harvest House Publishers, 1984.

Huxley Institute for Biosocial Research. *Concerned about Your Health?* Boca Raton, Fla., no date.

IAT, Ltd. *Immuno-Augmentative Therapy: Cancer Research and Treatment.* Freeport, Grand Bahama Island, no date.

Institute for Personal Transformation. *How Neuro/Cellular Repatterning Was Born.* Penryn, Calif., 1990.

International Association of Infant Massage Instructors. *Infant Massage: Your Chance to Make a Difference,* 1989.

International Bio-Oxidative Medicine Foundation. *Oxidative Therapy.* Dallas/Fort Worth, Tex., no date.

International Center for Release and Integration. *Be a Professional in Deep Bodywork.* Mill Valley, Calif., 1987.

International College of Applied Kinesiology. *An Historical Overview of Applied Kinesiology.* Shawnee Mission, Kans., no date.

International Foundation for Homeopathy. *Homeopathy: Healing the Whole Person.* Seattle, no date.

International Institute of Applied Physiology. *An Introduction to Applied Physiology.* Tucson, no date.

International Institute of Reflexology. *Facts about Foot Reflexology.* Ingham Publishing, 1987.

International Macrobiotic Shiatsu Society. *Macrobiotic Shiatsu.* Eureka, Calif., 1990.

———. *Macrobiotic Shiatsu: Comprehensive Training.* Eureka, Calif., 1989.

International Medical Center. *Chelation Therapy: The Common-Sense Alternative to Heart Disease.* El Paso, no date.

———. *H.B.O. (Hyperbaric Oxygenation) Defined.* El Paso, no date.

———. *Live Cell Therapy: A Natural Approach to Wellness.* El Paso, no date.

International Movement Therapy Association. *Movement Therapy.* Stanford, Calif., no date.

Infant Massage Northwest. *Infant Massage: Loving Touch Right from the Start.* Portland, Ore., no date.

Introduction to Dr. Vodder's Manual Lymphatic Drainage. Vol. 1, 3rd rev. ed. by Hildegard Wittlinger. Vols. 2 & 3 ed. by Ingrid Kurtz. Heidelberg, Germany: Karl F. Haug Publishers.

Jacobs, Susan. "Stephen Halpern: Exploring the Farther Reaches of Sound." *Yoga Journal,* November/December 1984.

Janov, Arthur. *The New Primal Scream: Primal Therapy Twenty Years On.* Wilmington, Del.: Enterprise Publishing, 1991.

Jaques, Jeannine. "Looyenwork: A New Era in Bodywork." *Massage News,* no date.

Jenkins, Richard Dean. "The Healing Power of Magnets." *Men's Fitness,* February 1992.

Jensen, Bernard. *Foods That Heal: A Guide to Understanding and Using the Healing*

Powers of Natural Foods. Garden City Park, N.Y.: Avery Publishing Group, 1988.

————. *Iridology Simplified.* Escondido, Calif.: Iridologists International, 1980.

Jin Shin Do Foundation for Bodymind Acupressure. *Directory of Authorized Teachers and Registered Acupressurists: Jin Shin Do Bodymind Acupressure.* Berkeley, Calif., no date.

Jin Shin Jyutsu, Inc. *Introducing Jin Shin Jyutsu.* Scottsdale, Ariz., no date.

Jordan, Kate, and Carole Osborne-Sheets. *Bodywork for the Childbearing Year.* La Jolla, Calif.: Somatic Learning Associates, 1987.

Juhan, Deane. *An Introduction to Trager Psychophysical Integration and Mentastics Movement Education.* Mill Valley, Calif.: Trager Institute, 1989.

————. *Job's Body: A Handbook for Bodywork.* Barrytown, N.Y.: Station Hill Press, 1987.

Karlins, Marvin, and Lewis M. Andrews. *Biofeedback: Turning on the Power of Your Mind.* New York: J. B. Lippincott, 1972.

Keowen, Gary D., and Tim Juett. "Myofascial Release: An Introduction for the Patient." *Physical Therapy Forum,* October 3, 1989.

King, Serge. *Kahuna Healing: Holistic Health and Healing Practices of Polynesia.* Wheaton, Ill.: Theosophical Publishing House, 1983.

Knaster, Mirka. "Premature Infants Grow with Massage." *Massage Therapy Journal,* Summer 1991.

————. "Ilana Rubenfeld: Our Lady of Synergy." *Massage Therapy Journal,* Winter 1991.

————. "Thomas Hanna: Mind over Movement." *Massage Therapy Journal,* Fall 1989.

Knutsen, E. Signy. "The Meaning of Meditation." *The Holistic Health Handbook,* 1978.

Kotzsch, Ronald. "Hoshino Therapy: Nothing Can Surpass the Hands." *East/West,* December 1988.

————. "Regain Grace: The Alexander Technique." *Natural Health,* March/April 1992.

Kowalchik, Claire, and William H. Hylton, eds. *Rodale's Illustrated Encyclopedia of Herbs.* Emmaus, Pa.: Rodale Press, 1987.

Krieger, Dolores. *The Therapeutic Touch: How to Use Your Hands to Heal or Help.* New York: Prentice-Hall, 1979.

Krumhausl, Bernice. *Opportunity in Physical Therapy.* Skokie, Ill.: VGM Career Horizons Division National Textbook, 1974.

Kunin, Richard. "Principles That Identify Orthomolecular Medicine: A Unique Specialty." *Journal of Orthomolecular Medicine,* vol. 2, no. 4 (1987).

Kushi Institute. *Macrobiotics: An Invitation to Health and Happiness.* Beckett, Mass., no date.

————. *Macrobiotics: Standard Dietary and Way of Life Suggestions.* Beckett, Mass., 1986.

Kushi, Michio. *The Macrobiotic Way: The Complete Macrobiotic Diet and Exercise Book.* Wayne, N.J.: Avery Publishing Group, 1985.

———. *The Macrobiotic Approach to Cancer: Towards Preventing and Controlling Cancer with Diet and Lifestyle.* Wayne, N.J.: Avery Publishing Group, 1982.

Laban/Bartenieff Institute of Movement Studios. *Laban Movement Analysis.* New York, 1992.

Lad, Vasant. *Ayurveda: The Science of Self Healing.* Santa Fe, N.M.: Lotus Press, 1985.

Landsdowne, Zachary F. *The Chakras and Esoteric Healing.* York Beach, Maine: Samuel Weiser, 1986.

Langone, John. *Chiropractors: A Consumer's Guide.* Reading, Mass.: Addison-Wesley, 1982.

La Patra, Jack. *Healing: The Coming Revolution in Holistic Medicine.* New York: McGraw-Hill, 1978.

"Lawrence Burton, Ph.D." *Health Consciousness,* August 1986.

Lawrence, D. Baloti, and Lewis Harrison. *Massageworks: A Practical Encyclopedia of Massage Techniques.* New York: Putnam Publishing Group, 1983.

Leboyer, Frederick. *Loving Hands: The Traditional Indian Art of Baby Massage.* New York: Alfred A. Knopf, 1976.

Le Cron, Leslie M. *The Complete Guide to Hypnosis.* New York: Harper & Row, 1971.

Lessman, Karen. "Getting to Know the U.S.S.R." *Massage Therapy Journal,* Winter 1991.

Le Strange, Richard. *A History of Herbal Plants.* New York: Arco Publishing, 1977.

Levine, Fred. "Holotropic Breathwork: More Than a Fantasy, Less Than a Reality." *Natural Health,* May/June 1992.

Lew, Share K., and Bill Helm. *Tui Na: Chinese Healing and Acupressure Massage.* 3rd ed. Fellowship of the Tao, 1988.

Lewis, Angelo John. "The Art of Aromatherapy: Healing with Essential Oils." *East/West,* October 1988.

Lilly, John C. *The Center of the Cyclone.* New York: Julian Press, 1972.

Lippman, Susannah. *The Truth about Subliminal Tapes.* Los Angeles: Alphasonics International, 1990.

Livingston Foundation Medical Center and Arthur D. Alexander III. *Livingston Foundation Medical Center: Patient Brochure.* San Diego, 1991.

Looyenwork Institute. *Looyenwork 535-Hour Certification Program.* Sausalito, Calif., no date.

"Looyenwork, Pain and The Body-Mind Connection." *Open Exchange,* April/May/June 1991.

Low, Jeffrey. "The Modern Body Therapies, Part IV: Aston-Patterning." *Massage Magazine,* October/November 1988.

Lowen, Alexander. *Bioenergetics.* New York: Penguin Books, 1976.

Luyties Pharmacal Company. *Homeopathic Primer.* St. Louis, 1976.

———. *Homeopathy.* St. Louis, no date.

Lyons, Albert S., and R. Joseph Petrocelli. *Medicine, An Illustrated History.* New York: Harry N. Abrams, 1987.

MacIvor, Virginia, and Sandra La Forest. *Vibrations: Healing through Color, Homeopathy and Radionics.* York Beach, Maine: Samuel Weiser.

McCabe, Ed. *Oxygen Therapies.* Morrisville, N.Y.: Energy Publications, 1988.

———. "Ozone Is Not Smog—Ozone Is Good and Natural." *ECHO Newsletter*, vol. 4, no. 2 (summer 1991).

Maharishi Ayurveda Medical Centers. *Maharishi Ayurveda: Natural Health Care for the Rejuvenation of Mind and Body.* No date.

Man-Ch'ing, Cheng. *T'ai Chi Ch'uan: A Simplified Method of Calisthenics for Health and Self Defense.* Berkeley, Calif.: North Atlantic Books, 1981.

Mann, Felix. *Acupuncture, the Ancient Chinese Art of Healing and How It Works Scientifically.* New York: Random House, 1971.

Mantell, Matthew E. *Applied Kinesiology: A New Drive for Total Health.* International College of Applied Kinesiology–USA, Shawnee Mission, Kans., no date.

Michaelsen, Johanna. *The Beautiful Side of Evil.* Eugene, Ore.: Harvest House Publishers, 1982.

Miesler, Dietrich W. "Geriatric Massage." *Massage Magazine*, September/October 1991.

———. *Teacher Training and Curriculum Development in Geriatric Massage.* Guerneville, Calif.: Day-Break Geriatric Message Project, no date.

———. *Day-Break Geriatric Massage Workshops.* Guerueville, Calif.: Day-Break Geriatric Massage Project, no date.

———. *The Use of Elderly Massage Volunteers in Day-Break Workshops.* Guerneville, Calif.: Day-Break Geriatric Massage Project, no date.

———. *Geriatric Massage Techniques.* Guerneville, Calif.: Day-Break Geriatric Massage Project, no date.

Miller, Michael M. *Therapeutic Hypnosis.* New York: Human Sciences Press, 1979.

Missett, Judi Sheppard. *The Jazzercise Workout Book.* New York: Charles Scribner's Sons, 1986.

Moore, Christine. "New Options for Feeling Better." *New Woman*, January 1989.

Murphy, Forest. "Schuessler's Biochemic Cell Salts." *Journal of the American Institute for Homeopathy (for Physicians and Surgeons)*, March 1980.

Murray, Michael, and Jospeh Pizzorno. "The Naturopathic Revolution." *Venture Inward*, July/August 1992.

Muscular Therapy Institute. *The Benjamin System of Muscular Therapy.* Cambridge, Mass., no date.

Myofascial Treatment Centers and Seminars. *Myofascial Release Treatment Center Brochure.* Paoli, Pa., no date.

Namikoshi, Toru. *Shiatsu Therapy, Theory and Practice.* Tokyo: Japan Publications, 1974.

National Association for Drama Therapy. *Drama Therapy.* New Haven, Conn., 1992.

National Association for Holistic Aromatherapy. *Aromatherapy and Essential Oils.* Boulder, Colo., no date.

National Association for Music Therapy. *Music Therapy Makes a Difference.* Silver Springs, Md., no date.

———. *NAMTA Fact Sheet.* Silver Springs, Md., no date.

National Cancer Institute. *Diet, Nutrition and Cancer Prevention: The Good News.* Bethesda, Md., 1986.

National Center for Homeopathy. *Homeopathy: Natural Medicine for the 21st Century.* Alexandria, Va., 1990.

Nelson, Dawn. "The Compassionate Touch for Those in the Later Stages of Life." *Geri News: Day-Break Geriatric Message Project Newsletter,* Spring 1992.

Netherton, Morris, and Nancy Shiffrin. *Past Lives Therapy.* New York: William Morrow, 1978.

Newhouse, Sandy, and John Amodeo. "Native American Healing." *The Holistic Health Handbook,* 1978.

New Mexico Association of Acupuncture and Oriental Medicine. *Acupuncture.* No date.

Norman, Laura. *Feet First: A Guide to Reflexology.* New York: Simon & Schuster, Fireside, 1988.

North American Society of Teachers of the Alexander Technique (NASTAT). *The Alexander Technique.* Champaign, Ill., no date.

North American Vegetarian Society. *Vegetarianism: Answers to the Most Commonly Asked Questions.* Dolgeville, N.Y. No date.

Ohsawa, George. *Essential Macrobiotics.* Oroville, Calif.: George Ohsawa Macrobiotic Foundation, no date.

———. *Macrobiotics: An Invitation to Health and Happiness.* Oroville, Calif.: George Ohsawa Macrobiotic Foundation, 1971.

Olsen, Kristin Gottschalk. *The Encyclopedia of Alternative Health Care.* New York: Pocket Books, 1989.

"On the Line ... Subliminal Technology: Taking the Struggle out of Personal Change." *American Council on Alcoholism Journal,* Spring/Summer 1990.

"The Original Save Your Life Diet." *Kempner Clinic Rice Diet News,* vol. 1, no. 1 (July 1992).

Orr, Leonard. *The Story of Rebirthing.* Chico, Calif.: Inspiration University, no date.

———, and Sondra Ray. *Rebirthing in the New Age.* Berkeley, Calif.: Celestial Arts, 1983.

Osborne-Sheets, Carole. *Deep Tissue Sculpting: A Technical and Artistic Manual for Therapeutic Bodywork Practitioners.* San Diego: International Professional School of Bodywork in collaboration with Integrative Bodywork Consultants, 1990.

———. "Healing Touch for ACS's (Adult Children of Alcoholics)." *Massage Magazine,* February/March 1989.

Overmyer, Luann. *Ortho-Bionomy.* Berkeley, Calif.: Society of Ortho-Bionomy International, no date.

"Ozone Therapy." *Healing and Renewal Newsletter,* vol. 6 (Spring 1992).

Painter, Jack W. *Postural Integration: Transformation of the Whole Self.* Mill Valley, Calif.: International Center for Release and Integration, 1986.

Pasternak, Rachel. "Dr. Alexander Lowen: Let Your Body Talk." *East/West,* April 1989.

Pati, Kumar. "Herbs as Medicine: Interview with Dr. Sharol Tilgner." *Health World,* September/October 1991.

Pearson, Durk, and Sandy Shaw. *Life Extension: A Practical Scientific Approach.* New York: Warner Books, 1982.

———. *The Life Extension Companion.* New York: Warner Books, 1984.

Perrenoud, Annelou. "Hydrotherapy in the Swiss Alps: The Old and the New." *Massage Therapy Journal,* Summer 1990.

Perrigoue-Messer, Terri. *Color Vision.* Diamond Springs, Calif., 1991.

Peterson, Rick. *Reiki: Tradition of Ancient Healing Art Continues.* No date.

Pfrimmer Association Deep Muscle Therapists. *Deep Muscle Therapy: Questions and Answers on Pfrimmer Technique.* Norristown, Pa., no date.

Pierce, Roger. *Rolfing.* Rolf Institute of Structural Integration, 1976.

Pinckney, Callan. *Callanetics: 10 Years Younger in 10 Hours.* New York: William Morrow, 1984.

Poleski, John S. "Link Crystalizes between Mind, Energy, Health." *New Visions Journal,* August 1992.

Pounds, Laraine. "Holistic Aromatherapy." *Beginnings,* March 1992.

Powers of Healing. Alexandria, Va.: Time-Life Books, no date.

Pritikin, Nathan. *Pritikin Program for Diet and Exercise.* New York: Grosset & Dunlap, 1979.

Pritikin, Robert. *The New Pritikin Program.* New York: Simon & Schuster, 1990.

Program Information (Rice Diet). Durham, N.C.: Duke University Medical Center: Kempner Clinic, no date.

Prudden, Bonnie. *Pain Erasure the Bonnie Prudden Way.* New York: M. Evans & Co., 1980.

Quinn, Janet. "Therapeutic Touch: The Empowerment of Love." *New Realities,* May/June 1987.

Radiance Technique Association International. *The Radiance Technique: A Transcendental Energy Science.* St. Petersburg, Fla., no date.

Raphaell, Katrina. "Crystals: The Next Step." *Body, Mind & Spirit,* November/December 1989.

Ray, Barbara. "The Radiance Technique." *Radiance Technique Journal,* January/March 1987.

Reiki Alliance. *The Usui System of Natural Healing.* Cotaldo, Idaho, no date.

Reiki Healing Institute. *Reiki: Healing Yourself and Others.* Encinitas, Calif., no date.

Reilly, Harold J., and Ruth Hagy Brod. *The Edgar Cayce Handbook for Health through Drugless Therapy.* New York: Macmillan Publishing, 1975.

"The Rice Diet: Forty Years of Progress." *Bulletin of the Walter Kempner Foundation,* vol. 5, no. 1 (October 1982).

Robbins, Jhan, and David Fisher. *Tranquility without Pills (All about Transcendental Meditation)*. New York: Peter H. Wyden, 1972.

Roberts, Nancy. *The Yoga Thing*. New York: Hawthorn Books, 1973.

Rockman, Stephen D. *Introduction to Bioenergetics and Character Structure*. Dana Point, Calif., no date.

Rodale, J. I., et al. *The Complete Book of Vitamins*. Emmaus, Pa.: Rodale Books, 1966.

Rogers, Sherry A. "Mechanisms of Macrobiotics: Thirty-two Scientific Validations." *Macrobiotics Today*, July/August 1990.

Rolf, Ida P. *What In the World Is Rolfing? An Introduction to Structural Integration: A Technique of Human Well Being*. Santa Monica, Calif.: Dennis-Landman, 1975.

Rolf Institute of Structural Integration. *Rolfing and Rolfing Movement Integration: The Whole Body Approach to Well-Being*. Boulder, Colo., 1991.

Rosenberg, Harold, and A. N. Feldzamen. *The Doctor's Book of Vitamin Therapy: Megavitamins for Health*. New York: G. P. Putnam's Sons, 1974.

Rosenfeld, Albert. "Teaching the Body How to Program the Brain is Moshe's Miracle." *Smithsonian*, January 1981.

Ross, Harvey. *Orthomolecular Psychiatry, Then, Now and Tomorrow*. Boca Raton, Fla.: Huxley Institute, no date.

Rossiter, Charles. *Why Poetry Therapy*. No date.

Rossman, Martin L. *Healing Yourself: A Step-by-Step Program for Better Health through Imagery*. New York: Walker and Company, 1987.

Rubenfeld, Ilana. "Beginner's Hands: Twenty-five Years of Simple Rubenfeld Synergy: The Birth of a Therapy." *Somatics*, Spring/Summer 1988.

———. "Ushering in a Century of Integration." *Somatics*, Autumn/Winter 1990–91.

Runck, Bette. *Biofeedback*. Rockville, Md.: U.S. Department of Health and Human Services Publication No. (ADM) 83-1273, 1983.

St. Helena Health Center. *The McDougall Program*. Deer Park, Calif., no date.

Sanders, Shell. "The Ancient Healing Benefits of Thai Massage." *Body, Mind & Spirit*, November/December 1989.

Schrader, Constance. "Modern Alchemy: Holistic High-Tech." *Harpers Bazaar*, April 1988.

Schultz, Linda. "New Age Shiatsu." *The Holistic Health Handbook*, 1978.

Schultz, William. *Shiatsu*. New York: Bell Publishing, 1976.

Scully, Tim. "Biofeedback and Some of Its Non-Medical Uses." *The Holistic Health Handbook*, 1978.

Shane, Richard. Review of *Hakomi Therapy*. *Association of Humanistic Psychology Newsletter*, February 1984.

SHEN Therapy Institute. *Information about SHEN for Health Professionals*. Sausalito, Calif., 1990.

———. *Information on Emotions, Your Body and SHEN Therapy*. Sausalito, Calif., 1990.

———. *SHEN PhysioEmotional Release Therapy*. Sausalito, Calif., no date.

Shone, Ronald. *Creative Visualization: How to Use Imagery and Imagination for Self-Improvement.* Rochester, Vt.: Destiny Books, 1988.

Siegel, Alan. "Dreams: The Mystery That Heals." *The Holistic Health Handbook,* 1978.

Silbey, Uma. *The Concept Crystal Guidebook.* San Francisco: U-Read Publications, 1986.

Sinclair, Marybetts. "A Look at Massage for Children in the United States." *Massage Therapy Journal,* Spring 1991.

Slagle, Priscilla. *The Way Up from Down.* New York: Random House, 1987.

Society of Ortho-Bionomy International. *Ortho-Bionomy: The Homeopathy of Bodywork.* Berkeley, Calif., no date.

Sorensen, Jacki. *Aerobic Dancing.* New York: Rawson, Wade Publishers, 1979.

Speeth, Kathleen Riordan. "The Healing Potential of Meditation." *The Holistic Health Handbook,* 1978.

Stamatakis, Manny. *Rebirthing: The Benefits and Principles of Conscious Connected Breathing.* Laguna Hills, Calif., 1992.

Standard Homeopathic Company. *Homeopathy: What It Is, How It Works.* Los Angeles, 1988.

Stern, Robert M., and William J. Ray. *Biofeedback.* Homewood, Ill.: Dow Jones–Irwin, 1977.

Straus, Charlotte Gerson. "The Gerson Therapy." *Cancer Control Journal,* vol. 3, nos. 1&2 (1975).

Sugrue, Thomas. *The Story of Edgar Cayce: There Is a River.* Rev. ed. Virginia Beach, Va.: A.R.E. Press, 1973.

Svoboda, Robert E. *Parkruti: Your Ayurvedic Constitution.* Albuquerque, N.M.: Geocom, Ltd., 1989.

Taber, Jerriann J. *Eye-Robics.* El Cajon, Calif.: Vision Training Institute, no date.

Tarshis, Barry. *DMSO: The True Story of a Remarkable Pain-killing Drug.* New York: William Morrow, 1981.

Teeguarden, Iona Marsaa. "Acupressure and Communication with the Unconscious Mind." *Jin Shin Do Acupressure Newsletter,* Fall/Winter 1991–92.

———. "Touch to Help Heal Abuse." *Jin Shin Do Acupressure Newsletter,* Fall/Winter 1991–92.

Thie, John F., with Mary Marks. *Touch for Health.* Santa Monica, Calif.: DeVross, 1973.

Thomson, Bill. "Assessing Alternative Practices." *Natural Health,* May/June 1992.

Tierra, Michael. *Planetary Herbology.* Santa Fe, N.M.: Lotus Press, 1988.

Touch for Health Association. *Touch for Health Is the Difference: What Is Touch for Health?* Pasadena, Calif., no date.

Toufexis, Anastasia. "The New Scoop on Vitamins." *Time,* April 6, 1992.

Trager Institute. *Trager Psychophysical Integration and Mentastics.* Mill Valley, Calif., 1984.

Travel, Janet. *Office Hours: Day and Night.* New York: World Publishing, 1968.

Tribe, Bill. "Naturopathic Medicine." *The Holistic Health Handbook,* 1978.

Ullman, Dana. *Homeopathy: Medicine for the Twenty-first Century.* Berkeley, Calif.: North Atlantic Books, 1988.

Upledger Institute. *CranioSacral Therapy I.* Palm Beach Gardens, Fla., no date.

————. *Discover the CranioSacral System.* Palm Beach Gardens, Fla., 1991.

————. *The Upledger Institute Comprehensive Brochure.* Palm Beach Gardens, Fla., no date.

Upledger, John E. *Somato-Emotional Release.* Palm Beach Gardens, Fla.: Upledger Institute, no date.

————. *The Therapeutic Value of the CranioSacral System.* Palm Beach Gardens, Fla.: Upledger Institute, no date.

Valentine, Tom. *Psychic Surgery.* Chicago: Henry Regnery, 1973.

Vallé, Esther, and John Veltheim. *Reiki Informational Brochure,* no date.

Van Straten, Michael. *The Complete Natural Health Consultant.* New York: Prentice-Hall, 1987.

Van Why, Richard P. "A Brief History and Exhortation Concerning Massage Therapy in America." *Massage Therapy Journal,* Winter 1992.

————. "Cornelius E. De Puy, M.D., Father of Massage Therapy in the United States." *Massage Therapy Journal,* Summer 1991.

Vega Study Center. *The Macrobiotic Dietary Approach.* Oroville, Calif., no date.

Villoldo, Alberto, and Stanley Krippner. *Healing States.* New York: Simon & Schuster, Fireside, 1986.

Vithoulkas, George. *Homeopathy: Medicine of the New Man.* New York: Arco Publishing, 1979.

Vlamis, Gregory. "Interview with Pierre Pannetier." *The Holistic Health Handbook,* 1978.

Wagenheim, Jeff. "Body Rebuilder." *New Age Journal,* November/December 1989.

Walker, Morton. *The Chelation Way: The Complete Book of Chelation Therapy.* Garden City Park, N.Y.: Avery Publishing Group, 1990.

Walker, Morton, with William Campbell Douglass. *DMSO: The New Healing Power.* Old Greenwich, Conn.: Devin-Adair, 1983.

Wallis, Claudia. "Why New Age Medicine Is Catching On." *Time,* November 4, 1991.

Warkentin, David, and Jonathan Shore. "Homeopathy." *Resonance,* vol. 12.

Wastrack-Tarnofsky, Yosel. "Thailand Medical Message." *Life Lines,* Fall 1991.

Weinman, Ric A. *Your Hands Can Heal: Learn to Channel Healing Energy.* New York: E. P. Dutton, 1988.

Weinstein, Emily. "A Healing Tool: Poetry Boosts Therapy." *ADVANCE: A Weekly News Exchange for Occupational Therapists,* vol. 3, no. 46 (November 16, 1987).

Weiss, Ann E. *Biofeedback: Fact or Fad.* New York: Franklin Watts, Impact Book, 1984.

Weiss, Brian L. "Many Lives, Many Masters." *Venture Inward,* July/August 1990.

Wellness Institute for Personal Transformation. *Personal Transformation Report.* Penryn, Calif., March 1992.

Wetherbee, Roberta J. "President's Message." *Dramascope*, Fall 1991.

"What Is Macrobiotics." *Solstice Magazine.*

Wheeler, Barbara, Iona Marsaa Teeguarden, D. V. Smith, and M. Stettler. *Learn the Secrets of Jin Shin Do Bodymind Acupressure.* Palo Alto, Calif.: Jin Shin Do Foundation for Bodymind Acupressure, 1991.

Whiton, Sherril. "Color Theory." *Interior Design and Decoration.* 4th ed. Philadelphia: J. B. Lippincott, 1974.

Wigmore, Ann. *The Wheatgrass Book: How to Grow and Use Wheatgrass to Maximize Your Health and Vitality.* Wayne, N.J.: Avery Publishing Group, 1985.

Willert, Gail. "The Practice of Physical Therapy and Massage Therapy: A Cooperative Approach." *Massage Therapy Journal*, Summer 1990.

Williams, Ellen G. "Soma Bodywork." *Massage Magazine*, October/November 1989.

Wine, Zhenya Kurashova. "From Russia with Love." *Massage Therapy Journal*, Fall 1989.

———. "Russian Massage: Putting It All Together." *Massage Magazine*, January/February 1992.

Winters, Catherine. "Guru on the Go; Is the Maharishi's Man a Visionary or Huckster?" *American Health*, January/February 1992.

Wooten, Sandra. "Relaxation of the Soul: My Experience in Russia." *RMPA Views*, March 1991.

———. *Rosen Method Bodywork.* Berkeley, Calif.: Halcyon Health Group, no date.

Wright, Pamela Amelia. "Chakra Clearing." *The Holistic Health Handbook*, 1978.

Wyrick, Dana L. "Dr. Vodder's Manual Lymph Drainage." *Ontario Massage Therapist Association Newsletter*, April/May 1988.

Yamamoto, Shizuko, with Patrick McCarty. "Revolutionary Health Care." *Healthways*, Fall/Winter 1991.

Zisk, Gary. *The Amino Acid Super Diet.* New York: G. P. Putnam's Sons, 1988.

❈ ❈ ❈

Further Reading

Books

Alternative Medicine: The Definitive Guide. Burton Goldberg Group (Future Medicine Publishing, 1993).

Alternative Medicine: Expanding Medical Horizons. National Institute of Health (Diane Publishing, 1995).

Aromatherapy: The Encyclopedia of Plants and Essential Oils and How They Help You (Bantam Books, 1993)   ·

Aromatherapy: A Lifetime Guide to Healing with Essential Oils. Valerie Gennari Cooksley (Prentice-Hall, 1995).

Acupressure's Potent Points: A Guide to Self-Care for Common Ailments. Michael Gach (Bantam Books, 1990).

Bach Flower Therapy: Theory and Practice. Mechthild Scheffer (Inner Traditions, 1987).

Back to Eden: The Classic Guide to Herbal Medicine: Natural Foods, and Home Remedies since 1939. Kloss Jethro (Back to Eden Books, 1989).

The Book of Massage. Lucy Lidell (Simon & Schuster, Fireside, 1984).

The Book of Sound Therapy. Olivia Dewhurst-Maddock (Simon & Schuster, Fireside, 1993).

Chinese Herbal Medicine. Daniel P. Reid (Shambala Publications, 1987).

Color Therapy, Ruben Amber (Aurora Press, 1993).

Conscious Breathing: Breathwork for Health, Stress Release, and Personal Mastery, Gay Hendricks, Ph.D. (Bantam, 1995).

The Consumer's Guide to Homeopathy: The Definitive Resource to Understanding

Homeopathic Medicine and Making It Work for You, Dana Ullman (Putnam, Jeremy P. Tarcher, 1996).

Encyclopedia of Homeopathy, 2nd ed., Trevor Smith (Atrium Publishers Group, 1994).

Encyclopedia of Natural Medicine, Michael Murray and Joseph Pizzorno (Prima Publishing, 1991).

Everybody's Guide to Homeopathic Medicines, Stephen Cummings and Dana Ullman, (Jeremy P. Tarcher, 1991).

The Family Herbal, Barbara Thesis and Peter Thesis (Inner Traditions, 1993).

Food, Your Miracle Medicine, Jean Carper (HarperCollins, 1993).

Healing and the Mind, Bill Moyers (Doubleday, 1993).

Healing Imagery & Music, Carol Bush (Rudra Press, 1995).

Healing with Whole Foods, Paul Pitchford (North Atlantic Books, 1993).

Healing Your Body Naturally, Gary Null (Four Walls Eight Windows, 1992).

Oriental Medicine: An Illustrated Guide to the Asian Arts of Healing, ed. by Jan Van Alphen (Shambala Publications, 1995).

Oxygen Healing Therapies for Optimum Health and Vitality, Nathaniel Altman (Inner Traditions, 1995).

Perfect Health: The Complete Mind-Body Guide, Deepak Chopra, M.D. (Harmony Books, 1991).

Qi Gong: The Chinese Art of Healing with Energy, Tzu Kou Shih (Station Hill Press, 1992).

Remarkable Recovery: What Extraordinary Healings Tell Us About Getting Well and Staying Well, Caryle Hirshberg and Marc Ian Barasch (Riverhead Books, 1996).

The Way of Herbs, 3rd ed., Michael Tierra (Pocket Books, 1990).

Videos

Healing and the Mind (Vols. 1–3). Bill Moyers

Body, Mind and Soul: The Mystery and the Magic (Vol. 1). Deepak Chopra, M.D.

Body, Mind and Soul: The Mechanics of Healing and Transformation (Vol. 2). Deepak Chopra, M.D.

Magazines

Natural Health

Body•Mind•Spirit

New Age Journal

The Natural Way: The Best Alternative Health News and Views

Herbs for Health

Massage Magazine

Yoga Journal

American Health

The Herb Quarterly

The Herb Companion

Total Health

Index

Abrams, Albert, 209, 210
Academy for Guided Imagery, 133, 313
Academy of Orthomolecular Medicine, 184, 317
acid ash, 23, 67, 275
Active Muscular Relaxation Techniques, 1–2
Acupressure Institute, 3, 305
Acupressure Massage, 2–3, 17, 18, 64, 214, 236, 252, 255, 263, 305
  acupoints in, 2, 3, 18, 251, 256
  Five Element Theory of, 20
  Jin Shin Do Bodymind, 138–39, 314
Acupressure Way of Health, The: Jin Shin Do (Teeguarden), 139
Acupuncture, xxi, 3–8, 55, 118, 175, 197, 199, 201, 219–20, 236, 252, 255, 265, 277, 278, 305–6
  acupoints in, 5–6, 18, 91, 123–24, 140, 141, 256, 264, 265
  needles in, 4, 5–6, 7, 92, 156
Adventure in Self-Discovery, The (Grof), 120
Aerobic Dance, 8–10, 50, 137–38, 206
Aerobic Dancing (Sorenson), 10
aerobics, 94–95, 204, 205–6
aging process, 14, 128, 143–44, 184, 186, 204, 270
Ahsen, Akhter, 133
AIDS, 6, 7, 67, 87, 184, 187, 188, 282
Albert Roy Davis Research Laboratory, 315

alcoholism, 6, 13, 14, 15, 17, 28, 131, 144, 184, 202
Alexander, Frederick Mathias, 11, 25, 99, 229
Alexander Technique, 10–12, 36, 99, 161, 166, 228, 229
Alexandria School of Scientific Therapeutics, 192, 318
alkali ash, 23, 67, 275
allergies, 35, 86, 87, 93-94, 180, 184, 245, 265, 282
allopathic medicine, Western, xvii, xx–xxi, 7, 64, 118, 144, 162, 163, 178, 184, 233, 236–37, 269
alpha state, 40–41, 165
Alsans, Ana, 144
American Academy of Medical Acupuncture, 8, 305–6
American Academy of Osteopathy, 186, 243, 317
American Apitherapy Society, 36, 307
American Art Therapy Association, 24, 25, 307
American Association for Music Therapy, 170, 316
American Association of Acupuncture and Oriental Medicine, 8, 305
American Association of Naturopathic Physicians (AANP), 176, 309, 316–17

American Biologics, 314

American Biologics Hospital, 306

American Botanical Council, 118, 311

American Cancer Society, 15, 17

American Center for the Alexander Technique, 12, 306

American Chiropractic Association, 309

American College of Advancement in Medicine, 58, 309

American College of Hyperbaric Medicine, 128, 312–13

American Council of Hypnotist Examiners, 131, 313

American Dance Therapy Association, 78, 79, 310

American Environmental Health Foundation, 94, 311

American Foundation of Traditional Chinese Medicine, 8, 59, 305, 319

American Health Sciences Institute, 101

American Herbalist Guild, 311

American Herb Association, 118, 311–12

American Holistic Medical Association, 119, 312

American Holistic Nurse's Association, 321

American Institute for Cancer Research, 16, 17

American Institute of Asian Studies, 202, 318

American Institute of Homeopathy, 122

American Journal of Medical Science, 58

American Magneto-Therapy Association, 315

American Massage Therapy Association, 160, 161, 162, 240, 241, 249, 315–16, 320

American Medical Association (AMA), 105, 106, 122, 125–26, 130, 210, 217

American Naprapathic Association, 172

American Natural Hygiene Society, 101, 173

American Oriental Bodywork Therapy Association (AOBTA), 3, 238, 252, 305, 317, 320

American Osteopathic Association, 186, 243, 317

American Physical and Physio Therapy Association, 194, 318

American Polarity Therapy Association, 199, 318

American Reflexology Certification Board & Information Service, 215, 319

American School of Ayurvedic Sciences, 307

American Yoga Association, 277, 322

amino acids, 56–58, 143
  free-form, 12–15

Amino Acid Super Diet, The (Zisk), 14

Amino Acid Therapy, 12–15, 270

Amino Revolution, The (Erdmann and Jones), 15

Amma, 236

Ancient Art of Color Therapy, The (Clark), 69

Andrews, Lynn V., 234

Angelica sinensis, 116

Ann Wigmore Foundation, 273, 322

Anticancer Diet, 15–17

antioxidants, 186

antiseptics, 22, 266

anxiety, 14, 158, 202, 203, 236, 260

Applied Kinesiology, 17–19, 64, 255

Applied Physiology, 19–20

Arabs, 113, 154, 193

ARE Medical Clinic, 52, 309

Are You Tense? The Benjamin System of Muscular Therapy (Benjamin), 37

Arica Institute, 81

Aristotle, 154, 195

armoring, 36–37, 215–16, 217

Armstrong, John W., 266–67

Aromatherapie (Valnet), 21

Aromatherapy, 20–23

Aromatherapy Institute of Research, 306

Arthritic's Cookbook, The (Dong), 87

arthritis, 6, 22, 63, 64, 80, 103, 104, 127, 146, 156, 158, 159, 182, 184, 204, 238, 245, 265, 282
  diets for, 23, 85–87, 179–80
  osteo-, 35, 124
  rheumatoid, 35, 98

Arthritis Diet, 23

Arthritis Foundation, 23, 35, 180

arthrosis, 124

Art Therapy, 23–25, 73–74

asanas, 276, 277

aspirin, 116

Associated Bodywork and Massage Professionals, 162, 249, 316

Association for Applied Psychophysiology and Biofeedback, 42, 308

Association for Humanistic Psychology, 318–19

Association for Network Chiropractic Spinal Analysis, 178, 317

Association for Past-Life Research and Therapies, 191, 318

Association for Research and Enlightenment (ARE), 52–53, 54, 309

Association for the Study of Dreams, 90, 310

asthma, 6, 98, 113, 265, 267, 282

Aston, Judith, 25–26

Aston-Patterning, 25–27, 148, 181, 244, 307

Aston Training Center, 27

atherosclerosis, 56–58, 104, 163

Aunty Margaret School of Hawaiian Lomilomi, 314

aura (etheric body), 201–2

Auto-Contractile Pain Response (ACPR), 235

Autogenic Discharge, 28

Autogenic Therapy (Luthe), 29

Autogenic Training, 27–29, 307

Autogenic Training: A Psychophysiologic Approach to Psychotherapy (Schultz and Luthe), 29

autointoxication, 66

autonomic nervous system, 28, 39–40, 188–89, 260

autopsies, 66

Avicenna, 21

Awareness Oriented Structural Therapy, 29–30, 307

Awareness Through Movement, 98, 108, 229

Ayurveda, 30–32, 69, 112, 114, 115–16, 117, 118, 157–58, 197, 307

Ayurveda: The Science of Self-Healing (Lad), 69

Ayurvedic Institute, 32, 307

Babylonians, 112, 126

Bach, Edward, 32–33

Bach Flower Remedies, 32–33, 307

back pain, 2–3, 4, 27, 50, 63, 91, 95, 103, 124, 139, 171, 202, 229, 243, 265, 283, 289

Baird, James, 130

Barefoot Shiatsu, 149, 150

Barefoot Shiatsu (video), 150–51

Bartenieff, Irmgard, 142

Baruch, Simon, 64

Bates, William Horatio, 33–34, 96

Bates-Corbett Method of Vision Training, 96, 311

Bates Method of Vision Training, 33–34, 96

Beasley, Ronald, 178

Becker, Robert O., 92

Bee Venom Therapy, 34–36, 307

Benjamin, Ben E., 36–37

Benjamin System of Muscular Therapy, 36–37, 307

bentonite, 67

beriberi, 269

Bernard Jensen International, 136, 275, 314, 322

Bernsworth, Frederick C., 57

beta-carotene, 16–17

Better Health Through Reflexology (Byers), 215

Beyond Sports Massage: Injury Prevention and Care Through Sports Massage (Hungerford), 241

Beyond the Brain: Birth, Death, and Transcendence (Grof), 120

Bible, 65, 97, 140, 201, 266

Bibliotherapy, 194

Bindegewebsmassage (Connective Tissue Massage), 29, 44, 70–71

Biochemical Way to Health and Happiness (Ishizuka), 151

Biochemic Handbook, The, 232

Bioenergetics, 37–39, 106, 281, 308

Bioenergetics (Lowen), 39

Biofeedback Certification Institute of America, 42, 308

Biofeedback Institute of Los Angeles, 308

Biofeedback Training, 19, 34, 39–42, 108, 132, 165, 179, 308

Biofeedback Training Associates, 308

Biokinesiology Institute, 306

Biomagnetic Therapy (Magnetic Therapy), 154–57, 315

Bio-Medical Center, 126, 312

Birth without Violence (Leboyer), 134

Blanton, Smiley, 195

Bodies in Revolt: A Primer in Somatic Thinking (Hanna), 108

body-care techniques, 37

Body-Centered Psychotherapy (Kurtz), 107

Body Electric, The (Becker), 29

Body Magnetic, The (Payne), 157

Bodywise (Heller and Henkin), 111

bodywork, meaning of term, 161

Bodywork for the Childbearing Year, 42–45, 82, 134, 308

bonesetting, 62–63, 185

Bonnie Prudden Myotherapy, 45–48, 308

Bonnie Prudden School for Physical Fitness and Myotherapy, 47–48, 308

Botanical Medicine, *see* Herbal Medicine

Bowers, Edwin, 213, 214

Bradshaw, John, 178

breathing, 37, 58–59, 119–20, 211–13, 217, 227, 228, 264, 265, 276–77, 312, 319

Brenner, Paul H., xvii–xviii

Bright's disease, 265, 266, 267

Brod, Ruth Hagy, 54

Brodmann, Korbinian, 27

broken bones, 92, 156

Buddhism, 59, 106, 139, 160, 164, 190, 236, 252

Buddhism (cont'd)
Zen, 28, 219, 249
Bulletin of Art Therapy, 24
Burmeister, Mary Ino, 140, 141
bursitis, 35, 63, 85, 124, 263, 284
Burton, Lawrence, 48–49
Burton Treatment (Immuno-Augmentative Therapy [IAT]), 48–49, 308–9
Byers, Dwight C., 214, 215

Caesar, Julius, 160
California Acupuncture Association, 8, 305
California Institute of Integral Studies, 88
Callanetics, 49–51
Callanetics: 10 Years Younger in 10 Hours (Pinckney), 50
cancer, 66, 84, 105, 133, 145, 146, 184, 186, 187, 188, 203, 222, 266, 267, 270, 284
Anticancer Diet and, 15–17
Burton Treatment for, 48–49, 308–9
Hoxsey Treatment for, 125–26, 312
as yin disease, 5
carpal tunnel syndrome, 91, 284
Castaneda, Carlos, 233
Caster, Paul, 63
candidiasis, 116, 284
cataracts, 33, 58, 284
cave paintings, 253
Cayce, Edgar, 52–54
Cayce (Edgar) Therapies, 51–53, 54, 309
Cayce/Reilly Massage, 53–54
cayenne pepper, 117
cellular memory, 178–79
Cellular Therapy (Live Cell Therapy), 144–45, 314
Center for Applied Physiology-Menninger Clinic, 308
Center for Biotherapeutics/Hoshino Therapy Clinic, 124, 312
Certification Board for Music Therapists, 170
Chakra Balancing, 54–56, 69, 76
chakras, 54–56, 69, 77, 201, 235
Chakra Samhita, 112
Chung San-feng, 249–50
character analysis, 39
Chelation Therapy, xxi, 56–58, 309
Chemical Theory of Longevity (Ishizuka), 151
Cheng Man-Ch'ing, 250, 251
chi, xxii, 2–3, 5–6, 58, 59, 140–41, 198, 201, 235, 236–38, 251, 264
Chia, Mantak, 60
Chi Kung (Qi Gong), 58–59, 264, 265, 319
Childers, Norman, 180

Children Massage, 60–61
China, 2–8, 62, 85–87, 97, 121, 126, 132, 139, 140, 160, 192, 197, 198, 235, 236, 269
Chi Kung in, 58–59
Color Therapy in, 68
Herbal Medicine in, 111, 112, 114–15, 116–17
Magnetic Therapy in, 154
Tai Chi Chuan in, 249–51
Tui Na Massage Therapy in, 263–65
see also Acupressure Massage; Acupuncture
Chi Nei Tsang (Chia), 60
Chi Nei Tsang (Internal Organ Massage), 59–60
Chinese College of Acupuncture, 277, 278
Chinese medicine, traditional, 2–8, 58–60, 86, 111, 112, 114, 115, 118, 123, 135, 149, 252, 264
Chiropractic, 2, 17–19, 52, 61–64, 118, 162, 172, 219, 255–56, 309
Network, 176–78, 317
chlorophyll, 271, 272
cholesterol, 56, 163, 204, 205, 221, 222
Chopra, Deepak, 158
Chua Ka, 80, 81
cinnamon, 112, 117
circulatory system, 8, 9, 22, 56, 79, 102–3, 128, 147–48, 155, 156, 186, 292
Clarity Productions, 213, 319
Clark, Linda, 69
Clarke, Norman E., 57–58
Clinical Ecology (Environmental Medicine), 93–94, 311
coffee enemas, 67, 105
Colon Health Handbook, The: New Health through Colon Rejuvenation (Gray), 67
Colon Therapy, 64–67, 309–10
Color Therapy, 55, 56, 67–69, 76, 310
Complete Herbal, The (Culpeper), 21, 113
Compression Massage, 79, 239, 240
connective tissue (fascia), 29, 74, 82, 110, 170–72, 199–200, 222–25, 244–45, 262–63
Connective Tissue Massage (*Bindegewebsmassage*), 29, 44, 70–71
Conquest of Cancer (Livingston), 146
constipation, 59, 168
Copeman, W. S. C., 261
Corbett, Margaret Darst, 96
core beliefs, 106
core issue, 149
cortisol, 3, 7
CranioSacral Therapy, 18, 71–73, 181, 186, 268, 310

CranioSacral Therapy (Upledger), 73
CranioSacral Therapy II (Upledger), 73
Creative Arts Therapy, 73–74
Cross-Fiber Friction Massage, 44, 74–75, 80, 148, 239, 240
Crown Zellerbach Corporation, 84
Cryotherapy (Ice Therapy), 75–76, 194, 239, 240
Crystal (Gem) Therapy, 55, 56, 76–78, 310
Culpeper, Nicholas, 21, 113
Curative Properties of Honey and Bee Venom (Yourish), 35
Cyriax, James H., 36, 74

Dance of the Deer Foundation, 234, 320
Dance Therapy, 73–74, 78–79, 142, 310
  see also Aerobic Dance
daoyin, 58–59
Dark Ages, 62, 113, 193
Davis, Roy Eugene, 164
Deal, Sheldon, 19
Deep Bodywork and Personal Development, Harmonizing Our Bodies, Emotions, and Thoughts (Painter), 201
Deep Compression Massage, 79, 239, 240
Deep Tissue Massage, 80, 109, 110
Deep Tissue Sculpting (Muscle Sculpting), 44, 80–83, 310
Deep Tissue Sculpting: A Technical and Artistic Manual for Therapeutic Bodywork Practitioners (Osborne–Sheets), 83
Deep Tissue Therapies, 29, 44, 74, 148
De Materia Medica (Dioscorides), 112–13
dementia, 14, 269
depression, 14–15, 32, 64, 68, 139, 184, 196, 203, 236, 270, 286
De Puy, Cornelius, E., 161
Dharuma, 249
diabetes, 17, 28, 58, 98, 156, 163, 203, 204–5, 267, 286
Diagnosis from the Eye (Liljequist), 136
Diamond, Harvey and Marilyn, 100–101, 173–74
Dicke, Elizabeth, 70, 71
diet, 4, 13, 65, 66, 67, 85, 97–98, 125, 199, 204, 255, 267
  Fit for Life Program and, 100–101, 173, 174
  rotary diversified, 94
  typical modern, 65, 86, 291
  vegan, 162
  vegetarian, 146, 267, 321
  see also specific diets
digitalis, 114
dimethyl sulfoxide (DMSO) Therapy, 83–85

Dinshah Health Society, 310
Dioscorides, 112–13
directos, 172
DMSO: The New Healing Power (Walker), 85
DMSO Therapy, 83–85
DMSO: The Remarkable Story of a Pain Killing Drug (Tarshis) 85
Do-In, 236
Dong, Colin H., 85–87
Dong Diet, 23, 85–87
doshas, 31, 69, 115–16
Drama Therapy, 73–74, 87–88, 310
dream incubation, 88
Dream Network: A Quarterly Journal Exploring Dreams and Myths, 90, 310
Dream Therapy, 88–90, 310
Dreamtime and Dreamwork (Krippner), 89
Drown, Ruth, 209–10
Dr. Vodder School–Walchsee, 315
Duggan, Joseph and Sandra, 54
Duke University Medical Center, 221–22, 319
dyslexia, 20, 72

Earp-Thomas, G. H., 271
eating disorders, 236, 282, 286
Ebers Papyrus, 65, 112
Edgar Cayce Handbook for Health through Drugless Therapy, The (Reilly and Brod), 52–53, 54
Edgar Cayce's Massage Hydrotherapy, and Healing Oils (Duggan and Duggan), 54
Edgar Cayce Therapies, 51–53, 54, 309
effleurage, 54, 160, 248
Egoscue, Pete, 90–91
Egoscue Method, 90–91, 310
Egoscue Method of Healing Through Motion, The (Egoscue), 91
Egypt, ancient, 20–21, 62, 65, 68, 88, 97, 126, 129, 154, 160, 192, 235, 253
  Herbal Medicine in, 111, 112
Ehret, Arnold, 167–68
Electrotherapy, 6, 62, 91–92, 156, 174, 194
Elizabeth I, Queen of England, 113
Elizabeth II, Queen of England, 123
Ellon U.S.A., Inc., 33, 307
emotional programs, suppressed, 178–79
emotional stress, 32–33, 36–37, 39, 81, 83, 87, 95, 110, 138, 139, 141, 182, 199, 202–4, 234–36, 238–39, 286
emphysema, 58, 286
endorphins, 3, 6–7, 15, 92
enemas, 65, 66–67, 105
energy cyst, 238–39

Energy: The Vital Principle in the Healing Art (Stone), 197

England, 21, 68, 113, 123, 210, 253, 259, 266, 269, 272, 278

Environmental Dental Association, 94, 311

environmental evaluation, 25, 27, 148

Environmental Medicine (Clinical Ecology), 93–94, 311

Enviro-Tech Products, 315

Epstein, Donald, 177

ephedra, 114

Erdmann, Robert, 15

Ericksonian Hypnotherapy, 106, 228, 229

Esalen Institute, 26, 223, 229, 257

Esalen Style Massage, 82, 189

Eskimos, 266

essential oils, 20–23

est (Erhard Seminar Training), 211

Estebany, Colonel Oscar, 253–54

etheric body (aura), 201–2

ethylenediaminetetraacetic acid (EDTA), 56–58

Exercise Therapy, 4, 17, 37, 52, 94–95, 127, 166, 175, 193, 265
    aerobic, 94–95, 204, 205–6; *see also* Aerobic Dance
    isometric, 1, 94
    see also specific Exercise Therapies

Expanded Reference Manual of the Radiance Technique, The (Ray), 208

Eydan, I., 155

Eye-Robics, 96, 311

Eye-Robics (Taber), 96

eyes:
    disorders of, 33–34, 58, 96, 284, 292–93, 311
    Iridology of, 135–36, 314

fascia (connective tissue), 29, 74, 82, 110, 170–72, 199–200, 222–25, 244–45, 262–63

Fasting, 97–98, 127, 167, 168, 174, 266, 267, 273

Feathered Pipe Ranch, 275

feet, 103, 127, 245, 282, 284
    Reflexology of, 44, 66, 147, 155, 213–15, 319

Feet First: A Guide to Reflexology (Norman), 215

Feldenkrais, Moshe, 25, 98–99, 108–9, 229

Feldenkrais Guild, 99–100, 311

Feldenkrais Method, 98–100, 106, 148, 161, 166, 181, 228, 311

Field, Tiffany, 134

"fight or flight" response, 27, 60, 188

Fischer, Hans, 272

Fit for Life, 316

Fit for Life (Diamond and Diamond), 101, 173

Fit for Life II—Living Health (Diamond and Diamond), 101, 173

Fit for Life Program, 100–101, 173–74

Fitzgerald, William H., 213, 214

Florida Institute of Natural Health & Florida Massage School, 29–30, 307

Flower Essence Society, 307

Food Alive: A Diet for Cancer and Chronic Disease (Livingston), 146

Food and Drug Administration, U.S. (FDA), 15, 85, 122, 126, 156, 188, 210, 217

Foods That Heal: A Guide to Understanding and Using the Healing Powers of Natural Foods (Jensen), 275

Foot Reflexology Awareness Association, 215, 319

free radicals, 186, 187

Freud, Sigmund, 38, 88–89, 130, 190, 195, 215, 216, 246

Fritz, Norman, 105–6

Fry, T. C., 173

Fuller, Buckminster, 229

Functional Integration, 98, 108, 229

Function of the Orgasm, The (Reich), 38

Furumoto, Phyllis Lei, 219

gag reflex, 217

Galen, 65, 112, 113, 116, 126, 154, 160

gangrene, 128, 266, 267

Garfield, Patricia, 89

gastrointestinal disorders, 2–3, 6, 22, 158, 245, 251, 287, 289

Gateway Research Institute, 320–21

Gattefossé, Rene M., 21

Gem (Crystal) Therapy, 55, 56, 76–78, 310

George Ohsawa Macrobiotic Foundation, 152, 154, 314

Geriatric Massage, 102–3

Germany, 22, 27, 34, 35, 57, 62, 70, 121, 160, 187, 195, 226

Gerovital (GH$_3$) Therapy, 144

Gerson, Charlotte, 105

Gerson, Max, 103–6

Gerson Institute, 106, 306, 311

Gerson Therapy, 67, 103–6, 311

Gerson Therapy Center of Mexico, 106, 188

Gestalt Therapy, 29, 81, 106, 199, 223, 228, 229

Getting Better, 184

Getting Started in Magnetic Healing (Payne), 157

Gindler, Elsa, 226
ginseng, 116, 117
Goodheart, George, 17–18, 255
gout, 35, 155, 204, 287
Graham, Sylvester, 173
Gram, Hans, 122
Gray, Robert, 67
Greece, ancient, 21, 62, 65, 68, 88, 97, 121, 126, 129, 140, 154, 160, 190, 192, 195, 265
  Herbal Medicine in, 112, 113, 114, 116
Greek language, 56, 108, 119, 120, 126, 149, 151, 170, 181, 182, 184
Green, Barry, 81, 82
Green, Elmer and Alyce, 41, 238
Green Pharmacy (Griggs), 118
Greifer, Eli, 195
Griggs, Barbara, 118
Grof, Christina, 119
Grof, Stanislav, 119, 120
Grof Transpersonal Training, Inc., 120, 312
gua sha, 4
Guru Dev, 259
gynecological disorders, 2–3, 6, 287, 290
  menstrual, 22, 202, 236, 265, 290, 291
Gypsies, 265

Hahn, Johann Siegmund, 127
Hahnemann, Samuel Christian, 32, 121
hair, graying, 128
Hakomi Bodywork, 106–7
Hakomi Institute, 107, 311
Hakomi Method of Body Mind Therapy, 29, 106–7, 218, 311
Hall effect, 156
Halpern, Steven, 169
hamma, 123
Hamilton, Richard, 242
Handbook of SHEN, The (Pavek), 236
Hanna, Thomas, 108
Hanna Somatic Education (Somatic Education), 107–9, 311
Harner, Michael, 233–34
Hatha Yoga, 30, 157, 276
Hawaiians, 146–48, 233
hawthorn berry, 116
headaches, 42, 72, 98, 116, 124, 139, 158, 171, 202, 287
  migraine, 2–3, 28, 41, 63, 103–4, 236, 238, 243
Healing Power of Dreams, The (Garfield), 89
Healing Power of Poetry, The (Blanton), 195
Healing States (Villoldo and Krippner), 234
Healing Within: The Complete Colon Health Guide (Weinberger), 67

Healing Yourself: A Step-by-Step Program for Better Health through Imagery (Rossman), 133
HealthPlex Clinic, 73
heart disease, 14, 17, 41, 56, 57, 64, 114, 116, 128, 163, 196, 203, 204–5, 221–22, 267, 270, 282, 288
heat, 76, 192, 194
  moxabustion, 4, 6, 150, 264
heavy metals, 56–58, 288
Heller, Joseph, 109–11, 224
Hellerwork, 80, 109–11, 161, 224, 244, 311
Hellerwork, Inc., 111, 311
Helm, Bill, 265
Henkin, William A., 111
Herbal Medicine, 4, 20–23, 32–33, 52, 64, 65, 66, 67, 111–18, 121, 125–26, 174, 175, 197, 264, 307, 311, 312
  in shamanism, 111, 232–33
herbals, 111, 112, 113
Herb Research Foundation, 118, 312
Herb Society of America, 118, 312
herpes, 14, 15, 288
Herschler, Robert, 84
Heyer, Lucy, 226
Hieronymus, T. G., 210
high blood pressure, 41, 58, 59, 63, 64, 95, 133, 158, 163, 203, 204, 205, 221, 222, 251, 288
Hinduism, 97, 126, 160, 190, 252
Hippocrates, 35, 62, 65, 75, 88, 112, 120, 160, 185, 269, 274
Hippocrates Diet and Health Plan, The (Wigmore), 273
histamine, 14, 35
History of Plants, A (Le Strange), 118
Hoffer, Abram, 183
Holistic Medicine, 13, 30, 52, 54, 98, 113, 118–19, 132, 150, 185, 245, 312
Holotropic Breathwork, 119–20, 312
Home Health Products, Inc., 309
Homeopathic Educational Services, 123, 312
Homeopathic Pharmacopoeia of the United States, 122
Homeopathy, 32, 118, 120–23, 174, 175, 220, 312
  Schuessler Cell Salts in, 231–32, 320
homeostasis, 2–3, 20, 157, 243, 256
Homer, 160
hormones, 13, 22, 35, 60, 95, 97
Hoshino, Tomezo, 25, 123–24
Hoshino Exercises, 124
Hoshino Therapy, 123–24, 312

Hoxsey, Harry M., 125–26
Hoxsey Treatment, 125–26, 312
Huang Fu, 46
Huang-ti, Yellow Emperor, 4, 112, 160, 236, 250
Huang-ti Nei-Ching (*The Yellow Emperor's Classic of Internal Medicine*), 2, 4, 112, 160, 252, 264
Huichol, 233
Hull, Charles, 130
humors, biological, 116
Hungerford, Myk, 240, 241
Huxley, Aldous, 11, 34
Huxley Institute for Biosocial Research, 184
Hyashi, Chujiro, 219
Hydrotherapy, 52, 126–28, 174, 175, 192, 194, 239
    Colon, 64–67, 309–10
Hyperbaric Oxygenation Therapy, 128, 312–13
Hypnosis and Suggestibility (Hull), 130
Hypnotherapy, 27–28, 128–31, 191, 313
    Ericksonian, 106, 228, 229
hypoglycemia, 183, 184

IAT, Ltd. Centre, 48, 49, 308–9
Ice Therapy (Cryotherapy), 75–76, 194, 239, 240
ICMA-Physician Referral, 318
Imagery and Visualization, xxi, 132–33, 313
immune system, 35, 48–49, 60, 95, 116, 145–46, 157, 165, 202, 272
Immuno-Augmentative Therapy (IAT) (Burton Treatment), 48–49, 308–9
Immunology Research Center, 49
impotence, 6, 289
In and Out of the Garbage Pail (Perls), 223
Incas, 62, 192
India, 43, 62, 68, 121, 133, 140, 154, 198, 232, 235, 236, 249, 253, 269
    Ayurveda of, 30–32, 69, 112, 114, 115–16, 117, 118, 157–58, 197, 307
    Herbal Medicine in, 111, 112, 114, 115–16, 118
    Massage Therapy in, 160, 252
    Vedas of, 21, 30, 112, 275
    Yoga of, 28, 30, 40, 54, 58–59, 157, 164, 197, 199, 206, 207, 252, 275–77, 322
Infant Massage, 43, 44, 45, 133–35, 313–14
Infant Massage: A Handbook for Loving Parents (Schneider-McClure), 134–35
influenza, 5, 285
Ingham, Eunice, 214–15

Inner Bridges, a Guide to Energy Movement and Body Structure (Smith), 279
insomnia, 2–3, 14, 15, 139, 158, 260, 289
Institute for Bioenergetics and Gestalt, 39, 308
Institute for Noetic Sciences, 316
Instituto Genesis West-Provida, 306
Integrative Bodywork Consultants, 83, 310
Internal Organ Massage (Chi Nei Tsang), 59–60
International Association of Holistic Health Practitioners, 119, 312
International Association of Infant Massage Instructors, 133, 134, 313
International Association of Professional Natural Hygienists, 101, 174, 316
International Association of Yoga Therapists, 277, 322
International Center for Release and Integration, 201, 318
International College of Applied Kinesiology, 19, 306
International Committee for Autogenic Training, 29, 307
International Foundation for Homeopathy, 123, 312
International Institute for Bioenergetic Analysis, 38, 39, 308
International Institute of Applied Physiology, 20, 306
International Institute of Reflexology, 215, 319
International Loving Touch Foundation, Inc., 134, 313
International Macrobiotic Shiatsu Society (IMSS), 150–51
International Medical and Dental Hypnotherapy Association, 131, 313
International Medical Center, 306
International Movement Therapy Association (IMTA), 165–66
International Ozone Association, 188, 318
International Professional School of Bodywork, 43, 82, 83, 310
International SHEN Therapy Association (ISTA), 236, 320
International Sports Massage Federation and Training Institute, 240, 241, 320
Introduction to Dr. Vodder's Manual Lymphatic Drainage, 160
Iridology, 135–36, 314
Ishizuka, Sagen, 151
isometrics, 1, 94
isotonics, 94
Issel, Christine, 215

Jacob, Stanley, 84
Jacobson, Edwin, 38
Jaguar Woman, The (Andrews), 234
Janov, Arthur, 202–4
Japan, 15, 123, 132, 138, 139–41, 150,
    151, 155, 156, 157, 160, 198,
    218–20, 236–38, 269
Jaques-Dalcroze, Emile, 38
Jazzercise, 137–38
Jazzercise Workout Book, The (Missett), 138
Jefferson, Thomas, 113
Jennings, Isaac, 173
Jensen, Bernard, 136, 273–74, 275
Jin Shin Do Bodymind Acupressure,
    138–39, 314
Jin Shin Do Foundation for Bodymind Acu-
    pressure, 139, 314
Jin Shin Jyutsu, 139–41, 314
Jin Shin Jyutsu, Inc., 141, 314
John Bastyr University, 175, 317
joint disorders, 6, 7, 12, 103, 156, 207, 251
    Bee Venom Therapy for, 34–36
    gout, 35, 155, 204, 287
    see also arthritis
joint mobilization therapy, 44
Jones, Lawrence, 181, 186, 243
Jones, Meirion, 15
Jordan, Kate, 43, 134
Journal of Orthomolecular Medicine, 184
Journal of the American Medical Association
    (JAMA), 125–26
Joy of Feeling, The: Bodymind Acupressure (Tee-
    guarden), 139
Jung, Carl, 89, 138

Kagan, Alfred, 36
kahunas, 147, 233
Kairos, 109–10
kapha, 31, 115, 116
Karni, Ziv, 238–39
Keble, John, 195
Kellogg, John Harvey, 127
Kempner, Walter, 221–22
Kempner Rice Diet, 220–22, 319
Kennedy, John F., 46, 261
kidney disease, 58, 265, 289
Killinger, John, 60
Kim, Christopher, 35
Kinesiology, Applied, 17–19, 64, 255
"King's Touch," 253
Kneipp, Father Sebastian, 126–27, 174
Kojiki, 140
Kong-Fu, 192
Kraus, Hans, 46
Krieger, Dolores, 253–54, 255

Krippner, Stanley, 89, 234
Kuhnau, Wolfram, 145, 314
Kunz, Dora, 253–54
Kurtz, Ron, 106–7, 218
Kushi, Aveline, 154
Kushi, Michio, 153–54
Kushi Institute of the Berkshires, 154, 314,
    315
kyphosis, 103

Laban, Rudolf, 142
Laban/Bartenieff Institute of Movement
    Studies, 142, 314
Laban Movement Analysis, 142, 314
labor massage, 43
Lad, Vasant, 69
Lancet, 15
Lange, Max, 46
Lao-Tzu, 250
laser light, 6
laying-on of hands, 208, 253
laying-on of stones, 77
Layne, Al, 51–52
Learning Strategies Corporation, 321
Leboyer, Frederick, 134, 135
Lee, Elmer, 64
Leedy, Jack J., 195–96, 197
Lerner, Arthur, 197
Le Strange, Richard, 118
Lew, Share K., 264, 265
Life Extension, 143–44, 265, 270, 289, 314
Life Extension: A Practical Scientific Approach
    (Pearson and Shaw), 14, 143
Life Extension Companion, The (Pearson and
    Shaw), 143
Life Extension Foundation, 144, 314
Life Science (Natural Hygiene), 98, 100,
    101, 172–74, 316
Lifestream Associates, 310
Liljequist, Nils, 136
Lillard, Harvey, 63
Lind, James, 269
Ling, Per Hendrik, 160–61, 193, 247–48
Linus Pauling Institute of Science and Medi-
    cine, 270, 321
Live Cell Therapy (Cellular Therapy),
    144–45, 314
Live Cell Therapy (Kuhnau), 145, 314
Livingston, Virginia Wuerthele-Caspe, 146
Livingston Foundation Medical Center, 146,
    314
Livingston Treatment, 145–46, 314
Lomilomi Massage, 146–48, 314
Loneliness of Children, The (Killinger), 60
Looyen, Ted, 148

LooyenWork, 148–49
lordosis, 83
Loving Hands: The Traditional Indian Art of Baby Massage (Leboyer), 135
Loving Relationships Training (LRT) International, 213, 319
Lowen, Alexander, 38–39, 218
lucid dreaming, 88, 89
Lucidity Association (Lucid Dreaming), 90, 310
lumbago, 35, 245
lupus, 104, 146, 289
Lust, Benedict, 174
Luthe, Wolfgang, 28, 29
Luyties Pharmacal Company, 232, 320
Lymphatic Drainage, Manual, 44, 158–60, 186, 189, 315

McCabe, Ed, 187, 188
McCarty, Patrick, 150
McDougall, John A., 162–64
McDougall, William, 130
McDougall Diet, 162–64, 221, 316
McDougall Program, The: Twelve Days to Dynamic Health (McDougall), 163–64
Machado, Margaret "Aunty," 146–47, 148, 314
Macrae, Janet, 255
Macrobiotic Approach to Cancer, The: Towards Preventing and Controlling Cancer with Diet and Lifestyle (Kushi), 153–54
Macrobiotics, 149–50, 151–54, 221, 314–15
Macrobiotic Shiatsu, 149–51
Macrobiotics Today, 154
Magnetic Therapy· (Biomagnetic Therapy), 154–57, 315
Maharishi Ayur-Veda, 157–58, 315
Maharishi Ayur-Veda Association of America, 158, 315
Maharishi Mahesh Yogi, 157, 259–61
Maharishi Vedic University, 261, 321
Manual Lymphatic Drainage, 44, 158–60, 186, 189, 315
Many Lives, Many Masters (Weiss), 191
Martin, Arthur H., 178–74
Massachusetts Institute of Technology, 155
Massage Therapy, 1, 2, 4, 21, 22, 36, 37, 52, 54, 64, 76, 160–62, 193, 194, 199, 217, 219, 263, 315–16
see also specific massage therapies
Materia Medica (Cullen), 121
Materia Medicia of Li-Shih-Chin, 112
Maya, 62, 121
Medicina Biologica, 160, 315

Meditation, 30, 34, 55, 164–65, 220, 233, 250, 316
Autogenic Training, 27–29, 307
guided, 191
Transcendental, 157, 207, 259–61, 321
menstrual disorders, 22, 202, 236, 265, 290, 291
mental health, 23–25, 73–74, 87–88, 95, 196, 290
Mentastics Movement Education, 257, 258
meridians, energy, 2, 5–6, 19, 77, 114, 115, 140–41, 237, 251, 252, 256, 264–65
Mesmer, Franz Anton, 129–30, 155
Michigan State University, 171, 238
midwives, 43
migraine headaches, 2–3, 28, 41, 63, 103–4, 236, 238, 243
Mill, John Stuart, 195
Miller, Neal, 41
mindfulness, 107
minerals, 12, 13, 14, 15, 127, 143, 268–69, 270, 271
Schuessler Cell Salts, 231–32, 320
Missett, Judi Sheppard, 137–38
Montague, Ashley, 135
Morrison, Morris, 196
movement education, 25, 26–27, 36, 109, 110, 148, 226, 256–58
Movement Therapy, 165–66
moxabustion, 4, 6, 150, 264
Muary, Margurite, 21
Mucusless Diet, 167–68
Mucusless Diet Healing System (Ehret), 168
mugwort, 6, 112
multiple sclerosis, 128, 165, 290
Munz, F., 57
Murai, Jiro, 140
muscle monitoring, 19–20
muscles, 1–3, 63, 75
pain in, 2–3, 12, 22, 36, 45–48, 80, 124, 182, 202, 226·
tension in, 10–12, 28, 34, 36–37, 39, 42, 60–61, 83, 110, 124, 138–39, 238
see also Massage Therapy
Muscle Sculpting (Deep Tissue Sculpting), 44, 80–83, 310
muscle testing, 17, 18, 19–20, 255, 256
muscular dystrophy, 20
Muscular Therapy Institute, 37, 307–8
Music Therapy, 73–74, 168–70, 316
Myofascial Release Centers, 171, 316
Myofascial Release Therapy, 170–71, 316
myofibrositis (rheumatism), 35, 103, 116, 265
Myotherapy, 45–48, 261, 308

Myotherapy: Bonnie Prudden's Complete Guide to Pain-Free Living (Prudden), 47
Myotherapy Institute, 47
My Water Cure (Kneipp), 127

Nakagawa, Kyoichi, 155
Namikoshi, Tokujiro, 237
Naprapathy, 171–72, 316
National Association for Drama Therapy, 87, 310
National Association for Music Therapy, 170, 316
National Association for Poetry Therapy, 196, 197, 318
National Association of Pregnancy Massage Therapists, 45, 308, 313
National Cancer Institute, 16, 17, 125
National Center for Homeopathy, 123, 312
National College of Naprapathy, 172, 316
National College of Naturopathic Medicine, 175, 317
National Commission for the Certification of Acupuncturists, 8, 305
National Institute on Alcohol Abuse and Alcoholism, 6
National Institute on Drug Abuse, 6
National Society of Hypnotherapists, 313
Native Americans, 76, 106, 121, 135, 164
  Chiropractic and, 62
  Fasting by, 97
  Herbal Medicine of, 116
  Hydrotherapy of, 126
  Shamanism of, 147, 232, 233, 234
Natural Gourmet Cooking School, 315
Natural Hygiene, Inc., 174, 316
Natural Hygiene (Life Science), 98, 100, 101, 172–74, 316
Naturopathic Medicine (naturopathy), 15, 64, 66, 118, 167, 174–76, 316–17
Naumburg, Margaret, 24
neck pain, 27, 63, 91, 103, 171, 243, 290
Netherton, Morris, 191
Network Chiropractic, 176–78, 317
Neuro/Cellular Repatterning, 178–79, 317
Neurolinguistic Programming (NLP), 106
Neuromuscular Therapy, St. John Method, 29, 241–43, 320
New Age music, 169
New Age Shamanism, 234
New Hope for the Arthritic (Dong), 87
New Primal Scream, The: Primal Therapy Twenty Years On (Janov), 204
New Pritikin Program, The (Pritikin), 205
Newton, Sir Isaac, 68
New York University, 88

Nicholson, Shirley, 234
Niehans, Paul, 144–45
night blindness, 270
Nikken Products, Inc., 157, 315
Nimmo, Raymond, 242
Nimmo technique, 242
No-Nightshade Diet, 23, 179–80
Norman, Laura, 215
North American Society of the Teachers of Alexander Technique, 12, 306
North American Vegetarian Society, 321
Novato Institute for Somatic Research and Training, 311
Novocain (procaine), 262–63
Nurse Healers-Professional Association, Inc., 321

obesity, 14, 17, 28, 95, 98, 131, 144, 222, 293
occupational therapy, 24
Odyssey (Homer), 160
Official Handbook of the Radiance Technique, The (Ray), 208
Ohashi Institute, 238, 320
Ohsawa, George, 151–52, 154, 314
oils, 82, 148, 160, 248–49
  essential, 20–23
One Thousand Notable Things, 265–66
ophthalmology, 34
Orcas Island Foundation, 321
Organon of the Rational Art of Healing, The (Hahnemann), 121
orgasm, 14, 215–16
orgone energy, 198, 216–17
Orgone Energy Accumulator (Reich), 218
Orgone Institute, 216
Ornish, Dean, 221
Orr, Leonard, 211–12
Ortho-Bionomy, 180–82, 317
Orthomolecular Medicine and Psychiatry, 183–84
Orthomolecular Therapy, 182–84, 268, 317
Osborne-Sheets, Carole, 43, 81–83, 134
Osler, Sir William, 4
Osmond, Humphrey, 183
osteoarthritis, 35, 124
Osteopathic Functional Technique, 181
Osteopathy, 2, 18, 52, 54, 64, 162, 172, 181, 184–86, 317
  CranioSacral Therapy in, 18, 71–73, 181, 186, 268, 310
  Strain-Counterstrain Therapy in, 186, 243
osteoporosis, 58, 290
Oxidative Therapy, 186–87, 317–18

Oxygen Therapies (McCabe), 187, 188
Ozone Therapy, 186, 187–88, 318

Pacific Institute of Aromatherapy, 307
pain, 1, 4–5, 6, 7, 29, 75, 85, 90, 127, 133,
    160, 225, 236, 238, 241–43, 254
    back, 2–3, 4, 27, 50, 63, 91, 95, 103,
        124, 139, 171, 202, 229, 243, 265,
        283, 289
    of bodywork, 148–49
    chronic, 2, 15, 165, 285
    muscular, 2–3, 12, 22, 36, 45–48, 80,
        124, 182, 202, 226
    neck, 27, 63, 91, 103, 171, 243, 290
    referred, *see* Trigger Point Therapy
Pain Erasure the Bonnie Prudden Way (Prudden), 47
Painter, Jack W., 199, 201
Palmer, Bartlett-Joshua, 63
Palmer, Daniel David, 63
Pannetier, Pierre, 197–98
Paracelsus, 120–21
Parasympathetic Massage, 188–89
Pare, Ambroise, 247–48
Parkinson, John, 113
Pasteur, Louis, 173
Past Lives Therapy, 131, 189–91, 318
Past Lives Therapy (Netherton and Shiffrin),
    191
Patanjali, 276
pau d'arco, 116
Pauling, Linus, 183, 269
Pauls, Arthur Lincoln, 181
Pavek, Richard R., 235, 236
Payne, Buryl, 157
Pearson, Durk, 14, 143, 270
peeling effect, 33
pellagra, 14, 183, 269
Pennsylvania School of Muscle Therapy,
    192
Pen Ts'ao (Shen-nung), 112
People's Republic of China, 264
peppermint, 22, 112
Perfect Health (Chopra), 158
Perls, Fritz, 223, 229
Persians, 21, 154–55, 160
petrissage, 54, 160, 248
Pfrimmer, Therese C., 191
Pfrimmer Technique, 191–92, 318
pharmacopeias, 112, 113, 116
phobias, 131, 202
Physical Dynamics of Character Structure, The
    (Lowen), 39
Physical Therapy, 2, 64, 74, 75, 92, 95,
    142, 192–94, 207, 219, 227, 241,
    318
Physicians Committee for Responsible Medicine, 317
Pierrakos, John C., 38, 39
Pinckney, Callan, 49–51
pink tourmaline, 77
pitta, 31, 115, 116
pituitary gland, 3, 55, 95
Planetary Herbology (Tierra), 118
plaque, arterial, 56–58, 163
Plutarch, 160
Poetry As Healer: Mending the Troubled Mind
    (Leedy, ed.), 197
Poetry in the Therapeutic Experience (Lerner,
    ed.), 197
Poetry Therapy, 73–74, 194–97, 318
Poetzel, O., 246
Polarity Therapy, 29, 197–99, 318
Polarity Therapy and Health Building: The Conscious Art of Living Well (Stone), 199
polio, 20, 291
Polo, Marco, 264
Polynesia, 62, 147
polypeptides, 13
Pomeranz, Bruce, 6–7
postpartum massage, 43, 45
Postural Integration, 148, 199–201, 244,
    318
posture, 10–12, 17, 27, 29, 36, 37, 58, 83,
    110, 180–82, 243, 276
prakruti, 31, 115
prana, 198, 201, 235, 251
Pranic Healing, 201–2, 318
Pranic Healing (Choa Kok Sui), 202
pregnancy massage, 43, 308, 313
Present-Centered Awareness and Therapy,
    29
preventive health care, 3, 176, 237
Primal Scream, The (Janov), 202
Primal Therapy, 81, 202–4
*Principles and Practice of Hydrotherapy, The: A
    Guide to the Application of Water in Disease* (Baruch), 64
Pritikin, Nathan, 163, 204–5
Pritikin, Robert, 205
Pritikin Diet, 95, 204–5, 206, 221, 318
Pritikin Exercise, 204, 205–6, 318
Pritikin Longevity Center, 204, 205, 206,
    318
Pritikin Program for Diet and Exercise (Pritikin),
    205
procaine (Novocain), 262–63
Proprioceptive Neuromuscular Facilitation
    (PNF Stretching), 206–7

proprioceptors, 74, 206
prostate gland, 270, 283, 291
Prudden, Bonnie, 45–48, 261
Psycheye: Self-Analytic Consciousness (Ahsen), 133
psychoneuroimmunology, 132
psychosomatic disorders, 28, 235
Psychosynthesis, 29
psychotherapy, 83, 89, 106–7, 130, 131, 142, 190, 220, 228
  Pranic, 202
  Primal, 81, 202–4
psyllium seed, 67
pumice, 67
Pyramid International, 315
Pythagoras, 68, 169, 190

Qi Gong (Chi Kung), 58–59, 264, 265, 319
Qi Gong Institute/East-West Academy of the Healing Arts, 59, 319
Quantum Healing: Exploring the Frontiers of Body-Mind Medicine (Chopra), 158
Quantum Quest, 321
quinine, 136

Radiance Technique, 207–8, 219, 319
Radiance Technique Association International, Inc., 208, 219, 319
Radiance Technique Journal, 208
"Radiant Health," 275
Radionics, 208–11
Rational Hydrotherapy (Kellogg), 127
Ray, Barbara, 208, 219
Reader's Digest Magic and Medicine of Plants, 118
Rebirthing, 211–13, 220, 319
Recovering Yourself (Martin), 179
Reflexology (Zone Therapy), 44, 66, 147, 155, 213–15, 319
Reflexology: Art, Science and History (Issel), 215
Regression Therapy, *see* Past Lives Therapy
Reich, Wilhelm, 36–37, 38, 39, 138, 198, 216–18
Reichian Therapy, 106, 199, 215–18
Reiki, 207, 218–20, 319
Reiki Alliance, 219, 220, 319
"Reiki" Factor, The: The Expanded Edition (Ray), 208
Reiki Healing Institute, 319
Reilly, Harold J., 52–54
Reilly Health Institute, 53
Reilly School of Massotherapy, 53, 54
reincarnation, 190
relaxation, 1–2, 27–28, 42, 96, 132, 227–28, 254

repression, 203
Reversal Diet, 221
rheumatism (myofibrositis), 35, 103, 116, 265
rheumatoid arthritis, 35, 98
Rice Diet (Kempner Rice Diet), 220–22, 319
rickets, 269
Rigveda, 112
Rilling, R., 187
Rinzler, Seymour H., 262
rishis, 30
Rocine, Victor G., 274
Rodale's Illustrated Encyclopedia of Herbs, 118
Rolf, Ida P., 25, 26, 110, 199, 222, 223–24, 226, 244, 257
Rolfing (Structural Integration), 26, 29, 44, 80, 82, 110, 148, 161, 199, 222–25, 226, 244–45, 257, 319
Rolfing Movement Integration, 226
Rolfing: The Integration of the Human Structure (Rolf), 224
Rolf Institute of Structural Integration, 110, 223, 224, 225, 226, 319
Rolling Thunder, 234
Roman Catholic Church, 113, 129, 253
Romans, 21, 62, 97
  enemas of, 65
  heat applied by, 192
  Herbal Medicine of, 112–13, 114, 116
  Hydrotherapy of, 126, 192
  Massage Therapy of, 160
Rosen, Marion, 226–27
Rosen Method, 226–28, 319
Rosen Method Practitioner Referral Service, 228, 319
rose quartz, 77
Rossman, Martin L., 133
Rubenfeld, Ilana, 228–30
Rubenfeld Center, 231, 320
Rubenfeld Synergy Method, 228–31, 320
Russia, 35, 92, 97, 155, 198, 240

St. Helena Health Center, 163, 164, 316
St. John, Paul, 241
St. John's Neuromuscular Pain Relief Institute, 243, 320
St. John's Neuromuscular Therapy, 29, 241–43, 320
Salmon's English Physician, 265
Samkhya, 30
Sanskrit, 30, 31, 54, 112, 126, 201, 219, 276
Saytzeff, Alexander, 84
Scheel, John H., 174

schizophrenia, 98, 183, 184, 196, 269, 270
Schnable, C., 271
Schneider-McClure, Vimala, 133, 135
Schuessler, Wilhelm Heinrich, 231
Schuessler Cell Salts, 231–32, 320
Schultz, Johannes, 27–29
Schweitzer, Albert, 104, 105
sciatica, 63, 124, 245, 291
Science and Fine Art of Food and Nutrition, The (Shelton), 173
Science and Practice of Iridology, The (Jensen), 136
sclerology, 135
scoliosis, 83, 103, 171, 245
sculpting, 80–83
scurvy, 265, 269
self-hypnosis, 27–28
self-massage, 58, 60, 81, 236
Selye, Hans, 108
sen meridians, 251
Sensory Awareness, 29
sensory-motor amnesia, 109
"Seven Guidelines for a Healthy Diet" (Arthritis Foundation), 23
sexual problems, 6, 14, 28, 131, 203
Shamanism, 129, 140, 232–34, 320
    Herbal Medicine in, 111, 232–33
    of kahunas, 147, 233
    Native American, 147, 232, 233, 234
    Poetry Therapy of, 194–95
Shamanism: An Expanded View of Reality (Nicholson, ed.), 234
Sharp Institute for Mind Body Medicine, 307
Shaw, Sandy, 14, 143, 270
shell shock, 130
Shelton, Herbert M., 173
Shen-nung, Emperor, 112
SHEN Therapy, 234–36, 320
Shiatsu, 147, 197, 236–38, 320
    Barefoot, 149, 150, 151
    Macrobiotic, 149–51
Shiatsu Handbook, The (Yamamoto and McCarty), 150
Shiffrin, Nancy, 191
Siberia, 232, 233
sinus disorders, 6, 28, 158, 159
skin disorders, 15, 20, 97, 127, 159, 265, 267, 273, 283, 288, 291–92
Slagle, Priscilla, 14–15, 270
Smith, Fritz Frederick, 277–78, 279
Smith, Oakley, 172
Society of Ortho-Bionomy International, Inc., 182, 317
Solomon, Paul, 178

Somatic Education (Hanna Somatic Education), 107–9
Somatic Learning Associates, 45, 308, 314
Somatics: Reawakening the Mind's Control of Movement, Flexibility, and Health (Hanna), 109
SomatoEmotional Release, 238–39, 320
SomatoEmotional Release and Beyond (Upledger), 73
Sorensen, Jacki, 8–10
sore throat, 5, 263, 265
Soviet Union, 156
"Spontaneous Release by Positioning" (Jones), 181
sports injuries, 171, 182, 239, 292
Sports Massage, 74, 75, 79, 83, 102, 161, 207, 239–41, 249, 320
Sports Massage Training Institute, 240, 241
spray and stretch, 46–47
Stevenson, Henry E., 173
Still, Andrew Taylor, 184–85
Stone, Randolph, 197, 198, 199
Strain-Counterstrain Therapy, 186, 243
stress, 6, 19, 32, 41–42, 132–33, 205, 226, 227–28, 260, 267–68, 270, 292
    in children, 60–61
    emotional, see emotional stress
    eye, 34
    held in the body, 28
stroke, 58, 128, 196, 204, 291
Structural Integration (Rolfing), 26, 29, 44, 80, 82, 110, 148, 161, 199, 222–25, 226, 244–45, 257, 319
structural myofascial massage, 43
Subliminal: The New Channel to Personal Power (Schulman and Schulman), 247
Subliminal Therapy, 246–47, 320–21
subtle body, 55
sugar, 15, 17, 23
suma, 116
Sumerians, 111–12
Sun Bear, 234
surgery, 4, 26, 37, 52, 95, 156, 292
Sutherland, William G., 71
Swedish gymnastics, 248
Swedish Massage, 44, 54, 80, 82, 160–61, 239, 247–49, 264
sympathetic nervous system, 188, 189

Taber, Jerriann J., 96
Tai Chi Chuan, 73, 82, 249–51
Tai Chi Chuan: A Simplified Method of Calisthenics for Health and Self Defense (Cheng Man-Ch'ing), 251
Takata, Hawayo, 208, 219

Taoism, 4, 5, 59, 106, 114, 138, 181, 236, 249–50
Taoist Institute of Los Angeles, 264, 265, 321
Taoist Sanctuary of San Diego, 265, 321
Tao-Yinn, 236
tapotement, 160, 248
Tarshis, Barry, 85
Technical Manual of Deep Wholistic Bodywork (Painter), 201
Teeguarden, Iona Marsaa, 138, 139
tei shin, 2
Temporomandibular Joint (TMJ) syndrome, 72, 243, 245
tendonitis, 6, 35, 75, 80, 85, 124, 263, 292
tennis elbow, 6, 91, 245
Thai Massage, 251–52
Theatrum Botanicum (Parkinson), 113
THE (Therapy, Health, Education) Clinic, 91, 310
Theophrastus, 113
Therapeutic Touch, 22, 80–81, 103, 253–55, 321
Therapeutic Touch: A Practical Guide (Macrae), 255
Therapeutic Touch: How to Use Your Hands to Heal (Krieger), 255
Thie, John F., 18, 255, 256
third eye, 55
thyme, 22
Tibet, 139, 207, 218, 253, 265
Tien-An, 236
Tierra, Michael, 118
Tivy, Desmond, 46, 47
tobacco, 13, 14, 17, 28, 144
Touch for Health, 18, 19, 255–56, 321
Touch for Health (Thie), 256
Touch for Health Association, 321
Touching, the Human Significance of the Skin (Montague), 135
Townsend Letter, 306
Trager, Milton, 82, 257, 258
Trager Approach, 256–58, 321
Trager Institute, 321
Trager Mentastics: Movement as a Way to Age-lessness (Trager), 258
Trager Psychophysical Integration, 257–58
Trall, Russell Thacher, 173
trance healing, 233
Transcendental Meditation (TM), 157, 207, 259–61, 321
transcutaneous electric nerve stimulator (TENS), 92
trauma, 20, 26, 37, 55, 72–73, 76, 83, 110, 148–49, 156, 177, 190, 202–4

Travel, Janet, 46, 261–63
Travel, Willard, 261
tridoshas, 31, 69, 115–16
Trigger Point Injection Therapy, 46–47, 262–63
Trigger Point Therapy, 44, 45–48, 70, 75, 186, 237, 239, 240, 242, 243, 261–63
tryptophan, 13, 14, 15
tuberculosis, 104, 126–27, 151
Tui Na: Chinese Healing and Acupressure Massage (Lew and Helm), 265
Tui Na Massage Therapy, 263–65, 321
Tungus, 232
Turkish bath, 126
Turner, Tina, 123
Twelve Schuessler Remedies, 231–32, 320

ulcers, 14, 59, 41, 98, 203, 292
Ulman, Elinor, 24
ultrasound, 64, 194
unwinding, 72–73, 268
Upledger, John E., 71–72, 73, 186, 238–39
Upledger Institute, 73, 239, 268, 310, 320, 321
urinary tract disorders, 6, 286, 292
Urine Therapy, 265–67
Use of Ozone in Medicine, The (Rilling and Viebahn), 187
Usui, Mikao, 218–19
Utt, Richard, 19

Valnet, Jean, 21
vata, 31, 115–16
Vedas, 21, 30, 112, 275
Vega Study Center, 154, 315
vegetotherapy, 217
verbal expression, 109, 110, 229
Viebahn, R., 187
Villoldo, Alberto, 234
viral infections, 14
Visceral Manipulation, 267–68, 321
vision, *see* eyes
Vision Training Institute, 96, 311
Visualization, Imagery and, xxi, 55, 132–33, 164
vital life energy, 177, 197–99, 201–2, 216–20, 233, 251–52, 253–55, 271
chakras and, 54–56
as *chi,* xxii, 2–3, 5–6, 58, 59, 140–41, 198, 201, 235, 236–38, 251, 264
meridians of, 2, 5–6, 19, 77, 114, 115, 140–41, 237, 251, 252, 256, 264–65
as orgone energy, 198, 216–17
as *tridoshas,* 31, 69, 115–16

vitamins (Vitamin Therapy), xxi, 12, 13, 14, 15, 64, 143, 268–70, 271, 321
  A, 16–17, 270
  B$_1$ (thiamin), 269
  B$_3$ (niacin), 14, 183, 269, 270
  B$_6$, 14, 270
  C, 16–17, 183, 269, 270
  D, 269
  E, 186
  folic acid, 270
  megadoses of, 182–83, 268
  pantothenate, 270
  recommended daily allowances (RDA) of, 268
Vodder, Emil and Estrid, 158–60, 315
Vodder School, 159
Vogt, Oskar, 27–28
voice, loss of, 11, 12, 51, 131
von Peczely, Ignatz, 135

Walker, Morton, 85
Walling, William B., 38
Warburg, Otto, 187
Water of Life, The: A Treatise on Urine Therapy (Armstrong), 266, 267
Wat Poh temple, 252
Way of the Shaman, The (Harner), 233–34
Way Up from Dawn, The (Slagle), 15, 270
Weeks, Virginia Travel, 261
weight-loss programs, 14, 100–101, 174
Weinberger, Stanley, 67
Weiss, Brian L., 191
Wellness Institute for Personal Transformation, 179, 317
Werner, Alfred, 57
Wesley, John, 126
What in the World Is Rolfing (Rolf), 224
wheatgrass, 67
Wheatgrass Book, The: How to Grow and Use Wheatgrass to Maximize Your Health and Vitality (Wigmore), 273
Wheatgrass Diet, 271–73, 322
whiplash injury, 63, 72, 83, 182, 243, 245
whirlpool spas, 127–28
Whistling Elk, Agnes, 234
Whole Foods Diet, 273–75, 322
Wiener, Norbert, 40
Wigmore, Ann, 271–72, 273
Withering, William, 114
Wittlinger, Gunther and Hildegard, 159
World Chiropractic Alliance, 309
World Health Organization, 6
World War I, 130, 271
World War II, 21, 84, 130, 155, 195, 204–5, 227
Wyrick, Dana, 315

Yale University, 95, 260
Yamamoto, Shizuko, 149, 150–51
Yellow Emperor's Classic of Internal Medicine, The (Huang-ti Nei-Ching), 2, 4, 112, 160, 252, 264
yin and yang, 5, 114–15, 153, 264
Yoga, 28, 30, 40, 54, 58–59, 157, 164, 197, 199, 206, 207, 252, 275–77, 322
Your Body Tells the Truth (Martin), 179
Yourish, Y., 35

Zen Buddhism, 28, 219, 249
Zero Balancing (ZB), 277–79, 322
Zero Balancing Association, 279, 322
Zin, A., 272
zinc, 270
Zisk, Gary, 14
Zone Therapy (Reflexology), 44, 66, 147, 155, 213–15, 319

❋ ❋ ❋

About the Authors

Mark Kastner was born in Yuma, Arizona; while a small child, his family moved to San Diego, California. Attracted to the healing arts field since the age of twelve, Mr. Kastner attended the University of California, San Diego, with the intention of becoming a physician. However, he became interested in nutrition and bodywork, which led him to leave UCSD and study with several holistic practitioners, including Ram Das and Dr. Bernard Jensen.

Under the tutelage of Dr. Jensen, Mr. Kastner became a certified iridologist. Dr. Jensen later introduced him to Oriental Medicine and Acupuncture, and with Dr. Jensen's encouragement, he attended the California Acupuncture College for three and one-half years.

Through a program supported by the United Nations and the World Health Organization, Mr. Kastner was chosen to participate in a clinical internship program at Guan An Min Hospital in Beijing, China, where he studied with Dr. Liu and Dr. Cheng-Gu Ye. Dr. Ye is considered one of the top acupuncturists in China. Upon completion of his internship, Mr. Kastner graduated from the Beijing School of Traditional Oriental Medicine.

Returning to the United States in 1985, he became licensed to practice acupuncture in the state of California and opened the Park Boulevard

Health Center, which became one of the largest and most successful acupuncture clinics in the United States.

In addition to acupuncture, Mr. Kastner incorporates other types of holistic healing into his practice, including herbal medicine and naturopathy. Currently, Mark Kastner lives in San Diego with his wife, Marie, also an acupuncturist, and sons Marcus and Christian.

Hugh Burroughs was born in Los Angeles, California, and graduated from California State University at Los Angeles with a B.S. degree in zoology. He began his professional career as an industrial chemist. Later, turning to writing, he authored several technical manuals and numerous other works.

Mr. Burroughs's first introduction to natural health care was around the age of five, when his maternal grandmother gave him honey and lemon juice to control a cough. Although always interested in alternative medicine, it was not until 1986 that his interest took a personal turn. While living in Sacramento, California, Mr. Burroughs began to suffer with debilitating headaches for several months. When prescription drugs had no effect on the pain, a friend recommended acupuncture. Within a relatively short period of time, with treatments of acupuncture and herbal medicine, his headaches were relieved.

After an automobile accident in 1989, Mr. Burroughs was left with neck and back pain. This led him to investigate and use other forms of alternative healing in his recovery, which further fueled his interest and knowledge of the field. In 1991, a recurrence of the headaches he had previously suffered led to his seeking acupuncture treatments once again. A friend recommended Mark Kastner, an acupuncturist she had been treated by. Ultimately Mr. Burroughs was cured of his headaches, and he and Mr. Kastner decided to collaborate and write this book. Hugh Burroughs lives in La Mesa, California, a suburb of San Diego.